Trauma-Informed Supervision

Survivors of trauma are disproportionately represented in agencies providing a broad range of behavioral, social, and mental health services. Practitioners in these settings must understand and be able to respond to survivors of trauma in ways that are empowering, normalize and validate their experiences and reactions, and minimize the risk of re-traumatization. Practitioners also will be indirectly traumatized as a result of their work with trauma survivors.

Practitioners' ability to help clients with histories of trauma depends upon clinical supervision that is trauma-informed. The trauma-informed supervisor has the dual responsibility of enhancing supervisees' skills as trauma-informed practitioners *and* helping them manage the impact their work has on them.

Nevertheless, many clinical supervisors only have limited knowledge and training in trauma and may not recognize either the needs of those whom they supervise or the clients their supervisees serve. This book compiles important recommendations from trauma-informed practitioners, supervisors, and researchers who share their professional reflections and personal stories based on their hands-on experiences across mental health and medical contexts.

This book was originally published as a special issue of *The Clinical Supervisor*.

Carolyn Knight is a professor of Social Work at the University of Maryland, Baltimore County, United States. She is a social worker with 30 years of experience, mostly pro bono, working individually and in groups with adult survivors of childhood trauma, particularly sexual abuse. She is the author of *Introduction to Working with Adult Survivors of Childhood Trauma: Strategies and Skills* (2008) and *Group Therapy for Adult Survivors of Child Sexual Abuse* (1996), co-editor of *Group Work with Populations at Risk* (with Geoffrey Grief, 4th ed., 2016), and co-author of a textbook on social work practice *The life model of social work practice, 4th ed.* Her recent presentations have focused on how to adopt a trauma-informed lens in clinical supervision and practice.

L. DiAnne Borders is the Burlington Industries Excellence Professor in the Counseling program at The University of North Carolina at Greensboro, United States. She teaches clinical supervision and supervises doctoral students' clinical supervision internships. Her current research focuses on supervision education and pedagogy as well as trauma-informed supervision. She is the author of several books and numerous empirical and conceptual articles on clinical supervision, and serves as editor of *The Clinical Supervisor*.

Trauma-Informed Supervision

Core Components and Unique Dynamics
in Varied Practice Contexts

Edited by
Carolyn Knight and L. DiAnne Borders

Routledge
Taylor & Francis Group

LONDON AND NEW YORK

First published 2020
by Routledge
2 Park Square, Milton Park, Abingdon, Oxon, OX14 4RN

and by Routledge
52 Vanderbilt Avenue, New York, NY 10017

Routledge is an imprint of the Taylor & Francis Group, an informa business

First issued in paperback 2021

British Library Cataloguing-in-Publication Data
A catalogue record for this book is available from the British Library

ISBN 13: 978-0-367-35280-6 (hbk)
ISBN 13: 978-1-03-208711-5 (pbk)

Typeset in Minion Pro
by codeMantra

Publisher's Note
The publisher accepts responsibility for any inconsistencies that may have arisen during the conversion of this book from journal articles to book chapters, namely the inclusion of journal terminology.

Disclaimer
Every effort has been made to contact copyright holders for their permission to reprint material in this book. The publishers would be grateful to hear from any copyright holder who is not here acknowledged and will undertake to rectify any errors or omissions in future editions of this book.

Contents

Citation Information   vii

Notes on Contributors   ix

Introduction: Trauma-informed supervision: Core components and unique
dynamics in varied practice contexts   1
Carolyn Knight and L. DiAnne Borders

1   Trauma-informed supervision: Historical antecedents, current practice, and
future directions   7
Carolyn Knight

2   Trauma-informed supervision and consultation: Personal reflections   38
Christine A. Courtois

3   Child welfare supervision: Special issues related to trauma-informed care in
a unique environment   64
Crystal Collins-Camargo and Becky Antle

4   Trauma-informed supervision: Counselors in a Level I hospital
trauma center   83
Laura J. Veach and Elizabeth Hodges Shilling

5   Trauma-informed supervision in deployed military settings   102
W. Brad Johnson, Matthew Johnson, and Kristin L. Landsinger

6   The intersection of identities in supervision for trauma-informed practice:
Challenges and strategies   121
Roni Berger, Laura Quiros, and Jamie R. Benavidez-Hatzis, LCSW

7   A personal narrative on responding to the tragedy at Pulse in Orlando:
A volunteer supervisor's perspective   141
John T. Super

8   Trauma-informed intercultural group supervision   157
Anthony Haans and Nora Balke

9   When religion hurts: Supervising cases of religious abuse   180
    Craig S. Cashwell and Paula J. Swindle

10 Attending to racial trauma in clinical supervision: Enhancing client and
    supervisee outcomes   202
    Alex L. Pieterse

11 Trauma-informed supervision in the disaster context   219
    Carole Adamson

    Index   239

Citation Information

The chapters in this book were originally published in the *The Clinical Supervisor* volume 37, issue 1 (January-June 2018). When citing this material, please use the original page numbering for each article, as follows:

Introduction

Trauma-informed supervision: Core components and unique dynamics in varied practice contexts
Carolyn Knight and L. DiAnne Borders
The Clinical Supervisor, volume 37, issue 1 (January-June 2018) pp. 1–6

Chapter 1

Trauma-informed supervision: Historical antecedents, current practice, and future directions
Carolyn Knight
The Clinical Supervisor, volume 37, issue 1 (January-June 2018) pp. 7–37

Chapter 2

Trauma-informed supervision and consultation: Personal reflections
Christine A. Courtois
The Clinical Supervisor, volume 37, issue 1 (January-June 2018) pp. 38–63

Chapter 3

Child welfare supervision: Special issues related to trauma-informed care in a unique environment
Crystal Collins-Camargo and Becky Antle
The Clinical Supervisor, volume 37, issue 1 (January-June 2018) pp. 64–82

Chapter 4

Trauma-informed supervision: Counselors in a Level I hospital trauma center
Laura J. Veach and Elizabeth Hodges Shilling
The Clinical Supervisor, volume 37, issue 1 (January-June 2018) pp. 83–101

Chapter 5

Trauma-informed supervision in deployed military settings
W. Brad Johnson, Matthew Johnson, and Kristin L. Landsinger
The Clinical Supervisor, volume 37, issue 1 (January-June 2018) pp. 102–121

Chapter 6

The intersection of identities in supervision for trauma-informed practice: Challenges and strategies
Roni Berger, Laura Quiros, and Jamie R. Benavidez-Hatzis, LCSW
The Clinical Supervisor, volume 37, issue 1 (January-June 2018) pp. 122–141

Chapter 7

A personal narrative on responding to the tragedy at Pulse in Orlando: A volunteer supervisor's perspective
John T. Super
The Clinical Supervisor, volume 37, issue 1 (January-June 2018) pp. 142–157

Chapter 8

Trauma-informed intercultural group supervision
Anthony Haans and Nora Balke
The Clinical Supervisor, volume 37, issue 1 (January-June 2018) pp. 158–181

Chapter 9

When religion hurts: Supervising cases of religious abuse
Craig S. Cashwell and Paula J. Swindle
The Clinical Supervisor, volume 37, issue 1 (January-June 2018) pp. 182–203

Chapter 10

Attending to racial trauma in clinical supervision: Enhancing client and supervisee outcomes
Alex L. Pieterse
The Clinical Supervisor, volume 37, issue 1 (January-June 2018) pp. 204–220

Chapter 11

Trauma-informed supervision in the disaster context
Carole Adamson
The Clinical Supervisor, volume 37, issue 1 (January-June 2018) pp. 221–240

For any permission-related enquiries please visit:
http://www.tandfonline.com/page/help/permissions

Contributors

Carole Adamson is a senior social work lecturer at the University of Auckland in Aotearoa, New Zealand.

Becky Antle is a marriage and family therapist practitioner. She specializes in the areas of parenting, divorce and depression, and has conducted 20 years of research, community-based practice.

Nora Balke is a psychologist, psychotherapist, and supervisor at the Center ÜBERLEBEN (formerly Berlin Center for Torture Victims) in Berlin, Germany.

Roni Berger is a professor at Adelphi University School of Social Work, United States.

Jamie R. Benavidez-Hatzis is in private practice and serves as the director of a program serving runaway and homeless youths.

L. DiAnne Borders is a professor at the Counseling and Educational Development (CED) department at The University of North Carolina at Greensboro, United States.

Craig S. Cashwell is a professor in the Department of Counseling and Educational Development at The University of North Carolina at Greensboro, United States.

Crystal Collins-Camargo is a professor and the associate dean of research at the Kent School of Social Work, University of Louisville, United States.

Christine A. Courtois is a psychotherapist, workshop leader, and consultant specializing in posttraumatic and dissociative conditions and disorders. She is a licensed psychologist in the District of Columbia (DC) and Maryland (MD), United States.

Anthony Haans works as a trainer and survivor at the Center ÜBERLEBEN in Berlin, Germany; Doctors Without Borders; and the War Trauma Foundation.

Matthew Johnson is a clinical psychologist in the Midshipmen Development Center at the United States Naval Academy.

W. Brad Johnson is a professor at the Department of Leadership, Ethics and Law at the United States Naval Academy, and a faculty associate at the Graduate School of Education at Johns Hopkins University, Baltimore, United States.

Carolyn Knight is a professor at the School of Social Work at the University of Maryland, Baltimore County, United States.

Kristin L. Landsinger is a clinical psychologist and a lieutenant commander in the United States Navy's Medical Service Corps.

Alex L. Pieterse is an assistant professor of Counseling at Lenoir-Rhyne University in Hickory, United States.

Laura Quiros is the associate dean for Academic Affairs and director of the Masters of Social Work Program at Adelphi University School of Social Work, United States.

Elizabeth Hodges Shilling is an assistant professor at the Wake Forest School of Medicine at Bowman Gray Center for Medical Education, Winston-Salem, United States.

John T. Super is a clinical assistant professor at the University of Florida, Gainesville, United States.

Paula J. Swindle is an assistant professor of Counseling at Lenoir-Rhyne University in Hickory, United States.

Laura J. Veach is a professor at the Wake Forest School of Medicine at Bowman Gray Center for Medical Education, Winston-Salem, United States.

Trauma-informed supervision: Core components and unique dynamics in varied practice contexts

Carolyn Knight and L. DiAnne Borders

ABSTRACT

The Co-Editors of the special issue on trauma-informed supervision describe the need for increased attention to this topic and their goals for this issue. They then provide an overview of each article, all written by persons with extensive practice and/or research experience around trauma-informed supervision. They conclude with brief observations of the similarities and unique aspects of trauma-informed supervision in the varied settings and situations included in the special issue, and invite future contributions to the journal that build on the knowledge and insights provided by the authors of the articles in this issue.

Trauma is ubiquitous in our world. Stories of trauma from around the world flood news sources daily: children abused by their parents, caregivers, and others in positions of authority; women killed by their partners; refugees fleeing civil wars and genocide at home; immigrants facing threat of deportation; military personnel facing the horrors of war and lasting memories when they return home; Black men killed by police; random terrorist attacks that kill and maim innocent individuals; individuals and entire communities displaced after hurricanes or other natural disasters; persons targeted—even murdered—because of the religious beliefs they practice or the people they love; and the thousands of individuals dying from gun violence, car accidents, and other random acts of violence. These tragedies affect not only those directly involved, but also those around them who witness the events, whether in person, through social media, or via other means. Indeed, research indicates that almost every adult has been exposed to at least one traumatic event in the course of their lifetime (Knight, 2018).

The short- and long-term impact of trauma exposure has been extensively investigated, and it is clear that survivors often face a number of challenges at the time of and long after their experience. Not surprisingly, efforts have been expended to identify appropriate and effective interventions that can be implemented in mental, physical, and behavioral health settings worldwide.

In 2001, Harris and Fallot introduced the term "trauma-informed" to refer to an orientation to clinical practice and organizational environment that takes into account the possibility that clients and consumers of services may have been exposed to one or more traumatic events. Since that time, clinicians, researchers, and educators alike have expanded upon and articulated what it means to engage in trauma-informed practice and offer trauma-informed treatment to survivors. Although clinical supervision consistently has been identified as a key vehicle for enhancing trauma-informed practice, far less attention has been devoted to articulating its core components. It is our hope that this special issue can begin to address that gap—*and* inspire new and ongoing explorations of trauma-informed supervision in research and practice.

We set out to produce a special issue that would include a range of practice contexts and situations that require both trauma-informed practice and trauma-informed supervision. Based on an extensive review of the literature, across several disciplines, we identified leading scholars from various parts of the world and invited them to submit an article in which they shared their knowledge, experience, and recommendations. Not all invitees were able to contribute to the special issue, but we believe we have assembled a collection of articles written by leaders in the trauma field that will assist our readers in understanding the nature and importance of trauma-informed supervision in a range of practice contexts.. We offer our sincere appreciation to our contributors for taking on the task of writing for the special issue and sharing their expertise with readers of *The Clinical Supervisor*.

First, drawing on her years of practice and scholarly attention to trauma, co-editor Knight sets the broad context for the special issue. She provides an overview of historical developments in understanding trauma and the evolution in thinking about trauma-informed practice and care. She then describes current views of indirect trauma—the impact that working with trauma survivors has on clinicians—along with characteristics of effective trauma-informed supervision identified by scholars and researchers. Knight concludes with her thoughts about future challenges for researchers, practitioners, and supervisors.

Knight's article is followed by one authored by Courtois (2018). Courtois also traces the development of the trauma-informed conceptualization, but her discussion is of a much more personal nature. Courtois truly is a pioneer in the field of trauma. She was one of the first clinicians to write about trauma work and she recognized early on the critical importance of knowledgeable supervision in this area. Her article provides an absorbing account of her personal and professional development as a trauma-informed clinician and supervisor. Readers will see how Courtois's observations resonate through many of the other contributions in this special issue.

Authors of the next three articles provide insider views from within specific settings requiring trauma-informed care and trauma-informed supervision. First, Collins-Camargo and Antle (2018) discuss the critical need for trauma-informed supervision in child welfare. They argue that the very nature of child welfare work creates trauma for the children who receive services and note that trauma also predominates in the lives of the children's families. Collins-Camargo and Antle provide a framework for understanding how supervisors can support their workers in this very challenging work, which includes managing the stress created by financial constraints placed upon public agencies and unfavorable media and public attention. A particularly important contribution is their discussion of the needs of child welfare *supervisors* who, like their supervisees, must manage intense stress and pressure associated with their roles.

Next, Veach and Shilling (2018) describe clinical services offered in their Level I trauma center in a large hospital and their approach to supervising students and practitioners who work in the acute care center. They highlight the startling costs of physical trauma, in both economic and psychological terms, and point to how substance use, especially alcohol, contributes to traumatic injuries and thus must be an integral part of their work. Their case descriptions vividly reflect the intensity of their setting and their work. Finally, Johnson, Johnson, and Landsinger (2018) depict the unique challenges that uniformed mental health care practitioners face when working in deployed military settings. These challenges include both the physical dangers of *in-extremis* practice as well as difficult ethical quandaries (e.g., allegiance to the military mission versus the service member client) practitioners encounter there. The authors include a compelling case example of the potential psychological impact this work can have on these military practitioners, and then conclude with a series of practical recommendations for clinical supervisors working in these settings.

The next five articles are focused on the interplay between trauma and culture and the need for trauma-informed supervision to be culturally relevant and competent. First, Berger, Quiros, and Benavidez-Hatzis (2018) explicate how the intersection of social and cultural identities influence trauma-informed supervision. They note how important it is for supervisors to understand the role that power and privilege play in the trauma-based supervisory relationship and, through the use of a compelling case example, identify skills that promote a more egalitarian and empowering experience for supervisees. Super (2018) provides a unique contribution through a chronicle of his personal involvement in the response to the June 2016 tragedy at the Pulse nightclub in Orlando, Florida. Super describes how events unfolded at a local agency that served gay, lesbian bisexual, transgender+ (GLBT+) clients, including his role there as a volunteer supervisor of volunteer helpers. His recollections and reflections, as a helping professional and a gay man, are at once distressing and inspiring. Haans and Balke (2018) describe their group supervision approach with practitioners who work with refugees who experienced torture and war in their home countries. These authors' international perspectives on trauma work and supervision with culturally diverse clients and therapists expand our understanding of what it means to be culturally competent. We want to note the challenges Haans and Balke faced in writing their piece, since English is not their first language. We deeply appreciate their perseverance in working with us to make sure their ideas and experiences were accurately translated.

Cashwell and Swindle (2018) focus on religious abuse, expanding the current definition of such abuse to include not only abuse by a religious leader but also abuse perpetrated by a religious community. They give particular attention to the unique aspects of religious abuse manifested as betrayal trauma conflated with "the sacred." In offering their suggestions for trauma-informed supervision around religious-based traumas, they provide informative case examples, particularly around attending to therapists' own histories with religious figures and institutions. Last in this section, Pieterse (2018) addresses racial trauma, a unique trauma response experienced by persons of color that seems particularly salient in the current social and political environment in the United States. Unlike other types of trauma, Pieterse explains, racial trauma is based on one's membership in a particular racial group, and includes both overt acts as well as microaggressions and invalidations, as well as connections to intergenerational racism. He both highlights the potential for supervisors to overlook or avoid racial trauma of supervisees and their clients, thus compounding their experiences of invalidation, and provides specific suggestions for effectively attending to racial trauma and racial dynamics in clinical work as well as supervision.

In the final contribution to the special issue, Adamson (2018) provides an in-depth description of the role of clinical supervision in the context of natural disasters. Writing from Aotearoa New Zealand, a country prone to earthquakes and tremors, Adamson emphasizes the need for a longitudinal focus in supervision and carefully outlines the supervisor's evolving roles through the phases of disaster risk reduction management. Of note, Adamson highlights the unique situation that practitioners often face after a natural disaster—as both disaster workers and disaster victims. She provides keen examples showing how these intertwining experiences may play out in supervision, as well as special considerations for clinical supervision with these workers.

Although we are pleased with the diversity of trauma situations reflected in the special issue, we would be remiss if we did not speak to its limitations. The articles primarily highlight supervisory responsibilities in settings that serve adults exposed to trauma. In addition, many other potentially traumatic situations are not included, either because an invited author was not able to participate and/or because of space limitations. These restrictions were not intentional, but we wish to acknowledge them. We hope readers who work in other areas (e.g., relationship, community, and domestic violence; sex trafficking; homelessness) will be inspired by this special issue to submit manuscripts for submission that report their own experiences and research. Also, an area of practice that is not adequately addressed is trauma-informed practice and supervision in contexts that serve traumatized children and adolescents. Moving forward, all of these are important areas requiring attention.

Throughout the articles in this special issue, readers will note some similarities in the experiences of clients and practitioners across trauma settings and trauma events. These are important commonalities that demand attention of practitioners and their supervisors. Importantly, however, the authors identify unique manifestations of specific traumas in both clients and supervisees/practitioners. We believe these more focused discussions of trauma-informed supervision illustrate the more nuanced examinations that are necessary for advancing our understanding of trauma-informed supervision in all the settings in which it should occur. We hope the articles, often poignant, sometimes intense, encourage readers to pursue additional explorations of trauma-informed supervision; for starters, the authors' reference lists provide a wealth of resources for further study and reflection that can inform readers' trauma-informed supervision practice. Building from there, we hope such study and reflection will inspire conceptual and empirical works that can further our understanding of both common, core elements and unique dynamics of trauma-informed supervision. We would welcome such submissions to *The Clinical Supervisor*.

References

Adamson, C. (2018). Trauma-informed supervision in the disaster context. *The Clinical Supervisor, 37*, 221–240.

Berger, R., Quiros, L., & Benavidez-Hatzis, J. R. (2018). The intersection of identities in supervision for trauma-informed practice: Challenges and strategies. *The Clinical Supervisor, 37*, 122–141.

Cashwell, C. S., & Swindle, P. J. (2018). When religion hurts: Supervising cases of religious abuse. *The Clinical Supervisor, 37*, 182–203.

Collins-Camargo, C., & Antle, B. (2018). Child welfare supervision: Special issues related to trauma-informed care in a unique environment. *The Clinical Supervisor, 37*, 64–82.

Courtois, C. A. (2018). Trauma-informed supervision and consultation: Personal reflections. *The Clinical Supervisor, 37*, 38–63.

Haans, T., & Balke, N. (2018). Trauma-informed intercultural group supervision. *The Clinical Supervisor, 37*, 158–181.

Harris, M., & Fallot, R. (2001). *Using trauma theory to design service systems: New directions for mental health services*. San Francisco, CA: Jossey Bass.

Johnson, W. B., Johnson, M., & Landsinger, K. L. (2018). Trauma-informed supervision in deployed military settings. *The Clinical Supervisor, 37*, 102–121.

Knight, C. (2018). Trauma-informed supervision: Historical antecedents, current practice, and future directions. *The Clinical Supervisor, 37*, 7–37.

Pieterse, A. L. (2018). Attending to racism and racial trauma in clinical supervision: Enhancing client and supervisee outcomes. *The Clinical Supervisor, 37*, 204–220.

Super, J. (2018). A personal narrative on responding to the Pulse tragedy in Orlando: An interdisciplinary supervisory perspective. *The Clinical Supervisor, 37*, 142–157.

Veach, L. J., & Shilling, E. H. (2018). Trauma-informed supervision: Counselors in a Level I hospital trauma center. *The Clinical Supervisor, 37*, 83–101.

Trauma-informed supervision: Historical antecedents, current practice, and future directions

Carolyn Knight

ABSTRACT

In this article, the author traces the development of the current emphasis on trauma-informed practice and care in behavioral and mental health treatment. Using the discrimination model of clinical supervision, the author then discusses the application of trauma-informed principles to supervision. Relevant research is cited, and case examples are employed to illustrate critical roles, responsibilities, and tasks. Challenges and future directions also are identified.

Over the past decade, increased attention has been devoted to articulating the nature and implications of trauma-informed care in mental health and related fields. Trauma-informed care is not "trauma therapy." The focus of treatment is not necessarily on the trauma and its aftermath. Trauma-informed practitioners are attuned to the multifaceted treatment needs of their clients and recognize the connection between present-day challenges and past trauma. Trauma-informed practice must address the differing contexts in which clients' trauma may surface. On the one hand, some clients seek assistance to address their responses to a traumatic experience, such as surviving a plane crash or natural or human-made disaster. In contrast, many clients seek, or are required to seek, treatment for current problems in living that reflect and stem from past trauma. Research suggests that it is this second scenario that is most common among clients seeking mental health services (Berthelot, Godbout, Hebert, Goulet, & Bergeron, 2014; Saunders & Adams, 2014). Trauma-informed practice also requires that clinicians recognize the impact that their work has on them personally and professionally, and be proactive in caring for themselves.

There is a notable dearth of literature available to guide supervisors in providing supervision that is sensitive to the implications that clients' histories of trauma have for them *and* those with whom they work. This special issue of *The Clinical Supervisor* begins to fill this gap. It is our hope that the articles in this special issue lead to increased emphasis on and inquiry into the nature and provision of knowledgeable supervision to those engaged—directly and indirectly—in trauma work.

In this introductory article, the author traces the evolution in thinking about and understanding of trauma and its effects. Based upon contemporary research and theory, the nature of trauma-informed practice (TIP) and trauma-informed care (TIC) are then explained. The suggested nature of trauma-informed supervision (TIS) is then discussed.

In the articles that follow, invited authors describe trauma-informed supervision in a variety of contexts. Trauma-informed care and supervision is necessary in any practice setting, including services to children and adolescents. In this special issue, we have focused primarily on treatment with adults. Although the core concepts, considerations, and competencies identified in this special issue are relevant with any client population, there also are significant differences.

Understanding trauma: A 40-year evolution

The past 40 years have seen an explosion in theoretical and empirical interest in trauma and its impact on those exposed to it and, more recently, the clinicians who work with trauma survivors.

Emphasis on precipitating events

In early literature, authors focused on the effects that potentially traumatic events had on individuals exposed to them, such as veterans of the Vietnam War and children exposed to interpersonal victimization, particularly sexual abuse (Courtois & Gold, 2009). Events such as the bombing of the federal building in Oklahoma City in 1995, the terrorist attacks in the United States in 2001, and the destruction from Hurricane Katrina in 2005 required researchers and clinicians alike to broaden their focus to include the traumatic impact of natural and human-induced disasters (Van Der Kolk, 2007). More recently, attention has been focused on the traumatic impact of socio-political occurrences, including civil wars, genocide, human trafficking, and community violence (Cook, Simiola, Ellis, & Thompson, 2017; Courtois & Gold, 2009; Wolf, Green, Nochajski, Mendel, & Kusmaul, 2014).

Emphasis on the effects of trauma

Throughout the 1980s and 1990s, attention turned to identifying common sequelae of trauma exposure. Numerous social, psychiatric, psychological, behavioral, and physical problems were identified. These included substance abuse, suicide and suicidal ideation, eating disorders, self-injury, chronic pain, and psychiatric conditions such as borderline personality disorder, depression, post-traumatic stress disorder (PTSD), somatization disorders, and dissociative identity disorder (Brown, Schrag, & Trimble, 2005; Garno, Goldberg, Ramirez, & Ritzler, 2005; Mulvihill, 2005; Randolph & Reddy, 2006). Childhood trauma survivors, in particular, were found to be at greater risk of subsequent victimization in the form of intimate partner violence and rape (Arata & Lindman, 2002; Yehuda, Halligan, & Grossman, 2001).

During this same 20-year period, a different line of inquiry focused on changes in cognitive schema. Researchers found that exposure to trauma often results in the belief that the world is unsafe and unpredictable, leading to a sense of powerlessness and reduced feelings of self-efficacy (Currier, Holland, & Malott, 2015; Jeavons, Greenwood, & Horne, 2000; Park, Mills, & Edmondson, 2012; Samuelson, Bartel, Valadez, & Jordan, 2017; Smith, Abeyta, Hughes, & Jones, 2015). Researchers observed that survivors of childhood trauma struggled with additional distortions in thinking about the self, characterized by feelings of worthlessness, and about others, in the form of mistrust (Cloitre, Miranda, & Stovall-McClough, 2005; Giesen-Bloo & Arntz, 2005; Ponce, Williams, & Allen, 2004; Smith, Davis, & Fricker-Elhai, 2004).

Risk and protective factors and post-traumatic/adversarial growth

Constructivist self-development theorists, including Lisa McCann, Karen Saakvitne, and Laurie Pearlman, were at the forefront of articulating the changes in cognition that resulted from trauma exposure. They argued that trauma was a uniquely individual experience (McCann & Pearlman, 1990a). The same event could produce very different responses in those who experienced it: "Constructivist self-development theory… emphasizes the importance of the individual as an active agent in creating and construing his or her reality" (McCann & Pearlman, 1990a, pp. 5–6).

The recognition that the experience of trauma is unique to the individual led to efforts to identify factors that either placed an individual at greater risk of being traumatized or minimized the impact that a stressful event had on the individual. Theorists and researchers alike also recognized that an individual's unique response to a stressful event reflected sociocultural influences and environmental context (Adams & Boscarino, 2005; Adeola & Picou, 2014; Elliott & Urquiza, 2006; Katerndahl, Burge, Kellogg, & Parra, 2005).

A particularly powerful factor found to be important is social support at the individual and community levels (Carlson et al., 2016; Evans, Steel, & DiLillo, 2013; Sattler, Boyd, & Kirsch, 2014; Smith, Felix, Benight, & Jones, 2017). Social support is important both at the time of exposure to trauma and long-term as the individual struggles with its after-effects (Sippel, Pietrzak, Charney, Mayes, & Southwick, 2015). This factor is multidimensional and includes validation and understanding, acceptance, affirmation, and availability of appropriate resources. The absence of support, which can consist of blame and/or accusation, continued exposure to the traumatic experience, and the lack of acknowledgment of the impact of the event, places the survivor at greater risk of being traumatized.

Prior emotional functioning is another factor that may either intensify or mitigate the impact of a stressful event (Carlson et al., 2016; Glad, Hafstad, Jensen, & Dyb, 2017; Lanctôt & Guay, 2014; Nickerson, Bryant, Rosebrock, & Litz, 2014). Individuals with preexisting mental health problems are at greater risk of being traumatized. Emotional, psychological, and psychiatric problems are common sequelae of trauma; researchers have suggested that these conditions may have preceded the exposure, or at least have been exacerbated by it.

The focus on risk and protective factors has been complemented by efforts to ascertain the ways in which individuals can grow and benefit from exposure to trauma. When individuals can identify positive aspects of their traumatic experience, they are likely to experience fewer negative long-term consequences (Burton, Cooper, Feeny, & Zoellner, 2015; Linley & Joseph, 2004; McLaughlin & Lambert, 2017; Poole, Dobson, & Pusch, 2017; Zalta et al., 2016).

Researchers have found that traumatized individuals may benefit in several ways; most notably, a reordering of priorities, an enhanced or new sense of spirituality, a deeper appreciation for life and for loved ones, and increased feelings of empathy and concern for others (Bonanno, 2004; Grasso et al., 2012; Mancini, Littleton, & Grills, 2016; Taormina, 2015). Adversarial growth also can lead to enhanced feelings of self-efficacy: "What doesn't kill you makes you stronger" (McMillen, 1999, p. 459). It does appear that survivors of interpersonal victimization in childhood, particularly sexual abuse, have a harder time identifying positive changes (Domhardt, Münzer, Fegert, & Goldbeck, 2015; Ulloa, Guzman, Salazar, & Cala, 2016).

Trauma and neurobiology

A more recent advancement in the understanding of trauma is a recognition of the neurobiological changes that result from exposure (Del Río-Casanova, González, Páramo, Van Dijkea, & Brenlla, 2016; Nemeroff & Binder, 2014; Sperry, 2016; Wilkinson, 2017). Biochemical changes in the developing brain have been found to interfere with the brain's ability to process trauma and affect the body's stress response systems. Delima and Vimpani (2011) explained, "The behaviours resulting from chronic stress include poor self-regulation, increased impulsive behaviours, and emotional responses such as high levels of experienced anxiety, aggression and suicidal tendencies and, in some, a learned helplessness from the constant impairment of self-regulation" (p. 45). Therefore, the long-term emotional, psychological, and cognitive effects of trauma often reflect maladaptive brain processes related to stress regulation.

Trauma and mental health disorders

The relationship between trauma exposure and later mental health issues was formally recognized in 1980 when the American Psychiatric Association's (APA) third edition of the *Diagnostic and Statistical Manual of Mental Disorders* (*DSM*) included two new diagnostic categories, Post-Traumatic Stress Disorder (PTSD) and Dissociative Disorder (DD) (Courtois & Gold, 2009). Trauma was assumed to occur in response to a specific event that was outside of the range of "usual human experience" (APA, 1980, p. 236). The definition of and requirements for PTSD, the most widely applied diagnosis for trauma-exposed individuals, have been refined over the years in response to ongoing research and the resulting refinement in thinking. In the most recent, fifth, edition of the *DSM* (APA, 2013), a new diagnostic category, Trauma and Stressor-Related and Dissociative Disorders, includes several specific disorders like PTSD and DD.

From the outset, controversy has surrounded the use of the PTSD diagnosis in cases of trauma exposure (McNally, 2009; Rosen & Lilienfeld, 2008). Even with the recent reconceptualization of stress disorders, no single diagnosis adequately accounts for the individual's unique interpretation of her or his exposure to trauma. Neurobiological changes and the changes in cognitive schema that typically accompany trauma exposure also are not adequately reflected (Wheeler, 2007).

Indirect trauma

A more recent line of inquiry has been focused on the impact that working with survivors of trauma, particularly interpersonal victimization, has on those engaged in the work. Imprecision in the use of terms to describe the effects of working with survivors has led to some confusion in the literature (Knight, 2015). Research substantiates three distinct but interrelated manifestations: vicarious trauma, secondary traumatic stress, and compassion fatigue. Theorists and researchers have agreed that indirect trauma is an inevitable consequence of working with survivors of trauma. Emphasis is placed on the practitioner being proactive in mitigating and managing its effects rather than prevention. Indirect trauma is different from burnout and countertransference, although it may lead to one or both phenomena (Berzoff & Kita, 2010; Pearlman & Saakvitne, 1995; Salston & Figley, 2003).

Secondary traumatic stress refers to a cluster of symptoms that mirror indicators of PTSD, analogous to those experienced by trauma survivors themselves. Manifestations include persistent, intrusive thoughts and images of clients, hypervigilance, reexperiencing the client's trauma in recollections and dreams, and hyperarousal (Bride, 2004). In response to these reactions, clinicians may adopt distancing strategies such as denial, detachment, emotional insulation, and disbelief. The *DSM-V*(APA, 2013) expanded the PTSD diagnosis to include this form of trauma.

The term vicarious trauma is often used to refer to the full range of professionals' reactions. In fact, it refers to a very specific manifestation, changes in cognitive schema, analogous to the distortions in thinking first noted by constructivist self-development theorists among individuals exposed to trauma. Like their clients, practitioners develop a worldview characterized by suspicion, pessimism, and powerlessness (Cunningham, 2004; McCann & Pearlman, 1990b; Pearlman & Saakvitne, 1995; Van Deusen & Way, 2006).

Compassion fatigue is not unique to working with trauma survivors, but it is particularly common among individuals who work with this population (Adams, Boscarino, & Figley, 2006; Berzoff & Kita, 2010; Figley, 1995). Listening to survivors' stories of trauma, coupled with witnessing the distress firsthand, can result in an inability to empathize with clients, particularly in those cases where the individual is difficult to engage or displays hostility toward the clinician.

Analogous to the study of direct exposure to trauma, researchers have sought to identify risk and protective factors. The risk of indirect trauma appears to be higher among professionals who have less education, are newer to their jobs, and have the most and least experience working with trauma survivors (Harr & Moore, 2011; Molnar et al., 2017). Findings regarding the influence of a personal history of trauma are mixed. There is some evidence that therapists who experienced childhood trauma are at higher risk of experiencing indirect trauma (Nelson-Gardell & Harris, 2003). It is unclear whether exposure to other forms of trauma predisposes therapists to indirect trauma, since empirical inquiry has been narrowly focused on the impact of childhood victimization.

An organizational climate that validates and normalizes workers' reactions mitigates the risk, while a climate that is perceived as unsupportive increases it (Brockhouse, Msetfi, Cohen, & Joseph, 2011; Dombo & Blome, 2016). Authors have agreed that proactive self-care is essential to managing the effects of indirect trauma (Bober & Regehr, 2006; Layne et al., 2011). Lower risk is associated with organizational and supervisory environments that promote self-care activities and convey to staff that mediating the impact of indirect trauma is an organizational responsibility as much as an individual one (Hensel, Ruiz, Finney, & Dewa, 2015; Sprang, Ross, Miller, Blackshear, & Ascienzo, 2017).

Analogous to the evolution in thinking regarding direct trauma exposure, the positive aspects of indirect trauma have been examined. "Vicarious resilience" or "vicarious posttraumatic growth" has been observed among therapists working in a variety of practice contexts (Barrington & Shakespeare-Finch, 2013; Cosden, Sanford, Koch, & Lepore, 2016; Frey, Beesley, Abbott, & Kendrick, 2017; Molnar et al., 2017). Positive outcomes include enhanced appreciation for one's advantages in life, a reordering of personal goals and priorities, increased sense of professional competence and resourcefulness, and heightened capacity for compassion and empathy. For those therapists with a history of trauma exposure, affirmation of their strengths and resilience also has been observed (Killian, Hernandez-Wolfe, Engstrom, & Gangsei, 2017).

Trauma-informed practice and care

The evolution in thinking about and the understanding of trauma and the impact on its victims has resulted in an appreciation for the role that this phenomenon plays in the lives of many of the individuals seeking or required to seek treatment. Studies of clinical populations consistently have demonstrated that adults with histories of childhood trauma are overrepresented among those seeking or required to seek treatment in mental health, substance abuse, forensic, domestic violence, child welfare, homeless, and sexual assault settings (Álvarez et al., 2011; Larsson et al., 2013; Rossiter et al., 2015). Furthermore, epidemiological studies have revealed that most adults have been exposed to at least one event that could be characterized as traumatic (Beristianos, Maguen, Neylan, & Byers, 2016; Courtois & Gold, 2009; Gillikin et al., 2016; McCall-Hosenfeld, Mukherjee, & Lehman, 2014). The increasing frequency of natural disasters, the escalation of terrorist attacks and gun and community violence, and ongoing wars underscore the requirement that practitioners be well-versed in understanding the needs of victims and survivors (Gil, 2015; Glad et al., 2017; Helpman, Besser, & Neria, 2015).

The terms *trauma-informed practice* and *trauma-informed care* began to appear in the mental health literature in 2001. Since that time, the nature of this approach has been refined and clarified. The underlying assumption is that "any person seeking services or support might be a trauma survivor.... [Treatment must] recognize, understand, and counter the sequelae of trauma to facilitate recovery" (Goodman et al., 2016, p. 748). The underlying assumption is that "any person seeking services or support might be a trauma survivor.... [Treatment must] recognize, understand, and counter the sequelae of trauma to facilitate recovery" (Goodman et al., 2016, p. 748).

The terms *practice* and *care* often are used interchangeably. However, it is more accurate to use the term practice when referring to the individual clinician and care when referring to an organizational approach to treating trauma survivors. Theorists and researchers have noted that trauma-informed practice cannot occur without organizational support in the form of assignment of caseloads, provision of supervision, and allocation of resources to manage indirect trauma (Bassuk, Unick, Paquette, & Richard, 2017; Conover, Sharp, & Salerno, 2015).

Trauma-informed practice

Authors (Berger & Quiros, 2016; Conover et al., 2015; Goodman et al., 2016) have agreed that trauma-informed practice must adhere to five principles: safety, trust, collaboration, choice, and empowerment. These principles reflect the considerable body of research that has documented the short- and long-term effects of trauma exposure. They also represent "the direct opposite conditions of persons who have experienced traumatic events. That is, the safety and experience of freedom and empowerment of those who have experienced trauma was compromised, leading to a distrust of others" (Hales, Kusmaul, & Nochajski, 2017, p. 318).

Trauma-informed practice also must avoid retraumatizing clients and, in cases of interpersonal victimization like childhood abuse, re-creating maladaptive social interactions in the therapeutic relationship. The ways in which these five principles are manifested will vary depending upon practice context. Survivors of human-made and natural disasters will often seek or be offered treatment at the time of the event. Intervention at this point is likely to be more crisis-oriented (Breckenridge & James, 2010; Courtois & Gold, 2009). Intervention in these cases may be more accurately referred to as trauma *specific* or *focused*. The intent is to help survivors make meaning of the traumatic event and develop ways of coping and managing the immediate emotional, behavioral, physiological, and cognitive effects (Gray & Litz, 2005). An additional—and important—focus is preventing or mitigating the long-term effects associated with exposure to trauma (Briere & Scott, 2014; Lopez Levers, Ventura, & Bledsoe, 2012; Manderscheid, 2009).

In contrast, many individuals seek or are required to seek services for current problems in living that stem from past trauma (Jones & Cureton, 2014; Knight, 2009). Most of the available literature on trauma-informed practice focuses on this context and these individuals. Intervention often emphasizes the resolution of the present-day difficulties, due to survivors' sense of urgency, a scarcity of resources, and narrowly defined agency focus. The trauma-informed clinician understands the "the ways in which current problems can be understood in the context of past victimization" (Knight, 2015, p. 26). The clinician also "recognizes the implications that being a survivor [of past victimization] have for the client's ability to enter into a working alliance... given core beliefs characterized by hostility towards others" (Knight, 2015, p. 26).

Safety

Survivors often experience the world—and, in many cases, other people—as unsafe. Creating a safe environment is multifaceted and includes both the physical and interpersonal environments. "The environment must not only *be* safe but also *feel* safe" (Berger & Quiros, 2014, p. 297). The location of furniture in the clinician's office can either promote safety or reinforce its absence. Clients should, for example, be able to avoid sitting with their backs to a door, window, or other potential source of anxiety. Furniture should be comfortable, and colors should be soothing. Privacy also must be ensured. The clinician creates a safe interpersonal environment by, among other things, normalizing and validating client reactions, displaying an understanding of the impact of trauma, and conveying empathy, understanding, and genuineness.

Trust

The elements that contribute to safety also contribute to trust. Harris and Fallot (2001), who were the first to write about trauma-informed practice and care, noted that trust also develops when the therapist maintains clear and appropriate boundaries, protects confidentiality to the extent that is possible (and informs clients when this is not possible), and interacts with the client in ways that are consistent, predictable, and transparent. Trustworthiness also depends upon cultural awareness, since cultural norms and traditions influence how individuals experience, interpret, and respond to traumatic exposure (Berger & Quiros, 2014; Mattar, 2011). Fostering trust in survivors of trauma requires clinicians to directly address and explain any mandates that might govern their interactions with clients (Becker-Blease, 2017; Knight, 2015).

Although not as widely discussed, trust also includes helping clients develop trust in themselves. Since survivors often feel overwhelmed by their reactions and believe their emotions are unmanageable, the clinician must create a therapeutic environment wherein clients learn to both express *and contain* feelings. This reduces the possibility that intervention will be retraumatizing (Knight, 2015).

Choice

Because feelings of powerlessness are prevalent among survivors of trauma, it is important that, to the extent possible, they have some degree of choice in deciding upon methods and modes of intervention. This leads to a need for the clinician to be schooled in a range of culturally relevant strategies and techniques and willing to employ those that respond to clients' stated needs. The clinician also adheres to principles of informed consent, advising clients of the advantages, disadvantages, and purpose of various courses of action.

Collaboration

Collaborative efforts between therapist and client reinforce the principles of choice and empowerment. "Clients [are encouraged] to play an active role in their treatment and providers acknowledge the expertise that clients bring to the treatment process" (Berger & Quiros, 2014, p. 298). A collaborative approach to treatment requires cultural competence and reinforces the notion that clients are the experts in their lives (Breckenridge & James, 2010; Mattar, 2011).

Empowerment

Adherence to the principles of choice and collaboration facilitate client empowerment, a particularly important therapeutic outcome, given the powerlessness that many trauma survivors experience. To the extent possible, clients should have an influential role in "planning, operating, and evaluating services" (Berger & Quiros, 2014, p. 298). The principle applies to an individual client's own course of treatment as well as to soliciting that client's input into the overall provision of services to clients in general. Empowerment also requires the clinician to introduce strategies that assist the trauma survivor in managing feelings and present-day challenges associated with their experience (Knight, 2015).

Status of trauma-informed practice

The findings of several studies have indicated that trauma-informed practice remains an ideal, rather than a reality, in many practice settings, even those that are widely viewed as and known for treating trauma survivors (Cook et al., 2017; Courtois & Gold, 2009; Layne et al., 2011; Mattar, 2011). It appears that opportunities are available to educate professionals and professionals-to-be about trauma and trauma-*specific* interventions (Smith, Hyman, Andres-Hyman, Ruiz, & Davidson, 2016; Valinejad, 2015; Zaleski, Johnson, & Klein, 2016). However, preparing clinicians to engage in trauma-*informed* practice, generally, is lacking (Berger & Quiros, 2016; Courtois & Gold, 2009).

Trauma-informed care

Numerous efforts have been undertaken to infuse trauma-informed care (TIC) into virtually all behavioral and mental health settings. However, TIC remains limited or nonexistent in many practice contexts (Becker-Blease, 2017; Bloom, 2010; Branson, Baetz, Horwitz, & Hoagwood, 2017). The reasons for this vary, but include limited financial resources, a lack of appreciation for the role that trauma plays in clients' lives, and an understanding of TIC and its principles. TIC is an "organizational change process that is structured around the presumption that everyone in the agency (from clients through agency management) may have been directly or indirectly exposed to trauma within their lifetime" (Wolf et al., 2014, p. 111). Trauma-informed care is guided by the same five principles that define practice; the additional consideration is that they apply both to clients and staff.

Safety

Considerations associated with the agency's exterior and interior appearance that promote safety for staff and clients include assessing the need for open versus locked doors and barred versus unbarred windows, comfortable and pleasant waiting areas, options for anonymity, and guaranteed privacy. Safety for clients requires organizational staff to be respectful, pleasant, and sensitive to signs of client distress.

Trust

An organizational climate and leadership that promotes respect among staff, clarifies expectations for performance, rewards excellence and supports employees' efforts to improve upon their work, and protects staff from external threats to job security and satisfaction (such as budget cuts, negative media attention, litigation) enhances trust among staff. Safety and trust among staff is engendered when self-care is not only promoted but provided and the existence of indirect trauma is normalized and validated (Bloom, 2010). Trauma-informed care also requires that organizations adhere to guidelines regarding the distribution of cases and the size of caseloads to prevent burnout and limit indirect trauma.

Collaboration, choice, and empowerment

Trauma-informed care means that staff are encouraged to provide input into policies that impact them and their clients. Like the clients who are served, agency personnel must believe they have a voice. At all levels within an organization, employees also must understand the needs of trauma-exposed clients, as well their own vulnerability to indirect trauma (Wolf et al., 2014).

Status of trauma-informed care

There appears to be consensus regarding what trauma-informed care should look like (Bassuk et al., 2017). However, the evidence suggests that, like trauma-informed practice, the implementation of TIC in most mental, behavioral, and physical health settings is limited (Branson et al., 2017; Conover et al., 2015; Lang, Campbell, Shanley, Crusto, & Connell, 2016; Wolf et al., 2014). Even in settings that provide trauma-*focused* services to clients, organizational policies and culture typically are not operating from a trauma-informed perspective (Bassuk et al., 2017).

Where it has been implemented, TIC has been found to enhance staff and client empowerment and client satisfaction with treatment services and reduce manifestations of indirect trauma (Sullivan, Goodman, Virden, Strom, & Ramirez, 2017). In contrast, lack of adherence to the principles of TIC, particularly trust and safety, has been found to be associated with higher rates of indirect trauma among staff, lower rates of vicarious resilience, and reduced overall quality of services to clients (Elliott, Bjclajac, Fallot, Markoff, & Reed, 2005; Frey et al., 2017).

Trauma-informed supervision

An essential element of trauma-informed care is trauma-informed supervision. It is only when therapists have knowledgeable and supportive supervision that they can operate from a trauma-informed perspective. The basic requisites of trauma-informed supervision include knowledge of trauma and its effects on clients, indirect trauma, core skills of clinical supervision, and core precepts of trauma-informed practice and care. Trauma-informed supervision requires the same five elements that comprise trauma-informed practice and care (Berger & Quiros, 2016).

A primary challenge to providing trauma-informed supervision is the lack of understanding among many clinical supervisors of the nature of trauma and its effects on victims, and a lack of familiarity with the principles of trauma-informed practice and care (Berger & Quiros, 2016; Courtois & Gold, 2009; Mattar, 2011). A second challenge reflects a common problem in the provision of clinical supervision generally. In many instances, the supervisor may have little or no training in or preparation for this role (Gray, Ladany, Walker, & Ancis, 2001; Mehr, Ladany, & Caskie, 2015). Furthermore, administrative responsibilities associated with both the clinician and supervisor roles often restrict the amount of time that can be devoted to supervisees' clinical practice (Knight, 2013; Sommer, 2008). Research findings continue to demonstrate that the topics that clinicians most need to discuss in supervision are the very topics that they avoid bringing up (Best et al., 2014; Mehr et al., 2015; Petrila, Fireman, Fitzpatrick, Hodas, & Taussig, 2015). In the case of therapists working with trauma survivors, this is likely to include manifestations of indirect trauma (Etherington, 2009; Furlonger & Taylor, 2013).

Although models of clinical supervision have proliferated over the past quarter-century, integration of trauma-informed principles is lacking, particularly when it comes to understanding how to address therapists' reactions to working with trauma survivors, a critical task of trauma-informed supervision (Bober & Regehr, 2006; Hernández, Engstrom, & Gangsei, 2010; Joubert, Hocking, & Hampson, 2013). When too much attention is paid to supervisees' reactions, it may take the form of quasi-therapy, which leads to boundary violations, distracts from supervisees' need for guidance, and undermines their self-efficacy (Berger & Quiros, 2016). When the clinician's reactions are ignored or minimized, this may intensify—rather than mitigate—the impact of indirect trauma (Yourman, 2003). The following example reveals the dele-terious effects of an uninformed response to manifestations of indirect trauma.

> Monica works in an outpatient substance abuse treatment program for women. Her primary purpose is to assist clients in remaining sober and address any challenges to their sobriety that may surface. She meets with her supervisor, Victor, monthly for supervision. Monica recently began working with Meghan, age 30, who has been using drugs and alcohol since she was 13. Meghan has been sober for one month. In their most recent weekly session, she disclosed to Monica that her father had molested her throughout her childhood. Starting at age 13, he began to "pimp her out" to his friends in exchange for money to support his own addiction to heroin. Meghan described violent and sadistic sexual and physical abuse and reported that her father often photographed the abuse and posted the photos to pornographic websites.

In her last supervisory session with Victor, Monica began to cry as she described Meghan's abuse; she also expressed her desire to "castrate" Meghan's father and her other perpetrators. Victor acknowledged Monica's feelings, but questioned if she was getting "triggered" by something in her own personal history. Monica replied, "I don't think so. Nothing comes to mind, at least." Victor then suggested that her "intense" affective response "strongly suggests" that she was experiencing countertransference. He gently suggested that she consider going into therapy to address her "unresolved issues," since as her supervisor it would be "inappropriate" for them to discuss this in supervision.

Victor's reaction to Monica revealed his lack of knowledge about the impact that her work had on her. Rather than normalizing and validating her responses to her client's victimization, he framed them as abnormal. Monica acknowledged that Victor's comments left her feeling confused and guilty. She was unable to identify something in her past that might have triggered her reaction, so she did not pursue therapy. But she continued to question why she had reacted so strongly and "inappropriately" to Meghan's disclosures. This supervision scenario was described in a workshop the author was conducting on trauma-informed practice. As Monica was dis-cussing her experience, numerous attendees acknowledged similar experi-ences in which manifestations of indirect trauma were either ignored or misinterpreted.

Integrating trauma-informed principles into the discrimination model of clinical supervision

Bernard's discrimination model of supervision is one of the more widely known, investigated, and utilized perspectives on supervision (Bernard & Goodyear, 2014). The supervisor helps supervisees "move from relatively passive learners to those who take an active role in enhancing their knowledge" (Knight, 2017, p. 3). The model readily lends itself to incorporating a trauma-informed lens. When the three discrimination model roles (i.e., teacher, counselor, consultant) are considered in a trauma-informed context, supervisory mistakes such as the one just described are avoided, and supervisees receive the guidance, education, and support they need.

In the teaching role, the supervisor assumes primary responsibility for supervisees' learning. This role is critical in those cases where supervisees are trainees, inexperienced, or encounter a clinical situation with which they are unfamiliar. The consultant role is appropriate when supervisees are more knowledgeable and confident in their abilities. The supervisor helps supervisees think more critically and analytically about their work. The counselor role remains constant throughout the supervisory relationship and fosters supervisees' understanding of and ability to manage their personal feelings and reactions as these surface in their work with clients. The intent is not to provide therapy. Rather, it is to help supervisees examine their reactions to clients and their work so as to minimize the potential for disruption in the therapeutic relationship.

Safety

Safety in trauma-informed supervision mirrors that which should exist in the therapeutic relationship. A supervisory alliance in which the following factors are present facilitates safety:

(1) Supervisees feel accepted and understood;
(2) the boundaries and expectations are clear; and
(3) supervisees are encouraged to take an active role in their learning and engage in honest and open discussion.

These requirements suggest the importance of the supervisor attending to the relational aspects of the supervisory relationship (Berger & Quiros, 2016).

Trauma-informed supervision normalizes supervisees' experiences and accommodates supervisees' unique learning needs and reactions to and understanding of their clients who are trauma survivors. Consistent with trauma survivors, supervisees will experience their work differently based upon personal and background characteristics and professional training and experience (Berger & Quiros, 2014; West, 2010). In describing what constitutes a safe place for supervisees working with trauma survivors, one supervisor in Berger and Quiros's (2016) study noted the need to "[create] an oasis within the chaos... [balance] being very attentive, gentle, supportive, and nurturing, while also nudging workers to challenge themselves, hold them accountable, and yet create a safe place to struggle toward professional growth" (p. 149).

The three roles associated with the discrimination model (Bernard & Goodyear, 2014) are relevant for this aspect of trauma-informed supervision. Supervisors should assist clinicians in minimizing the impact of their work and be proactive in taking care of themselves. As both teacher and consultant, the supervisor helps supervisees understand their reactions to their work. This knowledge normalizes and validates manifestations of indirect trauma which, in turn, makes these reactions easier to manage. Together, supervisee and supervisor work to identify strategies that minimize the impact of indirect trauma and allow the supervisee to engage in self-care.

The counseling role also may come into play as supervisors help therapists understand the source of countertransference and develop strategies to manage it. Indirect trauma is not countertransference, but these reactions are often co-occurring and can reinforce one another (McCann & Pearlman, 1990). In Berger and Quiros's study (2016), supervisors of clinicians who worked with trauma survivors noted the importance of "modeling vulnerability and process[ing] [supervisees'] own encounters with trauma" (p. 151) as a way of helping supervisees contain the pain that their work triggered. The supervisor's willingness to model transparency and vulnerability is essential for assisting supervisees in acknowledging and managing countertransference and indirect trauma.

Supervisors should consider routinely engaging in an "affective tuning in" in each supervisory session (Etherington, 2000). "Supervisees can be asked to reflect on any changes in their response to specific clients or to their work in general, since indirect trauma [and countertransference] vary in response to changing circumstances in supervisees' personal and professional lives" (Knight, 2013, p. 232). The use of a check-in normalizes supervisees' personal reactions and encourages them to be proactive around self-care and managing indirect trauma and countertransference.

Trust

As noted, trust and safety are interdependent. Trust is fostered when the supervisee views the supervisor as knowledgeable about trauma and its impact on survivors and therapists. This knowledge includes educating supervisees on appropriate intervention techniques and approaches. Of even greater importance is helping supervisees see how "the way [their clients] relate to the world and see themselves in context with the world around them has been significantly shifted by the traumatic events in their lives" (respondent quoted in Berger & Quiros, 2016, p. 150). As teacher and/ or consultant, the supervisor helps supervisees understand clients' core beliefs about self and others and appreciate how these beliefs influence their ability to engage in a therapeutic relationship. The supervisor also will need to assist supervisees in seeing manifestations of transference when these surface in the therapeutic relationship and understand how to use these dynamics to deepen the alliance and enhance clients' insight.

Bernard and Goodyear's (2014) teaching role takes on added significance in those practice contexts in which trauma survivors are seen for current problems in living, since many clinicians remain unfamiliar with the nature and effects of trauma exposure. In settings in which clients' present-day problems take precedence, clinicians may overlook or ignore signs and symptoms of underlying trauma, believing that their role prohibits exploration of the trauma (Knight, 2009). The supervisor helps supervisees understand that when they help clients better manage present-day challenges, this conforms to the trauma-informed principle of empowerment.

> James works in a mental health program that helps individuals leaving inpatient psychiatric facilities transition back into their local communities. He is young, 25, and a recent graduate of a master's program in counseling. His work typically is short-term, no more than eight sessions, and is focused primarily on helping clients secure resources that facilitate a successful transition into the community.

James recently began working with Al, a 42-year-old Army veteran. In their third session, James intended to discuss the various housing options available to Al. However, Al began to talk about his combat experiences, describing in detail how several of his friends and a commanding officer whom he respected were "blown apart" by an improvised explosive device. Al cried as he talked about being covered with "blood and guts" and also expressed a great deal of rage at the perpetrators and a desire to "cut them to shreds."

In his next supervision session with Elaine, James recounted his response to Al's disclosure. He expressed his shock at what Al had experienced, and told Elaine that he has said to the client, "This have must have been horrible for you. You must have been horrified, sick, disgusted, devastated. I can't even think of the words to describe what it must have been like." The following exchange with Elaine then occurred:

James: After he [Al] finished telling me all this, I was speechless. I felt helpless and totally unprepared to help him. I said the first thing that came out of my mouth. I wasn't even thinking. I know, I was inappropriate.

Elaine: At that moment, not thinking, but reacting spontaneously was a *good* thing. Al needed validation that what he had endured was indeed horrific, and you provided him with that.

James: But he needs so much more. He needs help with what happened to him and what he saw and experienced. And I can't help him. I'm only there to get him into community housing.

Elaine: You are right, sort of. But remember, you also need to find other resources in the community, like counseling, to support his move to community housing. In the meantime, you obviously created a safe place for him to disclose what happened to him in Afghanistan. He has developed enough trust in you to share this very deep and painful "secret."

James: Okay. But I'm not a therapist, I'm just a rehabilitation counselor.

Elaine: True, but how you responded to Al reassures him about how others will respond in the future. Your understanding and compassion lets him know that his reactions have merit and hopefully provide him with the courage he needs to make a connection with a therapist.

James: I just felt so unprepared, so out of my element.

Elaine: You did exactly what you needed to do. You listened and provided empathy. But, it sounds like you didn't encourage him to go into greater detail about what happened?

James: [Nods]

Elaine: That's exactly the right thing to do. Stripping away his defenses at this point would not be helpful to him and would undermine his stability and ability to go back to the community. Make sense?

James: Yes, actually it does. I never thought about my job this way.

Elaine: Good. Now, let me ask you something. How was it for you—how were you feeling, what was your reaction—as Al told you about his friends being blown up in front of him?

Even though her organization did not operate from a trauma-informed orientation, Elaine had gone through training in trauma-informed practice and she had many years of experience working with trauma survivors. In contrast, James had no such training and was quite inexperienced. Elaine adopted the teaching role and helped James understand how he could simultaneously work within his role as a case manager helping clients successfully transition into community housing and appropriately respond to clients with trauma histories. Elaine also utilized the counselor role when she normalized potential manifestations of indirect trauma by asking James about his reactions to Al's disclosures.

One area that often requires the supervisor's input is how to manage mandatory reporting requirements when the trauma involves interpersonal victimization (Knight, 2013). Mandatory reporting is presumed to contradict the trauma-informed practice principle of client empowerment. Clinicians often are ambivalent about adhering to the mandate, fearing the impact that their report will have on the therapeutic relationship (Pietrantonio et al., 2013). The supervisor may need to help supervisees understand how they can meet their legal obligations in a way that still provides clients with some measure of control (Henderson, 2013). Clinicians are required to report their adult clients' victimization as a child, but clients are not required to cooperate with authorities following the report. Therefore, the practitioner can encourage clients to disclose as little or as much information as they want when meeting with appropriate authorities (Daniluk & Haverkamp, 1993; Melton, 2005). Clinicians also can encourage clients to file a report themselves.

Trust also is established in the supervisory relationship when the supervisor addresses supervisees' affective reactions but clarifies and maintains appropriate boundaries. This approach reflects the appropriate use of the counselor role, limiting the possibility that the supervisory relationship will take on aspects of a therapeutic one (Bride & Jones, 2006). The supervisor's exploration of supervisees' personal reactions is intentional and designed to enhance self-awareness. Walker (2004) observed that the supervisor must be cognizant of the potential for retraumatization if there is too much focus on clients and their disclosures. An affective check-in centers on the *supervisees'* reactions, not the client's trauma. As the supervision session between James and Elaine continued, she engaged in a check-in, which was both liberating and validating:

James: [In response to Elaine's question about the impact of Al's disclosures] I'm not sure. I mean, it was sort of upsetting. But, I know that I need to not let my clients get to me.

Elaine: Where in the world did you learn that? [Laughs] Of *course* you are going to be affected by your clients! You're human. I suspect that hearing Al's story, thinking about or visualizing what he went through, must be upsetting?

James: Oh gosh, *yes*! It was so upsetting to me. I think almost more than what he shared with me, it was seeing this big, hulking, tattooed guy crying. I keep thinking about him, and about what he had to go through. Honestly, I've always wondered why we went to war over there, and now more than ever, I think it's wrong. It pisses me off.

Elaine: I'm so glad you could tell me this. If you are going to be there for your clients, you have to take care of yourself. That means being open with yourself—and with me—about your reactions. I'm not here to judge and I'm not playing therapist. I don't want to take that on. [Laughs] It's normal to think about your clients when they tell you the sorts of things Al shared. To worry about them. And we often start to see our world differently when we listen to our clients. Perhaps we can take a bit of time to talk about ways that you can take care of yourself?

Elaine made appropriate use of the counselor role as she encouraged James to discuss his reactions to his client and clarified the purpose of this discussion. The teacher and consultant roles also came in to play as she normalized James's reactions and urged him to consider ways he could take care of himself to minimize the impact that his work has on him.

Choice, collaboration, and empowerment

Inexperienced supervisees may need more guidance and instruction as they transition into trauma-informed practitioners, underscoring the teacher role. However, the trauma-informed supervisor recognizes and conveys to supervisees that "[their relationship] is a mutual one in which the knowledge and wisdom of the supervisor are not privileged over that of the supervisee…. Each learns from the other's experience and multiple realities are honored" (Berger & Quiros, 2014, p. 298). Trauma-informed supervisors must be able to balance the teaching role—in which they take on more of the role of the expert—with that of a consultant who fosters autonomy, independence, and empowerment.

An approach to supervision that has relevance for trauma-informed supervision was first described by Fontes (1995) and referred to as "sharevision." In this approach, supervisors create a more egalitarian relationship with supervisees; this in turn promotes more open and honest discussion. The concept of sharevision is consistent with relational approaches to supervision, which emphasize the attention that both parties pay to their relationship (Peled-Avram, 2017). This more egalitarian approach lessens the power differential between supervisor and supervisee that can impede honest discussion, particularly around the clinician's affective responses. As the previous example reveals, even though James is an inexperienced beginning clinician, Elaine treats him with respect, which is empowering to him.

An egalitarian approach is especially helpful when manifestations of parallel process surface in the supervisory relationship (Miehls, 2010). The existence of parallel process is acknowledged in the supervision literature, and it is presumed to be the result of supervisees reenacting in supervision a problematic dynamic from their practice (Goren, 2013). Therefore, when supervisees are helped to understand their reactions to their supervisor, they are learning more about their clients' reactions to them (Schamess, 2012).

Relational theorists have argued that parallel process may reflect transference on the part of *both* supervisee and supervisor (Miller & Twomey, 1999; Virtue & Fouché, 2009). Therefore, supervisors must promote and encourage honest discussion with their supervisees about their relationship. Miehls (2010) noted, "Supervision can be most helpful when supervisors and supervisees engage in an ongoing dialogue that explores difficulties and/or mutual transferences that occur during supervision" (p. 372). The discrimination model (Bernard & Goodyear, 2014) roles of teacher, consultant, and counselor will be instrumental in facilitating this sort of supervisory climate.

Supervisors often find themselves caught in the middle between organizational demands and their responsibilities to their supervisees and to their agency's clients (Knight, 2013). This challenge is particularly likely to occur in settings that do not adhere to a trauma-informed orientation (Becker-Blease, 2017). As supervisors acknowledge these reactions directly and actively seek to manage them, they are modeling how the supervisee can address countertransference in the therapeutic relationship.

In a workshop on trauma-informed practice led by the author, a participant, Maria, described an encounter she had with her supervisor, Tim. Maria worked in an outpatient mental health clinic. Most of her clients had a history of trauma exposure, typically childhood victimization. Maria reported the following:

> I met with my supervisor to discuss something that happened in a session I had with one of my clients, Nathan. Nathan had a long history of substance abuse and also was diagnosed with bi-polar disorder. I had been meeting with him for about two months, and we were making progress. He started trusting me, and had started to disclose his history of sexual abuse. We [her agency] had suspected he was a survivor, but so far there had been nothing in his record. I have worked with a lot of survivors, but not many men. In thinking back on it, I think that because he was a guy, his abuse just hit me harder. Not sure why, but it did. There were multiple perpetrators—a father, uncle, older siblings—the father forced them to sodomize Nathan. That probably also was why his case hit me so hard.

In supervision, I started to talk about the case. I don't usually get into too much detail with my cases because Tim doesn't really have a lot of time and is in a hurry. I started to describe what Nathan had told me about his abuse, and Tim sort of waved his hand at me, and said something like, "Okay, okay, so he was sexually abused. I get it. What is your question?" I couldn't believe it! He was so dismissive of me and Nathan. I made up some BS, and told him I'd handle it on my own. I know he knew I was angry, but he didn't say anything. But the next time we met for supervision, which was, like, two weeks later, he told me if I had an issue with him, I should tell him. But the way he said it, I could tell that wasn't a good idea. And in that supervision session, I could tell that he was pissed off at me. No way was I going to tell him how I felt!

As the author and seminar participants processed this exchange, it became clear to all, including Maria, that her supervisor's response to her presentation of Nathan's case triggered in her a great deal of anger at Tim's dismissive attitude and intensified her reactions to Nathan's abusers. Rather than using her reaction to deepen Maria's understanding of her and Nathan's feelings, Tim cut short the discussion, leaving Maria even angrier and feeling confused and isolated. Although it was unclear what may have triggered Tim's reactions and response, Maria speculated that he was extremely overworked and probably "burned out." Tim carried a small caseload himself, and Maria speculated that maybe he just could not handle hearing about someone else's cases.

In any supervisory relationship, interpersonal issues may surface that require attention. Given the power differential between supervisors and supervisees, it is the supervisor's responsibility to address these issues when they surface (Goren, 2013; Miehls, 2010). From relational and trauma-informed perspectives, bringing up relational challenges deepens the supervisory relationship and models what clinicians also must do in their practice when transference occurs (Becker-Blease, 2017; Miehls, 2010).

The supervisory relationship also is a place where posttraumatic and adversarial growth can be promoted (Brockhouse et al., 2011). This underscores the importance of the consultant role. A supervisory alliance that fosters choice, collaboration, and empowerment is one that, by definition, encourages the supervisee's growth. Research findings suggest that the supervisor should make a concerted effort to assist supervisees in identifying the ways in which they have grown—both personally and professionally—from their work (Killian et al., 2017). The supervisor can, for example, ask that supervisees come to supervision prepared to talk not only about their challenges, but also their successes and indicators of growth (Berger & Quiros, 2014). Encouraging this discussion in supervision also has the advantage of modeling for clinicians the conversations they should have in their therapeutic encounters with clients.

Challenges and future directions

An obvious challenge is the ongoing need to educate providers of mental health services at all levels about the nature and principles of trauma-informed practice and care. This education must include identifying strategies and techniques of intervention that are consistent with a trauma-informed orientation. The trauma literature is vast, but it remains somewhat bifurcated. There is abundant literature on the need for a trauma-informed orientation and what this means. But the intervention literature—which also is extensive—focuses primarily on trauma-*focused* interventions for trauma survivors.

Most clinicians practice in settings in which clients present for treatment with a current problem in living rather than a desire or intent to address underlying trauma. It is these settings that are most in need of a trauma-informed orientation. It also is in these practice contexts where specific practice guidelines and intervention strategies—beyond the five principles of trauma-informed practice—must be more clearly articulated. Future efforts must be directed toward merging the trauma-informed literature with the practice literature that outlines intervention strategies appropriate for both trauma-focused and trauma-informed settings.

In terms of supervision, three challenges are evident, in addition to those mentioned at the outset of the discussion of trauma-informed supervision. First, in many if not most settings, supervisors serve as a teacher, consultant, and counselor to their supervisees as well as an evaluator of their work. The supervisor's evaluative responsibilities may inhibit supervisees' willingness and ability to openly discuss challenges they face in their work or share with the supervisor observations about their working relationship. Authors have suggested that the evaluative function of supervision be separated from the clinical function (Mehr et al., 2015). For example, the supervisor could hold evaluative supervision meetings at a different time and context from those devoted to supervisees' clinical practice. Another option is to place responsibility for clinical supervision in the hands of individuals who do not have any associated administrative responsibilities for the supervisees (Heckman-Stone, 2004).

These two options require resources that may not be readily available. Therefore, it is noteworthy that the results of several studies have suggested that, when supervisors display genuineness and transparency, encourage supervisee feedback, clarify expectations associated with their clinical and administrative responsibilities, and create a supervisory climate characterized by mutual respect, the negative impact of their dual responsibilities is minimized (Kreider, 2014; Tromski-Klingshirn & Davis, 2007; Walsh, Gillespie, Greer, & Eanes, 2003). Each of these characteristics is inherent in trauma-informed supervision.

Second, trauma-informed supervision can only occur in an organizational context that is trauma-informed (Bassuk et al., 2017; Wolf et al., 2014). Trauma-informed supervision must be consistently available and ongoing. In many settings, more seasoned clinicians—who may be assigned the more challenging cases, including trauma survivors—receive little to no clinical supervision. Furthermore, trauma-informed supervisors must have access to the same sort of informed support and guidance as their supervisees. The requirements of trauma-informed care depend upon resources that may not be readily available.

Third, the trauma-informed literature assumes that trauma survivors are seen within an organizational context. In fact, many therapists who work with trauma survivors practice autonomously. The challenges associated with preparing individuals and agencies for trauma-informed practice and care are mirrored—and in fact amplified—in private practice settings. The application of trauma-informed practice and care in peer supervision has yet to be addressed.

Given the centrality of supervision to trauma-informed practice, far greater attention must be directed toward articulating specific supervisory techniques that are consistent with the principles of trust, safety, collaboration, control, and empowerment, but also account for the financial realities and the administrative responsibilities of the supervisor.

References

Adams, R. E., & Boscarino, J. A. (2005). Differences in mental health outcomes among Whites, African Americans, and Hispanics following a community disaster. *Psychiatry, 68*, 250–265. doi:10.1521/psyc.2005.68.3.250

Adams, R., Boscarino, J., & Figley, C. (2006). Compassion fatigue and psychological distress among social workers. *American Journal of Orthopsychiatry, 76*, 103–108. doi:10.1037/0002-9432.76.1.103

Adeola, F. O., & Picou, J. S. (2014). Social capital and the mental health impacts of Hurricane Katrina: Assessing long-term patterns of psychosocial distress. *International Journal of Mass Emergencies and Disasters, 32*, 121–156.

Álvarez, M., Roura, P., Osés, A., Foguet, Q., Solà, J., & Arrufat, F. (2011). Prevalence and clinical impact of childhood trauma in patients with severe mental disorders. *Journal of Nervous and Mental Disease, 99*, 156–161. doi:10.1097/NMD.0b013e31820c751c

American Psychiatric Association (APA). (1980). *Diagnostic and statistical manual of mental disorders* (3rd ed.). Washington, DC: Author.

American Psychiatric Association (APA). (2013). *Diagnostic and statistical manual of mental disorders* (5th ed.). Washington, DC: Author.

Arata, C., & Lindman, L. (2002). Marriage, child abuse, and sexual revictimization. *Journal of Interpersonal Violence, 17*, 953–971. doi:10.1177/0886260502017009003

Barrington, A. J., & Shakespeare-Finch, J. (2013). Working with refugee survivors of torture and trauma: An opportunity for vicarious post-traumatic growth. *Counselling Psychology Quarterly, 26*(1), 89–105. doi:10.1080/09515070.2012.727553

Bassuk, E. L., Unick, G. J., Paquette, K., & Richard, M. K. (2017). Developing an instrument to measure organizational trauma-informed care in human services: The TICOMETER. *Psychology of Violence, 7*, 150–157. doi:10.1037/vio0000030

Becker-Blease, K. A. (2017). As the world becomes trauma-informed, work to do. *Journal of Trauma & Dissociation, 18*, 131–138. doi:10.1080/15299732.2017.1253401

Berger, R., & Quiros, L. (2014). Supervision for trauma-informed practice. *Traumatology, 20*, 296–301. doi:10.1037/h0099835

Berger, R., & Quiros, L. (2016). Best practices for training trauma-informed practitioners: Supervisors' voice. *Traumatology, 22*, 145–154. doi:10.1037/trm0000076

Beristianos, M. H., Maguen, S., Neylan, T. C., & Byers, A. L. (2016). Trauma exposure and risk of suicidal ideation among older adults. *The American Journal of Geriatric Psychiatry, 24*, 639–643. doi:10.1016/j.jagp.2016.02.055

Bernard, J. M., & Goodyear, R. K. (2014). *Fundamentals of clinical supervision* (5th ed.). New York, NY: Pearson.

Berthelot, N., Godbout, N., Hebert, M., Goulet, M., & Bergeron, S. (2014). Prevalence and correlates of child sexual abuse in adults consulting for sexual problems. *Journal of Sex and Marital Therapy, 40*, 434–443. doi:10.1080/0092623X.2013.772548

Berzoff, J., & Kita, E. (2010). Compassion fatigue and countertransference: Two different concepts. *Clinical Social Work Journal, 38*, 341–349. doi:10.1007/s10615-010-0271-8

Best, D., White, E., Cameron, J., Guthrie, A., Hunter, B., Hall, K., & Lubman, D. I. (2014). A model for predicting clinician satisfaction with clinical supervision. *Alcoholism Treatment Quarterly, 32*, 67–78. doi:10.1080/07347324.2014.856227

Bloom, S. L. (2010). *Organizational stress as a barrier to trauma-informed service delivery.* Retrieved from https://www.nasmhpd.org/sites/default/files/Organizational%20Stress%202010%20formatted%20NTAC(1).pdf

Bober, T., & Regehr, C. (2006). Strategies for reducing secondary or vicarious trauma: Do they work? *Brief Treatment and Crisis Intervention, 6,* 1–9. doi:10.1093/brief-treatment/mhj001

Bonanno, G. (2004). Loss, trauma, and human resilience: Have we underestimated the human capacity to thrive after extremely aversive events?*American Psychologist, 59,* 20–28. doi:10.1037/0003-066X.59.1.20

Branson, C. E., Baetz, C. L., Horwitz, S. M., & Hoagwood, K. E. (2017). Trauma-informed juvenile justice systems: A systematic review of definitions and core components. *Psychological Trauma: Theory, Research, Practice, and Policy, 9,* 635–646. doi:10.1037/tra0000255

Breckenridge, J., & James, K. (2010). Educating social work students in multifaceted interventions for trauma. *Social Work Education, 29,* 259–275. doi:10.1080/02615470902912250

Bride, B. (2004). The impact of providing psychosocial services to traumatized populations. *Stress, Trauma, and Crisis, 7,* 29–46. doi:10.1080/15434610490281101

Bride, B. E., & Jones, J. L. (2006). Secondary traumatic stress in child welfare workers: Exploring the role of supervisory culture. *Professional Development, 9*(2/3), 38–43.

Briere, J., & Scott, C. (2014). Introduction to the second edition, *DSM*-5 update. In J. Briere & C. Scott (Eds.), *Principles of trauma therapy: A guide to symptoms, evaluation, and treatment* (2nd ed., pp. 1–5). Thousand Oaks, CA: Sage.

Brockhouse, R., Msetfi, R. M., Cohen, K., & Joseph, S. (2011). Vicarious exposure to trauma and growth in therapists: The moderating effects of sense of coherence, organizational support, and empathy. *Journal of Traumatic Stress, 24,* 735–742. doi:10.1002/jts.20704

Brown, R., Schrag, A., & Trimble, M. (2005). Dissociation, childhood interpersonal trauma, and family functioning in patients with somatization disorder. *American Journal of Psychiatry, 162,* 899–905. doi:10.1176/appi.ajp.162.5.899

Burton, M. S., Cooper, A. A., Feeny, N. C., & Zoellner, L. A. (2015). The enhancement of natural resilience in trauma interventions. *Journal of Contemporary Psychotherapy, 45,* 93–204. doi:10.1007/s10879-015-9302-7

Carlson, E. B., Palmieri, P. A., Field, N. P., Dalenberg, C. J., Macia, K. S., & Spain, D. A. (2016). Contributions of risk and protective factors to prediction of psychological symptoms after traumatic experiences. *Comprehensive Psychiatry, 69,* 106–115. doi:10.1016/j.comppsych.2016.04.022

Cloitre, M., Miranda, R., & Stovall-McClough, K. (2005). Beyond PTSD: Emotion regulation and interpersonal problems as predictors of functional impairment in survivors of childhood abuse. *Behavior Therapy, 36,* 119–124. doi:10.1016/S0005-7894(05)80060-7

Conover, K., Sharp, C., & Salerno, A. (2015). Integrating trauma-informed care principles in behavioral health service organizations. *Psychiatric Services, 66,* 1004. doi:10.1176/appi.ps.201400526

Cook, J. M., Simiola, V., Ellis, A. E., & Thompson, R. (2017). Training in trauma psychology: A national survey of doctoral graduate programs. *Training and Education in Professional Psychology, 11,* 108–114. doi:10.1037/tep0000150

Cosden, M., Sanford, A., Koch, L. M., & Lepore, C. E. (2016). Vicarious trauma and vicarious posttraumatic growth among substance abuse treatment providers. *Substance Abuse, 37,* 619–624. doi:10.1080/08897077.2016.1181695

Courtois, C., & Gold, S. (2009). The need for inclusion of psychological trauma in the professional curriculum: A call to action. *Psychological Trauma: Theory, Research, and Practice, 1,* 3–23. doi:10.1037/a0015224

Cunningham, M. (2004). Avoiding vicarious traumatization: Support, spirituality, and self-care. In N. Boyd Webb (Ed.), *Mass trauma and violence: Helping families and children cope* (pp. 327–346). New York, NY: Guilford Press.

Currier, J. M., Holland, J. M., & Malott, J. (2015). Moral injury, meaning making, and mental health in returning veterans. *Journal of Clinical Psychology, 71,* 229–240. doi:10.1002/jclp.2015.71.issue-3

Daniluk, J. C., & Haverkamp, B. E. (1993). Ethical issues in counseling adult survivors of incest. *Journal of Counseling & Development, 72,* 16–22. doi:10.1002/j.1556-6676.1993.tb02270.x

Del Río-Casanova, L., González, A., Páramo, M., Van Dijkea, A., & Brenlla, J. (2016). Emotion regulation strategies in trauma-related disorders: Pathways linking neurobiology and clinical manifestations. *Reviews in the Neurosciences, 27,* 385–395. doi:10.1515/revneuro-2015-0045

Delima, J., & Vimpani, G. (2011). The neurobiological effects of childhood maltreatment: An often overlooked narrative related to the long-term effects of early childhood trauma? *Family Matters, 89,* 42–52.

Dombo, E. A., & Blome, W. (2016). Vicarious trauma in child welfare workers: A study of organizational responses. *Journal of Public Child Welfare, 10,* 505–523. doi:10.1080/15548732.2016.1206506

Domhardt, M., Münzer, A., Fegert, J. M., & Goldbeck, L. (2015). Resilience in survivors of child sexual abuse: A systematic review of the literature. *Trauma, Violence, & Abuse, 16,* 476–493. doi:10.1177/1524838014557288

Elliott, D. E., Bjclajac, P., Fallot, R., Markoff, L. S., & Reed, B. G. (2005). Trauma-informed or trauma-denied: Principles and implementation of trauma-informed services for women. *Journal of Community Psychology, 33,* 461–477. doi:10.1002/jcop.20063

Elliott, K., & Urquiza, A. (2006). Ethnicity, culture, and child maltreatment. *Journal of Social Issues, 62,* 787–809. doi:10.1111/josi.2006.62.issue-4

Etherington, K. (2000). Supervising counselors who work with survivors of childhood sexual abuse. *Counseling Psychology Quarterly, 13,* 377–389. doi:10.1080/713658497

Etherington, K. (2009). Supervising helpers who work with the trauma of sexual abuse. *British Journal of Guidance & Counselling, 37,* 179–194. doi:10.1080/03069880902728622

Evans, S. E., Steel, A. L., & DiLillo, D. (2013). Child maltreatment severity and adult trauma symptoms: Does perceived social support play a buffering role? *Child Abuse & Neglect, 37,* 934–943. doi:10.1016/j.chiabu.2013.03.005

Figley, C. (1995). Compassion fatigue: Toward a new understanding of the costs of caring. In B. Stamm (Ed.), *Secondary traumatic stress: Self- care issues for clinicians, researchers, and educators* (pp. 3–28). Lutherville, MD: Sidran Press.

Fontes, L. (1995). Sharevision: Collaborative supervision and self-care strategies for working with trauma. *Family Journal, 3,* 249–254. doi:10.1177/1066480795033012

Frey, L. L., Beesley, D., Abbott, D., & Kendrick, E. (2017). Vicarious resilience in sexual assault and domestic violence advocates. *Psychological Trauma: Theory, Research, Practice, and Policy, 9,* 44–51. doi:10.1037/tra0000159

Furlonger, B., & Taylor, W. (2013). Supervision and the management of vicarious traumatisation among Australian telephone and online counsellors. *Australian Journal of Guidance and Counselling, 23,* 82–94. doi:10.1017/jgc.2013.3

Garno, J., Goldberg, J., Ramirez, P., & Ritzler, B. (2005). Bipolar disorder with comorbid cluster B personality disorder features: Impact on suicidality. *Journal of Clinical Psychiatry, 66,* 339–345. doi:10.4088/JCP.v66n0310

Giesen-Bloo, J., & Arntz, A. (2005). World assumptions and the role of trauma in borderline personality disorder. *Journal of Behavior Therapy and Experimental Psychiatry, 36,* 197–208. doi:10.1016/j.jbtep.2005.05.003

Gil, S. (2015). Personality and trauma-related risk factors for traumatic exposure and for posttraumatic stress symptoms (PTSS): A three-year prospective study. *Personality and Individual Differences*, *83*, 1–5. doi:10.1016/j.paid.2015.03.034

Gillikin, C., Habib, L., Evces, M., Bradley, B., Ressler, K. J., & Sanders, J. (2016). Trauma exposure and PTSD symptoms associate with violence in inner city civilians. *Journal of Psychiatric Research*, *83*, 1–7. doi:10.1016/j.jpsychires.2016.07.027

Glad, K. A., Hafstad, G. S., Jensen, T. K., & Dyb, G. (2017). A longitudinal study of psychological distress and exposure to trauma reminders after terrorism. *Psychological Trauma: Theory, Research, Practice, and Policy*, *9*(Suppl 1), 145–152. doi:10.1037/tra0000224

Goodman, L. A., Sullivan, C. M., Serrata, J., Perilla, J., Wilson, J. M., Fauci, J. E., & DiGiovanni, C. D. (2016). Development and validation of the Trauma-Informed Practice Scales. *Journal of Community Psychology*, *44*, 747–764. doi:10.1002/jcop.2016.44.issue-6

Goren, E. (2013). Ethics, boundaries, and supervision. Commentary on trauma triangles and parallel processes: Geometry and the supervisor/trainee/patient triad. *Psychoanalytic Dialogues*, *23*, 737–743. doi:10.1080/10481885.2013.851568

Grasso, D. J., Cohen, L. H., Moser, J. S., Hajcak, G., Foa, E. B., & Simons, R. F. (2012). Seeing the silver lining: Potential benefits of trauma exposure in college students. *Anxiety, Stress & Coping: An International Journal*, *25*, 17–136. doi:10.1080/10615806.2011.561922

Gray, L. A., Ladany, N., Walker, J. A., & Ancis, J. R. (2001). Psychotherapy trainees' experience of counterproductive events in supervision. *Journal of Counseling Psychology*, *48*, 371–383. doi:10.1037/0022-0167.48.4.371

Gray, M. J., & Litz, B. T. (2005). Behavioral interventions for recent trauma: Empirically informed practice guidelines. *Behavior Modification*, *29*, 89–215. doi:10.1177/0145445504270884

Hales, T., Kusmaul, N., & Nochajski, T. (2017). Exploring the dimensionality of trauma-informed care: Implications for theory and practice. *Human Service Organizations: Management, Leadership & Governance*, *41*, 317–325.

Harr, C., & Moore, B. (2011). Compassion fatigue among social work students in field placement. *Journal of Teaching in Social Work*, *32*, 350–363.

Harris, M., & Fallot, R. (2001). *Using trauma theory to design service systems: New directions for mental health services*. San Francisco, CA: Jossey Bass.

Heckman-Stone, C. (2004). Trainee preferences for feedback and evaluation in clinical supervision. *The Clinical Supervisor*, *22*, 21–34. doi:10.1300/J001v22n01_03

Helpman, L., Besser, A., & Neria, Y. (2015). Acute posttraumatic stress symptoms but not generalized anxiety symptoms are associated with severity of exposure to war trauma: A study of civilians under fire. *Journal of Anxiety Disorders*, *35*, 27–34. doi:10.1016/j.janxdis.2015.08.001

Henderson, K. L. (2013). Mandated reporting of child abuse: Considerations and guidelines for mental health counselors. *Journal of Mental Health Counseling*, *35*, 296–309. doi:10.17744/mehc.35.4.x35610245863n034

Hensel, J. M., Ruiz, C., Finney, C., & Dewa, C. S. (2015). Meta-analysis of risk factors for secondary traumatic stress in therapeutic work with trauma victims. *Journal of Traumatic Stress*, *28*, 83–91. doi:10.1002/jts.2015.28.issue-2

Hernández, P., Engstrom, D., & Gangsei, D. (2010). Exploring the impact of trauma on therapists: Vicarious resilience and related concepts in training. *Journal of Systemic Therapies*, *29*, 67–83. doi:10.1521/jsyt.2010.29.1.67

Jeavons, S., Greenwood, K. M., & Horne, D. L. (2000). Accident cognitions and subsequent psychological trauma. *Journal of Traumatic Stress*, *13*, 359–365. doi:10.1023/A:1007797904536

Jones, L., & Cureton, J. (2014). Trauma redefined in the *DSM-5*: Rationale and implications for counseling practice. *The Professional Counselor*, *4*, 257–271. doi:10.15241/lkj.4.3.257

Joubert, L., Hocking, A., & Hampson, R. (2013). Social work in oncology: Managing vicarious trauma-the positive impact of professional supervision. *Social Work in Health Care*, *52*, 296–310. doi:10.1080/00981389.2012.737902

Katerndahl, D., Burge, S., Kellogg, N., & Parra, J. (2005). Differences in childhood sexual abuse experience between adult Hispanic and Anglo women in a primary care setting. *Journal of Child Sexual Abuse*, *14*, 85–95. doi:10.1300/J070v14n02_05

Killian, K., Hernandez-Wolfe, P., Engstrom, D., & Gangsei, D. (2017). Development of the Vicarious Resilience Scale (VRS): A measure of positive effects of working with trauma survivors. *Psychological Trauma: Theory, Research, Practice, and Policy*, *9*, 3–31. doi:10.1037/tra0000199

Knight, C. (2009). *Introduction to working with adult survivors of childhood trauma: Strategies and techniques for helping professionals.* Monterey, CA: Thomson/Brooks-Cole.

Knight, C. (2013). Indirect trauma: Implications for self-care, supervision, the organization, and the academic institution. *The Clinical Supervisor*, *32*, 224–243. doi:10.1080/07325223.2013.850139

Knight, C. (2015). Trauma-informed social work practice: Practice considerations and challenges. *Clinical Social Work Journal*, *43*, 25–37. doi:10.1007/s10615-014-0481-6

Knight, C. (2017). The mutual aid model of group supervision. *The Clinical Supervisor*, *36*, 1–23. doi:10.1080/07325223.2017.1306473

Kreider, H. (2014). Administrative and clinical supervision: The impact of dual roles on supervisee self-disclosure in counseling supervision. *The Clinical Supervisor*, *33*, 256–268. doi:10.1080/07325223.2014.992292

Lanctôt, N., & Guay, S. (2014). The aftermath of workplace violence among healthcare workers: A systematic literature review of the consequences. *Aggression & Violent Behavior*, *19*, 492–501. doi:10.1016/j.avb.2014.07.010

Lang, J. M., Campbell, K., Shanley, P., Crusto, C. A., & Connell, C. M. (2016). Building capacity for trauma-informed care in the child welfare system: Initial results of a statewide implementation. *Child Maltreatment*, *21*, 113–124. doi:10.1177/1077559516635273

Larsson, S., Andreassen, O. A., Aas, M., Røssberg, J. I., Mork, E., Steen, N. E., & Lorentzen, S. (2013). High prevalence of childhood trauma in patients with schizophrenia spectrum and affective disorder. *Comprehensive Psychiatry*, *54*, 123–127. doi:10.1016/j.comppsych.2012.06.009

Layne, C. M., Ippen, C., Strand, V., Stuber, M., Abramovitz, R., Reyes, G.,... Pynoos, R. (2011). The core curriculum on childhood trauma: A tool for training a trauma-informed workforce. *Psychological Trauma: Theory, Research, Practice, and Policy*, *3*, 243–252. doi:10.1037/a0025039

Linley, P. A., & Joseph, S. (2004). Positive change following trauma and adversity: A review. *Journal of Traumatic Stress*, *17*, 11–20. doi:10.1023/B:JOTS.0000014671.27856.7e

Lopez Levers, L., Ventura, E. M., & Bledsoe, D. E. (2012). Models for trauma intervention: Integrative approaches to therapy. In L. Lopez Levers (Ed.), *Trauma counseling: Theories and interventions* (pp. 493–503). New York, NY: Springer.

Mancini, A. D., Littleton, H. L., & Grills, A. E. (2016). Can people benefit from acute stress? Social support, psychological improvement, and resilience after the Virginia Tech campus shootings. *Clinical Psychological Science*, *4*, 401–417. doi:10.1177/2167702615601001

Manderscheid, R. W. (2009). Trauma-informed leadership. *International Journal of Mental Health*, *38*, 8–86. doi:10.2753/IMH0020-7411380107

Mattar, S. (2011). Educating and training the next generations of traumatologists: Development of cultural competencies. *Psychological Trauma: Theory, Research, Practice, and Policy*, *3*, 258–265. doi:10.1037/a0024477

McCall-Hosenfeld, J. S., Mukherjee, S., & Lehman, E. B. (2014). The prevalence and correlates of lifetime psychiatric disorders and trauma exposures in urban and rural settings: Results from the National Comorbidity Survey Replication (NCS-R). *Plos ONE*, *9*(11), 1–11. doi:10.1371/journal.pone.0112416

McCann, I., & Pearlman, L. (1990a). *Psychological trauma and the adult survivor*. New York, NY: Brunner/Mazel.

McCann, I., & Pearlman, L. (1990b). Vicarious traumatization: A framework for understanding the psychological effects of working with victims. *Journal of Traumatic Stress, 3*, 131–149. doi:10.1007/BF00975140

McLaughlin, K. A., & Lambert, H. K. (2017). Child trauma exposure and psychopathology: Mechanisms of risk and resilience. *Current Opinion in Psychology, 14*, 29–34. doi:10.1016/j.copsyc.2016.10.004

McMillen, J. C. (1999). Better for it: How people benefit from adversity. *Social Work, 44*, 455–467. doi:10.1093/sw/44.5.455

McNally, R. (2009). Can we fix PTSD in *DSM-V*? *Depression and Anxiety, 26*, 597–600. doi:10.1002/da.v26:7

Mehr, K. E., Ladany, N., & Caskie, G. L. (2015). Factors influencing trainee willingness to disclose in supervision. *Training and Education in Professional Psychology, 9*, 44–51. doi:10.1037/tep0000028

Melton, G. (2005). Mandated reporting: A policy without reason. *Child Abuse and Neglect, 29*, 9–18. doi:10.1016/j.chiabu.2004.05.005

Miehls, D. (2010). Contemporary trends in supervision theory: A shift from parallel process to relational and trauma theory. *Clinical Social Work Journal, 38*, 370–378. doi:10.1007/s10615-009-0247-8

Miller, L., & Twomey, J. (1999). A parallel without a process: A relational view of a supervisory experience. *Contemporary Psychoanalysis, 35*, 557–580. doi:10.1080/00107530.1999.10746402

Molnar, B. E., Sprang, G., Killian, K. D., Gottfried, R., Emery, V., & Bride, B. E. (2017). Advancing science and practice for vicarious traumatization/secondary traumatic stress: A research agenda. *Traumatology, 23*, 129–142. doi:10.1037/trm0000122

Mulvihill, D. (2005). The health impact of childhood trauma: An interdisciplinary review, 1997–2003. *Issues in Comprehensive Pediatric Nursing, 28*, 115–136. doi:10.1080/01460860590950890

Nelson- Gardell, D., & Harris, D. (2003). Childhood abuse history, secondary traumatic stress, and child welfare workers. *Child Welfare, 82*, 5–26.

Nemeroff, C., & Binder, E. (2014). The preeminent role of childhood abuse and neglect in vulnerability to major psychiatric disorders: Toward elucidating the underlying neurobiological mechanisms. *Journal of the American Academy of Child & Adolescent Psychiatry, 53*, 395–397. doi:10.1016/j.jaac.2014.02.004

Nickerson, A., Bryant, R. A., Rosebrock, L., & Litz, B. T. (2014). The mechanisms of psychosocial injury following human rights violations, mass trauma, and torture. *Clinical Psychology: Science & Practice, 21*, 172–191.

Park, C. L., Mills, M. A., & Edmondson, D. (2012). PTSD as meaning violation: Testing a cognitive worldview perspective. *Psychological Trauma: Theory, Research, Practice, and Policy, 4*, 66–73. doi:10.1037/a0018792

Pearlman, L., & Saakvitne, K. (1995). *Trauma and the therapist: Countertransference and vicarious traumatization in psychotherapy with incest survivors*. New York, NY: Norton.

Peled-Avram, M. (2017). The role of relational-oriented supervision and personal and work-related factors in the development of vicarious traumatization. *Clinical Social Work Journal, 45*(1), 2–32. doi:10.1007/s10615-015-0573-y

Petrila, A., Fireman, O., Fitzpatrick, L. S., Hodas, R. W., & Taussig, H. N. (2015). Student satisfaction with an innovative internship. *Journal of Social Work Education, 51*, 121–135.

Pietrantonio, A. M., Wright, E., Gibson, K. N., Alldred, T., Jacobson, D., & Niec, A. (2013). Mandatory reporting of child abuse and neglect: Crafting a positive process for health professionals and caregivers. *Child Abuse & Neglect, 37*, 102–109. doi:10.1016/j.chiabu.2012.12.007

Ponce, A., Williams, M., & Allen, G. (2004). Experience of maltreatment as a child and acceptance of violence in adult intimate relationships: Mediating effects of distortions in cognitive schemas. *Violence and Victims, 19*, 97–108. doi:10.1891/vivi.19.1.97.33235

Poole, J. C., Dobson, K. S., & Pusch, D. (2017). Anxiety among adults with a history of childhood adversity: Psychological resilience moderates the indirect effect of emotion dysregulation. *Journal of Affective Disorders, 217*, 144–152. doi:10.1016/j.jad.2017.03.047

Randolph, M., & Reddy, D. (2006). Sexual abuse and sexual functioning in a chronic pelvic pain sample. *Journal of Child Sexual Abuse, 15*, 61–78. doi:10.1300/J070v15n03_04

Rosen, G., & Lilienfeld, S. (2008). Posttraumatic stress disorder: An empirical evaluation of core assumptions. *Clinical Psychology Review, 28*, 837–868. doi:10.1016/j.cpr.2007.12.002

Rossiter, A., Byrne, F., Wota, A. P., Nisar, Z., Ofuafor, T., Murray, I., & Hallahan, B. (2015). Childhood trauma levels in individuals attending adult mental health services: An evaluation of clinical records and structured measurement of childhood trauma. *Child Abuse & Neglect, 443*, 36–45. doi:10.1016/j.chiabu.2015.01.001

Salston, M., & Figley, C. R. (2003). Secondary traumatic stress effects of working with survivors of criminal victimization. *Journal of Traumatic Stress, 16*, 167–174. doi:10.1023/A:1022899207206

Samuelson, K. W., Bartel, A., Valadez, R., & Jordan, J. T. (2017). PTSD symptoms and perception of cognitive problems: The roles of posttraumatic cognitions and trauma coping self-efficacy. *Psychological Trauma: Theory, Research, Practice, and Policy, 9*, 537–544. doi:10.1037/tra0000210

Sattler, D. N., Boyd, B., & Kirsch, J. (2014). Trauma-exposed firefighters: Relationships among posttraumatic growth, posttraumatic stress, resource availability, coping and critical incident stress debriefing experience. *Stress and Health: Journal of the International Society for the Investigation of Stress, 30*, 356–365. doi:10.1002/smi.2608

Saunders, B., & Adams, Z. (2014). Epidemiology of traumatic experiences in childhood. *Child and Adolescent Psychiatry Clinics of North America, 23*, 167–184. doi:10.1016/j.chc.2013.12.003

Schamess, G. (2012). Mutual influence in psychodynamic supervision. *Smith College Studies in Social Work, 82*, 142–160. doi:10.1080/00377317.2012.693012

Sippel, L. M., Pietrzak, R. H., Charney, D. S., Mayes, L. C., & Southwick, S. M. (2015). How does social support enhance resilience in the trauma-exposed individual?*Ecology & Society, 20*, 136–145. doi:10.5751/ES-07832-200410

Smith, A. J., Abeyta, A. A., Hughes, M., & Jones, R. T. (2015). Persistent grief in the aftermath of mass violence: The predictive roles of posttraumatic stress symptoms, self-efficacy, and disrupted worldview. *Psychological Trauma: Theory, Research, Practice, and Policy, 7*, 179–186. doi:10.1037/tra0000002

Smith, A. J., Felix, E. D., Benight, C. C., & Jones, R. T. (2017). Protective factors, coping appraisals, and social barriers predict mental health following community violence: A prospective test of social cognitive theory. *Journal of Traumatic Stress, 30*, 245–253. doi:10.1002/jts.2017.30.issue-3

Smith, D., Davis, J., & Fricker-Elhai, A. (2004). How does trauma beget trauma? Cognitions about risk in women with abuse histories. *Child Maltreatment, 9*, 292–302. doi:10.1177/1077559504266524

Smith, J. C., Hyman, S. M., Andres-Hyman, R. C., Ruiz, J. J., & Davidson, L. (2016). Applying recovery principles to the treatment of trauma. *Professional Psychology: Research and Practice, 47*, 347–355. doi:10.1037/pro0000105

Sommer, C. (2008). Vicarious traumatization, trauma-sensitive supervision, and counselor preparation. *Counselor Education and Supervision, 48*, 61–71. doi:10.1002/ceas.2008.48.issue-1

Sperry, L. (2016). Trauma, neurobiology, and personality dynamics: A primer. *Journal of Individual Psychology, 72*, 161–167. doi:10.1353/jip.2016.0014

Sprang, G., Ross, L., Miller, B. C., Blackshear, K., & Ascienzo, S. (2017). Psychometric properties of the Secondary Traumatic Stress–Informed Organizational Assessment. *Traumatology, 23,* 65–171. doi:10.1037/trm0000108

Sullivan, C. M., Goodman, L. A., Virden, T., Strom, J., & Ramirez, R. (2017). Evaluation of the effects of receiving trauma-informed practices on domestic violence shelter residents. *American Journal of Orthopsychiatry.* doi:10.1037/ort0000286

Taormina, R. J. (2015). Adult personal resilience: A new theory, new measure, and practical implications. *Psychological Thought, 8,* 35–46. doi:10.5964/psyct.v8i1.126

Tromski-Klingshirn, D., & Davis, T. E. (2007). Supervisees' perceptions of their clinical supervision: A study of the dual role of clinical and administrative supervisor. *Counselor Education and Supervision, 46,* 294–304. doi:10.1002/ceas.2007.46.issue-4

Ulloa, E., Guzman, M. L., Salazar, M., & Cala, C. (2016). Posttraumatic growth and sexual violence: A literature review. *Journal of Aggression, Maltreatment & Trauma, 25,* 286–304. doi:10.1080/10926771.2015.1079286

Valinejad, C. (2015). Delivering efficient psychotherapy. *Clinical Psychology Forum, 271,* 33–35.

Van Der Kolk, B. (2007). The history of trauma in psychiatry. In M. Friedman, T. Keane, & P. Resick (Eds.), *Handbook of PTSD: Science and practice* (pp. 19–36). New York, NY: Guilford Press.

Van Deusen, K., & Way, I. (2006). Vicarious trauma: An exploratory study of the impact of providing sexual abuse treatment on clinicians' trust and intimacy. *Journal of Child Sexual Abuse, 15,* 69–85. doi:10.1300/J070v15n01_04

Virtue, C., & Fouché, C. (2009). Multiple holding: A model for supervision in the context of trauma and abuse. *Aotearoa New Zealand Social Work Review, 21/22*(4/1), 64–72.

Walker, M. (2004). Supervising practitioners working with survivors of childhood abuse: Countertransference; secondary traumatization and terror. *Psychodynamic Practice, 10,* 173–193. doi:10.1080/14753630410001686753

Walsh, B. B., Gillespie, C., Greer, J. M., & Eanes, B. E. (2003). Influence of dyadic mutuality on counselor trainee willingness to self-disclose clinical mistakes to supervisors. *The Clinical Supervisor, 21*(2), 83–98. doi:10.1300/J001v21n02_06

West, A. (2010). Supervising counsellors and psychotherapists who work with trauma survivors: A Delphi study. *British Journal of Guidance and Counselling, 38,* 409–430. doi:10.1080/03069885.2010.503696

Wheeler, K. (2007). Psychotherapeutic strategies for healing trauma. *Perspectives in Psychiatric Care, 43,* 132–141. doi:10.1111/ppc.2007.43.issue-3

Wilkinson, M. (2017). Mind, brain, and body. Healing trauma: The way forward. *The Journal of Analytical Psychology, 6,* 526–543. doi:10.1111/1468-5922.12335

Wolf, M. R., Green, S. A., Nochajski, T. H., Mendel, W. W., & Kusmaul, N. (2014). "We're all civil servants": The status of trauma-informed care in the community. *Journal of Social Service Research, 40,* 111–120. doi:10.1080/01488376.2013.845131

Yehuda, R., Halligan, S., & Grossman, R. (2001). Childhood trauma and risk for PTSD: Relationship to intergenerational effects of trauma, parental PTSD, and cortisol excretion. *Development and Psychopathology, 13,* 733–753. doi:10.1017/S0954579401003170

Yourman, D. (2003). Trainee disclosure in psychotherapy supervision: The impact of shame. *Journal of Clinical Psychology, 59,* 601–609. doi:10.1002/(ISSN)1097-4679

Zaleski, K. L., Johnson, D. K., & Klein, J. T. (2016). Grounding Judith Herman's trauma theory within interpersonal neuroscience and evidence-based practice modalities for trauma treatment. *Smith College Studies in Social Work, 86,* 377–393. doi:10.1080/00377317.2016.1222110

Zalta, A. K., Tirone, V., Siedjak, J., Boley, R. A., Vechiu, C., Pollack, M. H., & Hobfoll, S. E. (2016). A pilot study of tailored cognitive-behavioral resilience training for trauma survivors with sub-threshold distress. *Journal of Traumatic Stress, 29,* 268–272. doi:10.1002/jts.2016.29.issue-3

Trauma-informed supervision and consultation: Personal reflections

Christine A. Courtois

ABSTRACT

This contribution is focused on the provision of supervision and consultation that is trauma-informed, following the Trauma-Informed Care (TIC) model. TIC requires a specialized knowledge base and skill set, not just for the clinician but also for the supervisor. Its core emphasis is the use of a theoretical model of traumatic stress and its many aftereffects, including the use of specialized evidence-based and evidence-supported techniques within a relationship-based and responsive treatment. Supervisors need a broad understanding of the risks and benefits that accompany work with the traumatized and must have the ability to support and protect their supervisees and their clients.

In addition to the Trauma-Informed Care initiative now being applied in social service agencies and medical settings across the United States and in many other countries, major efforts by professional organizations and behavioral health facilities are underway to add issues pertaining to trauma to the formal training curriculum. These issues include research on trauma, its effects, and the efficacy of various treatment approaches; care of traumatized clients and the treatment of their symptoms and associated problems; the well-being of the practitioner; and the philosophical alignment of the agency or organization in which services are provided. Several major professional organizations have taken on these topics. The Council on Social Work Education (CSWE) identified the competencies needed across all types of social work (i.e., administrative, supervisory, treating, researching, teaching) and at different levels of expertise and outlined a training curriculum (Strand, 2009). The International Society for the Study of Trauma and Dissociation (ISST-D; www.ISSST-D.org) developed a set of treatment competencies and a hierarchical set of courses (basic to expert) on the treatment of dissociative conditions and disorders and complex trauma for adults and children.

In 2010, Division 56 (Trauma Psychology) of the American Psychological Association (APA) initiated an ongoing survey of graduate psychology training programs that offer specializations or courses on trauma as a core part of their curriculum and how (and if) they prepared their graduates to work with trauma. Division 56 undertook the development of a set of trauma-related core competencies at three different levels of training, each with more sophisticated knowledge and skills: (a) for generalist professionals and administrative and support staff, (b) for staff offering direct services, and (c) for those with expertise in trauma research and treatment. The process undertaken in the development of these competencies and the listing of competencies can be found in Cook and Newman; the New Haven Trauma Competency Work Group (2014).

The field of traumatic stress studies is now robust with research findings and suggested approaches to treatment published on almost a daily basis. Many specialized areas of research and practice (acute and disaster trauma, refugee trauma, sexual abuse and assault trauma, etc.) have developed. In recent years, several major trauma treatment organizations, such as the Veterans Administration and The Trauma Center in Boston, and the founders of various trauma-focused treatments, such as cognitive processing therapy (CPT) and eye movement desensitization and reprocessing (EMDR) therapy, have organized comprehensive training programs that include practica and ongoing supervision post-training. These initiatives give therapists the opportunity to gain certification in these specialized treatments and this dedicated area of practice. For these and other reasons, namely, the overwhelming number of traumatized clients seeking help in behavioral health settings, it is expedient for professional training programs to follow these leaders. Specifically, they need to modify their core training curricula and applied training to incorporate trauma and research findings; stay updated and assist students and trainees in evaluating the new research, the various sub-specialties, and emerging treatments; and stay abreast of clinical practice and professional practice guidelines for trauma disorders. (See Appendix for a listing of clinical practice and professional practice guidelines for posttraumatic stress disorders.)

Supervision/consultation in trauma treatment

Against this background, I now address the main issues of this contribution: trauma-informed supervision and consultation. My focus is on addressing several sub-issues: How do supervisors/consultants establish a workable contract that protects both parties? How do they provide a secure base for therapists to support a parallel relationship between supervisees and their traumatized clients? How do they educate therapists about trauma, its effects, and its treatment, while supporting them as they provide treatment to what can be a most challenging population? These issues relate to the content of the treatment and the treatment approaches that are implemented, but, more importantly, to the treatment relationship itself as a mechanism of change. How do supervisors/consultants assist therapists with the foundational information they need, hone their skills, and support them as they experience the countertransference responses, counter-trauma, and vicarious traumatization that accompany this work, while also promoting vicarious resilience and posttraumatic growth?

First, some of my history in the field: I began my work with traumatized clients in 1972 when, as a graduate student in college counseling, I co-founded the Women's Rape Crisis Center at the University of Maryland, College Park. I wrote both my master's thesis and dissertation on rape and incest survivors, respectively, and therapeutic approaches to their healing. In those days, as there was limited and often outdated literature on those topics, my peers and I learned by reading authoritative texts, by conducting research and studying the findings of other researchers, and by doing therapy—often by trial and error—and learning from our successes and mistakes. And, I'm sorry to say, many of us made every mistake in the book (or close to it) because we had no road map and no guideposts, and certainly no specialized information on these and other trauma-related topics in our training or in supervision. But we did learn a lot as we went along, as did our peers in similar settings across the country. We read one another's writings, consulted with one another at professional conferences and in continuing education offerings, and gradually came to understand more about the population we were working with, their needs, and what approaches worked or did not. We also came to understand that the personal toll of the work on the therapist could be overwhelming, and that burnout was a constant challenge in some settings and organizations. It didn't help that insurance companies sometimes refused to pay for treatment when the diagnosis was post-traumatic stress disorder (PTSD) or for trauma-focused work (having determined it made patients worse and in need of more care), and managed care placed major limitations on the number of sessions insurance would cover. These constraints often put more pressure on therapists and on their therapeutic endeavors.

Early on, I became a supervisor of volunteers in my position as the Director of the Rape Crisis Center and of trainees as a staff psychologist working in university counseling centers. In these settings I began to understand that I had attained specialized knowledge by virtue of my studies and my direct application of what I had learned in treating trauma survivors. Although I was trained in an eclectic and psychodynamic psychotherapy tradition within the medical model, I came to realize I was working from a different perspective (what I then called "trauma-referenced treatment"). I was increasingly sought out for that very expertise because, as trauma achieved extensive media coverage and associated public recognition during the 1980s and 1990s, more and more victim/survivors disclosed their trauma histories and sought psychotherapy to address and resolve the consequences. The need and the resources were asymmetrical: a vast new treatment population emerged for therapists who had little or no training to treat them. To fill the need, books were published and continuing education offerings proliferated. I published *Healing the Incest Wound* (Courtois, 1988, 2010) and a number of colleagues authored books on other traumatized populations and on posttraumatic conditions such as dissociation. We cross-referenced and cross-pollinated one another's works, thereby achieving some peer consensus in how to proceed.

Supervision competencies: A neglected professional issue

Up until fairly recently, with the exceptions of social work, counseling. and counseling psychology, supervision of trainees as a specific skill did not receive a great deal of attention in the mental health professions. This gap has now been recognized as one that has many ramifications, some quite negative, for trainees and for practicing clinicians, as well as for their clients. In 1996, the American Psychological Association (APA) adopted *Guidelines and Principles of Accreditation*, which required training programs to provide students and interns with at least some training in supervision, identified supervision as one of the eight core competency domains of psychologists, and articulated those competencies related to supervisory practice (American Psychological Association, 1996). Since then, other professional disciplines in the United States and in other countries have developed best practices in supervision. In 2014, the *Guidelines for Clinical Supervision of Health Service Psychologists* were approved as APA policy (American Psychological Association, Board of Educational Affairs Task Force on Supervision Guidelines, 2014). These are based on a competency-based approach rather than a particular theoretical (psychotherapy) approach, and are applicable to a wide range of activities (e.g., psychotherapy, assessment, consultation services). These guidelines include a set of foundational assumptions and competencies and encourage ongoing self-assessment by the supervisor, for which they provide a self-assessment instrument as an aid to ongoing education.

As a counseling psychology intern in the late 1970s, I was fortunate to have received an early form of training called "supervision of supervision." It proved to be very useful in getting me to think about what differentiates supervision from treatment and how to approach it but, again, the topic of trauma was never mentioned. It occurred to me then (as it has since then) that it would be up to those of us in the emerging field of traumatic stress studies to develop a supervision model that took trauma into account and that provided basic education on the topic and the dynamics of treatment to supervisees/consultees. Since that time, I have attended a large number of training sessions on trauma treatment where I have been able to develop and expand my own knowledge base and hone my skills on an ongoing basis, and have also presented workshops on the treatment of trauma and related topics to thousands of therapists. I am routinely sought out as a consultant/supervisor and have run peer consultation groups for decades. I have had the good fortune to engage with other trauma-informed therapists, especially Laurie Anne Pearlman and Kay Saakvitne, as they began to develop their model of a theoretically based supervision for trauma treatment. I largely follow their model that can be found in their classic text, *Trauma and the Therapist* (Pearlman & Saakvitne, 1995), and numerous other publications and training workshops, and in the trauma-focused curriculum they wrote with colleagues titled *Risking Connection* (Saakvitne, Gamble, Pearlman, & Lev, 2000).

Beginning trauma-informed supervision and consultation: Ensuring security

I begin by presenting a prototypical case that includes various issues that usually come up in requests for supervision/consultation pertaining to a trauma case, and then provide an overview of how I've learned to address and manage this type of presentation and to conduct trauma-informed supervision. It should be noted that I do conduct supervision/consultation of more general non-trauma-focused treatments (some of which turn out to be based on trauma that has gone unrecognized or undisclosed), but, even in more generic cases, I work from a trauma-informed perspective (along with other theoretical models, discussed later), since I believe it to be pertinent to all mental health care.

> *Therapist X calls to make an appointment for supervision of a case that has become quite a problem and that involves a client with a history of trauma. He/she would like to meet as soon as possible. I inquire whether supervision or consultation is being sought, as there is a huge difference in responsibility in each (discussed later). Therapist X is confused by my question so we first talk about what is needed or sought and what would be provided. Then, following a verbal synopsis of the case, I ask the therapist to write up a brief description for me to read with specific questions before we meet.*
>
> *Quite often, the client was in treatment long before the trauma was disclosed (often surprising the therapist, who now may not trust the client and may wonder what else hasn't been disclosed, or who may now feel tricked or incompetent), but, in some cases, the client sought treatment specifically for a trauma history and trauma-related symptoms. Therapist X accepted the case (whether or not the trauma was disclosed) without specific knowledge, interest, or training as he/she is new in private practice and is in need of clients or because the client was the next up on the clinic's waiting list. The treatment is usually at some sort of impasse or crisis when*

supervision/consultation is sought and/or the therapist is seeking to transfer the client to someone else with more experience with trauma. Maybe I would be interested once I hear about the case?

The responsibilities and liabilities associated with *supervision and consultation* vary substantially so it is important to clarify the nature of the relationship right from the start. Although this contribution is on the topic of supervision, I rarely agree to formally supervise the work of another professional unless I am required to do so by the terms of my employment, if clinical trainees or associates need to acquire hours of formal case supervision for licensure, or if an individual practitioner approaches me. Whatever the context or circumstance, each must develop a formal supervision contract with me detailing our agreement to work together and the rights and responsibilities of each party (and such a contract may be required by a training program or a licensing body). My consultation work generally follows the same process I use in supervision, described later; however, the major difference is who is responsible for what.[1] In a formal supervision relationship, responsibility for that individual's case or caseload belongs to the named and registered supervisor. The supervisee has an obligation to take the supervisor's directives or recommended courses of action and/or to discuss them if in disagreement or uncertain about them. In the event that something goes wrong, the supervisor can be held liable by a licensing board or a court of law, even as the treating therapist is not, especially if that therapist is not yet licensed. On the other hand, a consultant does not have the same direct responsibility or liability and has much less to say about the consultee's chosen course of action than does a supervisor. In a consultation relationship in most jurisdictions in the United States, the therapist trainee/consultee is not formally attached to the supervisor's license; therefore, there is no formal responsibility for the treatment offered. The primary distinction in these relationships, in my experience, is unfortunately an area that many clinicians and trainees are not aware of, and this can lead to problems if a client chooses to take legal or licensing board action against a therapist that then extends to the supervisor/consultant of record.

Due to the degree of responsibility in supervision, I first make sure the potential supervisee is clear about the distinction between supervision and consultation and get as much personal and professional information as possible ahead of time. I explain that the setup for supervision might take several weeks' time as I routinely ask for references from current or past professors and supervisors, get paperwork signed, and get to know something about the potential supervisee. This can be difficult for someone like Therapist X, who waited too long to seek outside help and who is in the midst of a crisis. In a case such as this, I may give a general consultation before putting a contract into place, but I indicate that I expect to have one as a condition of continuing to consult. Sometimes a one-time consultation is all that is needed to identify any issues or an impasse. If that is the case, then the paperwork involved in an ongoing relationship is not required.

I also make sure the supervisee understands the gravity and responsibility of working under my license and the concept of vicarious liability, which means that I carry direct liability for what they do or don't do. At present, whether for supervision or consultation, I generally start by discussing that an exchange of information is important in order for informed decision making about working together. It is not an automatic thing that supervisor and supervisee will be a good "fit," something that should be explored. I also stress the need for mutual honesty and trust and the need for clear boundaries in the relationship. For example, I make clear that I will not take over the client's treatment, but I will help with referrals to other experienced providers, as needed. I also will not provide psychotherapy for the supervisee, but will provide appropriate referrals if I recommend he or she receive psychotherapy.

I routinely ask consultees about their previous experience, what is being sought, why and for what purpose, personal and professional goals, any time frame, and history of their training and provision of psychotherapy or counseling services (including setting and previous supervision).[2] I want to know about the quality of any past supervision and how the supervisee responded to it. I also ask something about the individual's personal and developmental history (including a trauma history) and if there have been any difficulties in previous professional endeavors that I should be aware of, including any legal or ethical actions taken by or against the supervisee (or any that are under consideration). I have learned that some supervisees have had problems with their training programs that were not described to me by the program director and only became obvious due to my inquiry. I specifically ask whether the individual has had trauma-specific education and supervision and whether she/he has worked with cases of trauma previously.

In turn, I offer general information about myself, especially about my history as a psychologist and the philosophy and strategies I use in psychotherapy and consultation. I work from an eclectic, psychodynamic, developmental, and trauma-informed perspective, with special emphasis on the treatment relationship. I also am more self-disclosing than I would be with clients, wanting my consultees to know more of me as a person and about aspects of my life (Pearlman & Courtois, 2005). My approach includes asking personal questions of consultees and encouraging them to self-explore (meta-analyze) in order to understand more about themselves in relation to clients and the treatment relationship. Right from the start of any consultation or supervision, I want to gently test out individuals as to their openness and how my inquiries and explorations might be received. The individuals' previous training might play a part in how open they are. For example, those taught in a strictly cognitive-behavior paradigm may have had less opportunity or initiative to engage in a relational approach or one involving psychodynamically based use of self or self-exploration, so my way of supervising might feel invasive and unappealing to them. From another perspective, shame is an emotion that has been identified as keeping important information out of therapy. In parallel form, I believe the same occurs in consultation/supervision and strive to inform potential consultees up front that I am aware of this and that I will move cautiously and take it into consideration in our relationship. I also explain that what might be kept out or unaddressed in psychotherapy or supervision due to shame might be the most important information to be addressed. What we do and how we relate in our supervisory relationship may thus provide modeling for the psychotherapy that is under review.

This provision of information and a signed contract are not guaranteed methods, as I've learned the hard way over the course of my career, but they do underscore the mutual nature of the responsibility and provide rationale in the event supervision is not going well and the supervisor decides to terminate it for cause. As an example, a colleague decided to terminate a supervision relationship after he found out "through the psychotherapy grapevine" that the supervisee was a very unstable individual who had confided to a friend that she spent her weekends at home deciding whether she should commit suicide. She had her own history of trauma that she had minimized in her self-introduction and in supervision. Her treatment of traumatized clients was overwhelming her emotionally and she was continuously being triggered into posttraumatic and dissociative responses and suicidal ideation, both in and out of session. She was also drinking heavily. She kept the information about the severity of her history, her ongoing stress, and her suicidality from the supervisor and refused to discuss them when the supervisor broached the topics.

Following extensive discussion and the supervisee's continued refusal to disclose much about herself (citing her right to privacy), the supervisor first determined that she was in adequate treatment and had outside support (he called her therapist to consult on her safety and to notify the therapist about his pending actions, which were likely to further destabilize the supervisee/client), notified her training program director and the licensing board of her impairment and sought their assistance (they mandated that she continue in treatment and suspended her from her training program and from treating clients), arranged for her clients to be transferred to different therapists, and terminated the supervision contract between them.

In such cases, great discretion is obviously called for due to the sensitivity of the issues as play. The supervisor was required to spend much time in all of these efforts and in documenting all that transpired. The supervisee was assured that, once her mandated treatment was well underway or major issues resolved, her therapist would be required to assess her as to her ability to continue as a therapist. Her training program and the licensing board would receive the therapist's recommendation along with the evaluation and recommendation of another outside and more neutral therapist in determining her suitability for reinstatement. This was a very sad case for all involved; however, it was not an uncommon one. Many adult survivors of abuse enter the mental health professions in order to help others, often in identification with them and due to their own "unfinished business." They may do very well and have no problems with the academic part of their program, but falter when they are faced with symptomatic clients. This is not to say that survivors cannot be effective or even exemplary therapists—many are. It is necessary for them to have addressed their own issues so those issues are not routinely revived as they treat their clients. It may benefit survivor therapists to have ongoing consultation and supervision in order to keep an outside perspective on their work and have a confidential and safe source of support.

Related to matters like those raised in this case and other types of concerns and issues that may arise, I require all of my supervisees/consultees to carry professional liability insurance that applies to me and our work together. If he or she is a student or trainee in a particular program, I also require a placement and supervisory contract with the program that all parties co-sign and that spells out terms such as duration of the contract, rights and responsibilities of all parties, methods of resolving any problems or disputes that might arise, and the provision of liability insurance that extends to supervisors/consultants. I have learned that I cannot be too careful with regard to professional safeguards and personal and professional self-protection, and this stance models for the trainee the need to give attention to professional issues before engaging in practice. With the benefit of hindsight and some highly negative experiences, I now know that early in my career I was not careful enough with these issues. I did not clearly make the distinction between supervision and consultation, did not require a signed placement contract as a condition of working with a student in a training program or meeting requirements for licensing, nor did I learn enough about the individual who was to become my consultee/supervisee *before* agreeing to either (see discussion by Fox, 1983, about contracting in supervision). These issues had not been part of my supervisory training.

When goals and methods are compatible, for purposes of *informed consent*, I introduce the idea of an individually developed *consultation* or *supervision contract* (different from any placement contract with a training program or site) that specifies rights, responsibilities, and boundaries/limitations of the relationship, along with methods for mediating any difficulties or disputes. The contract is not designed to be a legally binding document, but could be used in the event of a major breach or if a particular issue needs to be clarified. Included in the contract are such issues as purpose, term, general understandings about what is being provided and responsibilities of each party (record keeping, any form of recording, listening to tapes or reading reports, maintenance of confidentiality, duration of the contract, etc.), whether consultation is general or related to a particular case or issue, malpractice coverage of both parties, billing and payment arrangements (as needed), documentation, back-up support, avoidance of dual relationships, and other issues as indicated. Model contracts can be found in Sutter, McPherson, and Geeseman (2002) and Osborn and Davis (1996).

There needs to be specific recognition of the power differential in the supervisory relationship in general, but more particularly when supervision is part of trainees' practicum internship, other training placement, or a requirement of their employment or licensure. There is less of a power imbalance in consultation, especially when it occurs between relative peers. As noted earlier, there is no obligation for the consultee to follow the consultant's recommendations. This does not mean that there should be a hidden agenda between the parties. As an example, a colleague reported an experience with a long-term consultee who surprised him with the announcement that she had only sought his consultation over the course of many years mostly for "CYA" ("cover your ass") purposes. She rarely did as the consultant suggested because she was quite certain her own way of working was the right way. This perspective had never been shared and was very contrary to the consultant's philosophy and mode of working. He was quite offended by the cavalier attitude exhibited by the consultee. They soon parted ways over this discrepancy of purpose and the mistrust that developed.

Although it is advisable not to have dual relationships in any way (for example, student/professor/supervisee; employer/supervisee), there are times and locations when this is not possible. This should be discussed openly, with boundaries and methods of working together articulated and remediation discussed in the event of any problems. Other boundaries and limitations of the relationship should also be noted. The relationship must remain on professional and collegial terms. Romantic/sexual relationships or any form of sexual harassment or intimidation by either party (especially the supervisor due to the power differential) are forbidden, in accordance with professional codes of ethics and state licensing laws. Reasons for termination of the relationship or making recommendations for personal psychotherapy should also be discussed. Friendships between peer consultants are a different matter, but should also be kept distinct from the clinical relationship and discussions. A romantic/intimate relationship is not explicitly prohibited between peers, but obviously the professional relationship should be ended if one were to be contemplated or developed.

The process in trauma-informed supervision

Once all of these issues are attended to and the contract is developed and co-signed, supervision begins. I again stress the seriousness of the endeavor that is being undertaken and propose working to develop a relationship of safety, support, and trust that is both collaborative and growth-producing for all parties (therapist-client, supervisee-supervisor). I share that, as much as I expect the client and consultee to have a growth experience, I, too, hope to self-analyze and grow over the course of our work together. Within the established boundaries, I want to convey my enjoyment of consulting and my hope that it results in growth for all involved. Such an approach is designed to model the stance to be taken by the consultee with the client and can work to lessen the power imbalance. It emphasizes the vibrant and collaborative nature of the relationship and the work, and makes the consultee (and, by extension, the client) responsible for his or her own development and growth. Supervisee/consultee behaviors and expectations are discussed. Toward this end, a listing of such behaviors developed by Vespia, Heckman-Stone, and Delworth (2002) can be useful. More recently, a special issue of the journal *Psychotherapy*, published in 2015, was devoted to the topic of (general, not trauma-specific) supervision process, and includes articles on the supervisory relationship and its quality, an article on evidence-based supervision that tracks outcomes and principles of change, and one on using client outcome monitoring as a tool for supervision. These and other resources show how supervisory practice has received increased attention and research in recent years. As of yet, there are a limited number of articles devoted to supervision of trauma treatment or from a trauma-informed perspective. For example, even the recently published two-volume *APA Handbook of Trauma Psychology* (Gold, Cook, & Dalenberg, 2017) does not have a chapter devoted to supervision of trauma treatment, although one by Saakvitne (2017) can be found in Gartner (2017).

We might then spend the first couple of sessions getting to know more about each other while also beginning to talk in more detail about what the consultee is seeking and how its achievement will be determined. Then we can begin the discussion of specific cases and issues. The supervision model that I use is a developmental one that increasingly moves the responsibility to the supervisee as I move from providing direct teaching to guidance and discussion to consultation. A foremost expectation is for the supervisee to learn about trauma and its treatment, but also to learn to self-assess, not only psychologically, but also in terms of physiological reactions as well. This stance is in keeping with the recent findings in neurobiology and attachment about stress and trauma that suggest it as a psychophysiological event and that clients and therapists (and by extension supervisees and supervisors) must attend to their physical responses as a way of gauging their emotional responses. Schore (2003) and others working from a neuroscience perspective stress therapist (and, by extension, supervisor) attention to the physiological reactions, which might give clues to implicit material via somatosensory channels. I have had times when my physical and psychological reactions have provided clues to the emotions of the therapist and from there to those of the client. When this happens and is noticed, we are usually able to develop insights into client dynamics. As an example, a consultee had pressured speech and was quite emotionally activated during our sessions and pushed me to come up with immediate solutions. When I reflected on how pressured I felt, she acknowledged she did as well. The client had inundated her with information and demands for an instant "cure" that she was transferring to me. This opened the discussion of dependency needs and unrealistic expectations on the part of the client and how to address them.

The supervisee is expected to develop knowledge and skills over the course of the work and to become increasingly adept at discussing case assessment, conceptualization, content and process issues, relational dynamics, treatment plans, and application, as well as increased capacity to attune to the client and increased ability to self-reflect. I make clear that the supervisee is not expected to be perfect, but is expected to be as honest as possible about the specifics of the case and issues and interactions that take place that evoke strong feelings and reactions. We explicitly discuss the issue of shame. All of the material is "grist for the mill"—that is, opportunities for exploration, reflection, and mutual problem solving. For this and other purposes, I often suggest that supervisees read the enlightening article by Chu (1988) on common traps in the treatment of trauma. In it, the author normalized a series of difficulties that are usual in trauma treatment and offered ways to deal with them. He also stressed that learning about these difficulties doesn't necessarily stop them from happening, but that therapists will get out of them sooner and with less damage if they are cognizant of them ahead of time. I share with my supervisees that this article was important to my own development as a trauma therapist and one that I often reread, as it has an enormous amount of wisdom and provides comfort and desensitization.

Early on, I also ask in detail what education supervisees have received about trauma, how knowledge was acquired, whether it was included in professional training and previous casework and supervision, whether they have treated clients with a trauma history of some sort, and how the treatment went. I further inquire about how they *feel* about trauma and working with the traumatized, whether they want to or are comfortable treating trauma survivors, and whether any major misconceptions or stigmatized views are part of the picture (for example, a supervisee casually referring to a difficult female client as a "borderline" or "bad borderline"; callously describing a client as a "cutter" rather than as someone who self-injures; indicating that the client is to blame for what has transpired—past or present —or is faking symptoms; stigmatizing the client in some way; suggesting the client has to "put it behind her or him or just get over it"; along with other reactions indicative of denial, detachment, dislike, and other countertransference reactions or vicarious traumatization). Attitudes such as these are obviously in need of remediation, so the starting point is education. I might begin by suggesting specific reading on the topic or the viewing of online or other digital materials that provide visuals and other information about trauma, along with follow-up discussions. The intention here is for the supervisee not only to learn specific objective information about trauma and its aftereffects, but also to begin to learn about victims' more personal and subjective responses in order to foster empathy and to desensitize the therapist. We also discuss possible blocks the individual may have to hearing about trauma, due to his or her own trauma history, misinformation or prejudice, or more personal or general issues.

In terms of supervisees' own trauma history, this is an area to be approached gently and with empathy by a supervisor. As noted earlier, the most important question is whether such a history has been recognized, addressed, or resolved. Researchers have indicated that a high percentage of mental and behavioral health workers have a personal trauma history (often, although not always, from childhood) that, in part, accounts for their choice of profession (Elliott & Guy, 1993). That history may also have resulted in their having an insecure attachment style that may cause them to over-respond to or to detach from their clients. Many such "wounded healers" are highly invested in helping others as part of their own "survivor mission," whether they understand the motivation for what they do or not. Supervision and consultation can bring to the fore some of these unconscious and "hidden-from-self issues" of how a trauma history relates to choice of profession and attachment style and ability to emotionally self-regulate. It can also lead to discussion about some of the more common therapeutic errors and pitfalls that might accompany such a history, such as getting too involved with the client and attempting to rescue (associated with the anxious preoccupied insecure attachment style), becoming detached from or overly angry with the client (associated with the avoidant/detached insecure attachment style), or becoming emotionally dysregulated in response to the client (associated with the disorganized/disoriented/dissociated attachment style).

The supervisee should be advised that a personal trauma history does not mean he or she is unable to successfully treat this population; in fact, such a history may be an asset in providing the client with deep empathic attunement. However, the therapist must have addressed his or her own issues in personal psychotherapy so as not to be triggered into emotional dysregulation by the client's story and presentation. Such triggering is not totally avoidable, but the therapist's awareness of this pitfall can help to identify and manage it without overly compromising the treatment or burdening the client. Analyses of this sort provide a template about how some of these issues might arise in the treatment process. In cases where it appears that supervisees' history (including attachment style and ability to self-regulate in response to the client) is interfering with the ability to provide effective treatment, or when they are exhibiting reactions and symptoms suggestive of PTSD or a dissociative disorder (or other condition such as depression, anxiety, or a personality disorder), personal therapy can be recommended. I note again that consultation and supervision are not stand-ins for personal therapy: their goals and purposes are entirely different. Blending them constitutes a dual relationship and is unethical, per the ethical codes of professional organizations.

Even if the therapist previously has been in supervision/consultation and is generally cognizant of the process, it can still evoke anxiety, especially with a new supervisor or one who works from a different theoretical or therapeutic approach. Determining expectations as clearly as possible and explaining one's philosophy and theoretical orientation are useful. Regarding trauma therapy, I share and discuss my assumption that the work will change the therapist in profound ways that can be both positive and negative. The demands associated with the treatment of trauma are complex and often challenging. Those demands can cause strong reactions and countertransference in the therapist, who must listen to the trauma story and interact with a client whose ability to relate to others may be limited due to the trauma. Therapists must learn to sit with their own emotions and stay emotionally regulated, even as they feel upended, turned off or disgusted, or overwhelmed by what they hear. Consultation is a place to identify and discuss these responses and any personal transformation/vicarious traumatization responses they arouse. It is also the place to discuss and analyze transference and countertransference, vicarious traumatization, and traumatic reenactments for the implicit information they often convey. Finally, it is the place to have personal support over the course of self-analysis and self-monitoring and for engaging in self-care.

Defining trauma

So, education is the starting point of trauma-informed supervision. With the less knowledgeable supervisee, I basically start from scratch with attention to how trauma is defined and what it is. I want him or her to understand the many types of trauma and their different objective and subjective dimensions, in addition to understanding that reactions can be highly idiosyncratic due to the particulars of the event or experience and the victim's individual risk and protection and resilience factors. I provide education during sessions and also give consultees pamphlets and other sources of information. It is also important to note that not all traumatized individuals (especially adults) develop PTSD at the time of the trauma or later, but that some exhibit delayed-expression PTSD, often in response to a present-day trauma or traumatic reminders or triggers (both of which might be out of the client's awareness). A search for triggering events and experiences can help make a connection where none previously existed and the therapist can then help the client to anticipate and to manage triggers when they occur. Many symptomatic trauma clients enter therapy thinking they are crazy. They either do not know their trauma history or do not realize how it is connected to their symptoms. When they learn of the connection, it can be very relieving and can lead to the lessening of self-blame or other emotions that underlie symptoms.

Following this introduction to trauma and traumatic stressors, I utilize Pearlman and Saakvitne's (1995, 1996) listing of five essential elements of trauma consultation, which I share with consultees (and describe in more detail later):

(1) Information about the effects of trauma—developmental, physiological, psychological
(2) Information about working with common trauma adaptations, symptoms, and crises
(3) A focus on the therapeutic relationship, not just the client
(4) Relational safety to address countertransference response
(5) Attention to vicarious traumatization

Effects of trauma and common adaptation, symptoms, and crises

Again, depending on the consultee's degree of knowledge and previous education, I recommend various readings on the effects of trauma, emphasizing all the developmental, physiological, and psychological possibilities and nuances, and discuss how trauma adaptations later can become symptoms of posttraumatic distress and other mental health and medical concerns. We also discuss how the effects of trauma relate to clients; attachment history and resultant primary attachment style, how clients typically cope, and how they present for treatment. Various assessment issues and assessment instruments can also be brought into the discussion. In particular, supervisees might need to learn how to take a trauma history, how to ask in a supportively neutral way about a trauma, and how to respond to a client's trauma disclosure. We also discuss that not all clients are able to disclose their histories or are even aware of having been traumatized at the outset of treatment (often due to dissociative compartmentalization of information, normalization, denial, or minimization). This does not mean the client is being dishonest or uncooperative—just that they don't know or are not ready. This can also lead into a discussion of dissociation as a common response to trauma, especially when the trauma is chronic and occurs over the course of childhood, a time when dissociative process is the most available to humans. Dissociative process may have helped the victim cope in the midst of ongoing abuse, but leaves the client with gaps in his or her personal history, sense of self, and sense of continuity. Teaching supervisees about how to identify dissociative process through the observation of behavioral and physiological cues, and teaching them how to ground clients who are in a state of hyper-reactivity or activation or the opposite, hypo-reactivity or shutdown, is also useful at this point. Knowing about these various styles, symptoms, and processes ahead of time and not being surprised by them in the moment can be an enormous comfort that works against therapist anxiety and sense of being unskilled. Supervisors might engage in role-plays with supervisees with regard to education and skill building. Finally, supervisees might be advised about issues pertaining to traumatic memory and be educated in ways to neutrally support a client who has absent or hazy memory, while not being suggestive (Courtois, 1999).

Different philosophies of treatment and modes of intervention can be generally discussed at this point, with choices dependent on the supervisee's training or experience with certain modalities or the development of new skills. Obviously, for any specialized method, focused training and possibly additional supervision in that method (and associated certification) is needed before it is used. At the present time, a number of treatments, most of which are cognitive behavioral, have an evidence base and are recommended in clinical guidelines. Consultees should know that, despite the evidence, there is controversy in the field regarding application of some of these strategies with clients with complex trauma histories, and there are questions about the use of a sequenced or stage-oriented treatment that is the current standard of care for complex trauma. Critics question whether such a treatment sequence, and especially a stabilizing phase, is a necessary precursor to trauma-focused treatments (i.e., those with the strongest evidence base; Courtois & Ford, 2009, 2013; DeJongh et al., 2016). The supervisor can provide information about issues such as these and help supervisees to discern the most useful type of treatment and whether to apply it in a specific sequence, according to the assessment, needs, and preferences of the client. Supervisees can be made aware of a growing number of short-term and manualized strategies that have an evidence base. These may be especially useful in settings with a limited number of sessions allotted per client or with clients who have limited personal or financial resources. Group and family system treatment models and applications (free-standing or concurrent with individual therapy) are also available and can be explored (see Ford & Saltzman, 2009).

Supervisees, like psychotherapists in general, are likely to be confused by all of the novel treatments that are being advertised for trauma. Since most have acronyms, I describe them as the "alphabet soup" of trauma treatment. How to make sense of all of them and how to choose what to try or learn? Optimally, the trauma-informed supervisor has an awareness of these various approaches (or strives to be updated on most of them) and so can assist the supervisee in discriminating between them. I suggest that supervisees refer to the clinical practice treatment guidelines (CPG) for PTSD, Complex Posttraumatic Stress Disorder (CPTSD), and the Dissociative Disorders (DDs) published by various professional organizations (see Appendix for a listing) to learn of those methods that have an evidence base, but to be aware that the definition of what constitutes an "evidence base" varies according to the organization that publishes the guidelines or lists treatments based on different standards for the research base and methods of analysis that were used. Clinicians should also be aware of available professional practice guidelines (PPGs) that are based on clinician consensus and research. These can be found in professional organizations such as the American Psychological Association and the American Psychiatric Association[3] and are also contained in some books and journal articles and special issues. These are available on a wide array of patient populations (i.e., women, gay, lesbian, bisexual, transgender [GLBT]) and diagnoses (i.e., anxiety disorders, depression) that have been published regarding the particulars of that group and recommendations (pro and con) regarding treatment approaches.

I also suggest that they get training and certification in at least one primary evidence-based treatment for trauma from among those recommended in several of the most methodologically robust and recent clinical practice guidelines. These include prolonged exposure therapy (Foa & Kozak, 1986), cognitive processing therapy (Resnick & Schnicke, 1992), cognitive therapy (Ehlers, 2013), brief eclectic psychotherapy (Lindauer et al., 2005), the aforementioned EMDR therapy (Shapiro, 2017), and narrative exposure therapy (Schauer, Neuner, & Elbert, 2005). I also suggest that they choose which treatment approach best matches their preferred way of working. They are also encouraged to maintain awareness of the evidence-base status of emerging treatments (Metcalf et al., 2016) and to consider training in some of the emerging methods that appeal to them and that have a strong theoretical base and evidence support. Many of these, such as acupuncture and yoga, are experiential and include a somatosensory emphasis, something being encouraged by the foremost experts in trauma treatment (Van Der Kolk, 2014).

Focus on the treatment relationship and not just the client

Supervision obviously attends to the content of the sessions; however, it also attends to the interaction between the treatment dyad (and its unique intersubjective relationship) and the self of the therapist. This self-focus may feel foreign or overly intrusive to the supervisee, who may be much more comfortable with the focus on the client and their interaction and on the content rather than process. Attention to relational issues in supervision needs careful discussion and negotiation. These issues are not privacy incursions or attempts to shame the supervisee, nor are they personal psychotherapy, and attention to them is in the interest of developing a broader understanding of the unique therapy relationship that is being undertaken and, in parallel process, allow a more multifaceted understanding. I routinely recommend the books *Principles of Trauma Treatment* (Briere & Scott, 2006), *Countertransference and the Treatment of Trauma* (Dalenberg, 2000), *Trauma and the Therapist* (Pearlman & Saakvitne, 1995), and *Treating the Adult Survivor of Childhood Sexual Abuse* (Davies & Frawley, 1994), and other works on relational psychotherapy and psychoanalysis for those supervisees who wish to explore these topics (along with transference and countertransference and different relational patterns) in more depth or as they struggle with particular issues or impasses in the treatment.

Safety to address the countertransference responses

One aim of the supervision relationship is to provide enough safety to surface and examine countertransference responses to the client, the trauma narrative, and the treatment. Countertransference and vicarious traumatization are understood in the literature as different processes. Countertransference refers to the response to a particular client and the unique therapeutic relationship that exists based upon the self of the therapist and their life history. In her book, Dalenberg (2000) noted that countertransference is often quite charged and challenging for therapists treating the traumatized, more so than the non-traumatized. It may involve aversive feelings such as disempowerment, hopelessness, anger, rage, contempt, sadness, dislike, discomfort, and so on, as well as a spectrum of positive and altruistic feelings, including a strong urge to remediate and save survivor clients from their distress. Countertransference is not something bad per se and not something to hide; rather, its identification can lead to a better understanding of the client's dynamics and the interaction between therapist and client. When used this way, countertransference sheds light on unconscious processes and can thus deepen the work by helping supervisees become aware of implicit material (in the same way the supervisee hopes to do with the client).

Attention to vicarious traumatization, compassion fatigue, and secondary traumatic stress

Vicarious traumatization (VT) refers to negative personal transformation of the therapist that results from close engagement with traumatized clients and their stories, and that is believed to be cumulative (McCann & Pearlman, 1990; Saakvitne & Pearlman, 1996). It is not necessarily a bad thing but rather an expectable response to the work. Put another way, psychotherapy of traumatized individuals cannot be effectively conducted without the therapist being personally affected or changed in some way, sometimes minor and rather inconsequential and sometimes major and life-altering. Until identified and managed, VT can result in less emotional resilience and other resources with which to respond to clients. The developers of this conceptualization (Saakvitne & Pearlman, 1995, 1996) posited that, when countertransference is strong and unmanaged, it can lead to more vulnerability to vicarious traumatization. If left unaddressed, countertransference and associated VT can be corrosive to the therapy and the stability of the relationship, as it may cause the therapist to become disheartened, lose hope and optimism, or detach as a means of self-protection.

A related but separate concept is compassion fatigue (Figley, 1995), which refers to the therapist's emotional exhaustion from empathizing (and often over-empathizing and over-engaging) with the client (or a number of clients) whose needs may feel insatiable to the therapist. Compassion fatigue, a form of burnout, can also lead to detachment, withdrawal, and hostility toward the client, among other responses, usually after a period of intense empathy or involvement and possibly due to disillusionment with the pace of the treatment or the ongoing variety of issues and crises that emerge over time. Compassion fatigue can result in feelings of incompetence or impotence. These feelings, in turn, can lead to cynicism in therapists, causing them to withdraw more and more from the work and, in some cases, to leave the work altogether.

The importance of attending to these issues cannot be stressed enough. If left unaddressed, they can result in secondary traumatic stress in the therapist with symptoms that resemble those of PTSD/DD and their associated features. Thus, the therapist's mental health is at risk and deteriorates. Posttraumatic symptoms such as hyperarousal, numbing, and hypervigilance may be accompanied by personal and professional alienation from others, increased depression and anxiety, blame or rage directed at clients and the mental health professions as major sources of stress, the use of substances or behaviors to excess to numb out or to feel, to name but a few of the most common symptoms. When these occur, treatment of the therapist is mandated.

Saakvitne and Pearlman (1996) recommended strategies with the acronym ABC as a means of self-management and as antidotes to VT, along with compassion fatigue and secondary traumatic stress: **A**wareness, **B**alance, and **C**onnection, **C**ontainment, and Self-**C**ompassion.

- *Awareness.* Routine and ongoing feelings of being overwhelmed, dispirited, and hopeless can challenge the meaning of the work for therapists. These therapists may be reacting to the toxicity of the trauma and carrying many of their clients' emotions (traumatized clients are often very accomplished at not feeling their own feelings and projecting them onto others). As noted earlier, they may begin to react in secondary or vicarious posttraumatic ways (and relieve themselves of the pain through denial and by detaching and engaging in other self-protective strategies). It is useful to engage supervisees in self-exploration, starting with their own physical responses, to glean information about their reactions and emotions. Tracking physical responses, such as chest tightness, jaw clenching, nausea, and an urge to run or to cry, may give clues to unacknowledged and unaddressed feelings and issues, some of which might mimic or parallel those of the clients. In the safety of the supervision space, these can be explored, identified, normalized, emoted, verbalized, and addressed away from the client. Therapist self-awareness can help the therapist return to personal self-regulation that, in itself, is a potent therapeutic strategy that undergirds and contains the treatment

- *Balance.* This is the second recommendation for self-management of VT. Therapists likely have gotten out of balance in carrying too much of the client's material (emotions, intrusions) or they may be caught up in enactments. They may need to give more attention to self-care and work-life balance to counteract this enmeshment. Therapists may need to implement specific strategies to become more balanced and supervisors can help them with self-assessment and brainstorming ideas. For example, taking time to exercise, having breaks in the day, doing an in-office yoga practice or meditation between sessions, rebalancing a caseload, and engaging in a spiritual practice might all be useful in relieving some of the stress and gaining more perspective on the work. Also, attention to vicarious growth, counterresilience, posttraumatic growth, and the satisfaction of the work can counteract VT. Long-term therapies can be very challenging in terms of being able to identify client growth and improvement. A rebalancing of goals or expectations might be in order, and the use of a process of change model or client outcome measures by which to evaluate and assess outcome might prove to be useful to both therapist and client.*Connection, containment, and self-compassion.* These factors also go a long way toward helping therapists with their various responses. Many writers have advised that trauma work should not be conducted in conditions of personal isolation. Conditions of isolation and detachment from others limit outside perspective and support from others when it is most needed. As we advise and teach our clients to engage with others and to build support systems, we therapists should do the same. Connection with others, including supervision and consultation, provides the space for personal exploration exposure through discussion and containment of what is toxic and for the provision of support and other interpersonal enrichments. Therapists are also called upon to do another thing that they are working with their clients to develop: to have self-compassion that counters the self-contempt and self-alienation that many survivor clients exhibit. Self-understanding and compassion can be modeled by the consultant to the consultee and then to the client, a major transformation of self that provides hope and optimism for the future.

Attention to vicarious resilience, counterresilience, and posttraumatic growth

It has become ever more apparent over the years that psychotherapy of traumatized individuals can also be uniquely rewarding and satisfying for therapist and client. Just as counter-trauma can occur, so can counter-resilience. Therapists come to identify with their clients' resilience and perseverance and often the spirituality and humanity their clients exhibit, despite all of their hardships. As they learn from their clients, therapists themselves may become more personally resilient. They may also experience posttraumatic growth in parallel with their clients as the therapy progresses and takes hold. Another parallel process can occur at the consultant/supervisory level, as they are also affected by the lessons learned and the achievements of the supervisee in conducting a successful treatment.

Summarizing comments

Against the backdrop of lack of training in even the basics of trauma and trauma treatment that remains widespread in professional curricula, both the therapist who treats the traumatized and the supervisor/consultant have their work cut out for them. Treatment of traumatized clients is often highly complicated and challenging, as clients present with posttraumatic symptoms as well as a host of other difficulties and comorbidities. Moreover, they may be difficult to relationally engage due to their trauma history. Especially when the trauma involves relational betrayal by someone of significance to them, the trauma may result in mistrust of others and an expectation of being abused or exploited by anyone in a position of authority or anyone they get close to, including the therapist. Mistrust and anger may be ongoing challenges to the therapist, who must maintain some equanimity in dealing with them and who must assist the client in understanding their origin. Elsewhere, I have written that the therapeutic relationship is a catalyst and container of these relational challenges (Courtois & Ford, 2013; Kinsler, Courtois, & Frankel, 2009; Pearlman & Courtois, 2005), a position that has recently received a great deal of support in the relational psychoanalytic writing on the treatment of trauma. Supervision/consultation can greatly assist the therapist in understanding and responding to these relational challenges in a regulated way, and can also help decode implicit information in the transference and countertransference.

I have not said enough about dissociation in this contribution. It is a common response to chronic childhood abuse and traumatization, and therapists not trained to identify it will be hard-pressed to understand how it presents and how to treat it. It can tremendously complicate treatment and the burden on the therapist until it is identified, understood, and treated. A thorough focus on this topic is beyond the scope of this contribution; however, specialized education of the therapist is needed when the client is highly dissociative or carries a dissociative disorder diagnosis.

A trauma-informed philosophy and perspective on treatment can be very helpful to clinicians in treating both the traumatized and a more general population, as it has an open and exploratory stance toward the client and his or her distress and symptoms. It can be applied according to the needs of the supervisee and hopefully fills in the training gaps. My intent, these many years, in considering what supervision of trauma treatment has to offer, is to keep therapists from making the mistakes that were made in the early years of contemporary trauma treatment. It is well-known that treatment can help or it can harm, both therapist and client, and it can also impact the supervisor who holds vicarious liability as well as other third parties (for example, the client's family members, friends, and colleagues). Through the provision of education and active support of the therapist's growth and exploration, it is my hope to provide improved services to clients who enter treatment with a trauma history. Posttraumatic growth is a joy to behold for the client, the therapist, and the supervisor, but it requires client resilience as well as a cognizant and emotionally responsive therapist and supervisor to achieve.

Notes

1. The APA *Guidelines for Clinical Supervision in Health Service Psychology* (2014) note that supervision is distinct from consultation, personal psychotherapy, and mentoring.
2. The terms "consultee" and "supervisee" are used interchangeably in the remainder of this article with the understanding of the differences between supervision and consultation as articulated earlier.
3. This CPG and PPG terminology is used by the American Psychological Association.

References

American Psychological Association. (1996). *Guidelines and principles of accreditation.* Washington, DC: Author.

American Psychological Association, Board of Educational Affairs Task Force on Supervision Guidelines. (2014). *Guidelines for clinical supervision in health service psychology.* Retrieved from http://www.apa.org/about/policy/guidelines-supervision.pdf

Briere, J., & Scott, C. (2006). *Principles of trauma therapy: A guide to symptoms, evaluation, and treatment.* Thousand Oaks, CA: Sage.

Chu, J. A. (1988). Ten traps for therapists in the treatment of trauma survivors. *Dissociation, 1*(4), 24–32.

Cook, J. M., & Newman, E.; the New Haven Trauma Competency Work Group. (2014). A consensus statement on trauma mental health: The New Haven competency conference process and major findings. *Psychological Trauma: Theory, Research, Practice and Policy, 6,* 300–307.

Courtois, C. A. (1988). *Healing the incest wound: Adult survivors in therapy.* New York, NY: Norton.

Courtois, C. A. (1999). *Recollections of sexual abuse: Treatment principles and guidelines* New York, NY: W. W. Norton.

Courtois, C. A. (2010). *Healing the incest wound: Adult survivors in therapy* (2nd ed.). New York, NY: Norton.

Courtois, C. A., & Ford, J. D. (Eds.). (2009). *Treating complex traumatic stress disorders: An evidence-based guide.* New York, NY: Guilford Press.

Courtois, C. A., & Ford, J. D. (2013). *Treatment of complex trauma: A sequenced, relationship-base approach.* New York, NY: Guilford Press.

Dalenberg, C. (2000). *Countertransference and the treatment of trauma.* Washington, DC: American Psychological Association.

Davies, J. M., & Frawley, M. G. (1994). *Treating the adult survivor of childhood sexual abuse: A psychoanalytic perspective.* New York, NY: Basic Books.

DeJongh, A., Resick, P. A., Zoellner, L. A., Van Minnen, A., Lee, C. W., & Bicanic, I. A. E. (2016). Critical analysis of the current treatment guidelines for complex PTSD in adults. *Depression and Anxiety, 33*(5), 1–11.

Ehlers, A. (2013). Trauma-focused cognitive behavior therapy for posttraumatic stress disorder and acute stress disorder. In G. Simos & S. G. Hofman (Eds.), *CBT for anxiety disorders: A practitioner book* (pp. 161–190). London, England: Wiley. doi:10.1002/9781118330043

Elliott, D. M., & Guy, J. D. (1993). Mental health professionals versus non-mental-health professionals: Childhood trauma and adult functioning. *Professional Psychology: Research and Practice, 24,* 83–90.

Figley, C. R. (1995). Compassion fatigue: Towards a new understanding of the costs of caring. In B. Stamm (Ed.), *Secondary traumatic stress: Self-care issues for clinicians, researchers, and educators* (pp. 3–28). Lutherville, MD: Sidran Press.

Foa, E. B., & Kozak, M. J. (1986). Emotional processing of fear: Exposure to corrective information. *Psychological Bulletin, 99,* 20–35.

Ford, J. D., & Saltzman, W. (2009). Family system therapy. In C. A. Courtois & J. D. Ford (Eds), *Treating complex traumatic stress disorders: An evidence-based guide* (pp. 391–414). New York, NY: Guilford Press.

Fox, R. (1983). Contracting in supervision: A goal oriented process. *The Clinical Supervisor, 1* (1), 37–49.

Gartner, R. B. (Ed.). (2017). *Trauma and countertrauma, resilience and counterresilience: Insight from psychoanalysts and trauma experts.* New York, NY: Routledge, Taylor & Francis Group.

Gold, S. N., Cook, J. M., & Dalenberg, C. (Eds.). (2017). *APA handbook of trauma psychology.* Washington, DC: American Psychological Association.

Kinsler, P. J., Courtois, C. A., & Frankel, A. S. (2009). Therapeutic alliance and risk management. In C. A. Courtois & J. D. Ford (Eds.), *Treating complex traumatic stress disorders: An evidence-based guide* (pp. 183–201). New York, NY: Guilford Press.

Lindauer, R. J. L., Gersons, B. P. R., Van Meijel, E. P. M., Blom, K., Carlier, I. V. E., Vrijlandt, I., & Olff, M. (2005). Effects of brief eclectic psychotherapy in patients with posttraumatic stress disorder: Randomized clinical trial. *Journal of Traumatic Stress, 18,* 205–212.

McCann, I. L., & Pearlman, L. A. (1990). Vicarious traumatization: A framework for understanding the psychological effects of working with victims. *Journal of Traumatic Stress, 3,* 131–149.

McLean, C. P., Asnaani, A., & Foa, E. B. (2015). Prolonged exposure therapy. In U. Schnyder, M. Cloitre, U. Schnyder, & M. Cloitre (Eds.), *Evidence based treatments for trauma-related psychological disorders: A practical guide for clinicians* (pp. 143–159). Cham, Switzerland: Springer. doi:10.1007/978-3-319-07109-1_8

Metcalf, O., Varker, T., Forbes, D., Phelps, A., Dell, L., DiBattista, A.,... O'Donnell, M. (2016). Efficacy of fifteen emerging interventions for the treatment of posttraumatic stress disorder: A systematic review. *Journal of Traumatic Stress, 29*, 88–92.

Osborn, C. J., & Davis, T. E. (1996). The supervision contract: Making it perfectly clear. *The Clinical Supervisor, 1*(4), 121–134.

Pearlman, L. A., & Courtois, C. A. (2005). Clinical applications of the attachment framework: Relational treatment of complex trauma. *Journal of Traumatic Stress, 18*, 449–459.

Pearlman, L. A., & Saakvitne, K. W. (1995). *Trauma and the therapist: Countertransference and vicarious traumatization in psychotherapy with incest survivors.* New York, NY: Norton.

Resnick, P. A., & Schnicke, M. K. (1992). Cognitive processing therapy for sexual assault victims. *Journal of Consulting & Clinical Psychology, 60*, 748–756.

Saakvitne, K. W. (2017). Clinical consultation to help transform vicarious traumatization. In R. B. Gartner (Ed.), *Trauma and countertrauma, resilience and counterresilience: Insight from psychoanalysts and trauma experts* (pp. 236–250). New York, NY: Routledge, Taylor & Francis Group.

Saakvitne, K. W., Gamble, S. G., Pearlman, L. A., & Lev, B. T. (2000). *Risking connection: A training curriculum for working with survivors of childhood abuse.* Lutherville, MD: Sidran Press.

Saakvitne, K. W., & Pearlman, L. A. (1996). *Transforming the pain: A workbook on vicarious traumatization.* New York, NY: Norton.

Schauer, M., Neuner, F., & Elbert, T. (2005). *Narrative exposure therapy: A short-term intervention for traumatic stress disorders after war, terror, or torture.* Cambridge, MA: Hogrefe.

Schore, A. N. (2003). *Affect regulation and the repair of the self.* New York, NY: Norton.

Shapiro, F. (2017). *Eye movement desensitization and reprocessing: Basic principles, protocols, and procedures.* (3rd ed.). New York, NY: Guilford Press.

Strand, V. (2009, November, 9). *Preparing graduate social work students for evidence based trauma intervention.* Symposium presented at the annual meeting of the Council on Social Work Education, San Antonio, TX.

Sutter, E., McPherson, R. H., & Geeseman, R. (2002). Contracting for supervision. *Professional Psychology: Research and Practice, 33*, 495–498.

Van Der Kolk, B. (2014). *The body keeps the score: Brain, mind, and body in the healing of trauma.* New York, NY: Viking.

Vespia, K. M., Heckman-Stone, C., & Delworth, U. (2002). Describing and facilitating effective supervision behavior in counseling trainees. *Psychotherapy: Theory/Research/ Practice, 39*, 56–65.

Appendix

Trauma Treatment Guidelines

American Psychiatric Association. (2004). *Practice guideline for the treatment of patients with acute stress disorder and posttraumatic stress disorder.* Washington, DC: Author.

American Psychological Association. (2017). *Clinical practice guideline for the treatment of PTSD in adults.* Washington, DC: Author. Retrieved from www.apa.org/ptsd-guideline

Australian Centre for Posttraumatic Mental Health, University of Melbourne. (2007, 2013). *PTSD guidelines.* Melbourne, Australia: Author.

Clinical Resource Efficiency Support Team (CREST). (2003). *The management of posttraumatic stress disorder in adults.* Belfast, Ireland: Author.

Cloitre, M., Courtois, C. A., Charuvastra, A. Carapezza, R., Stolbach, B. C., & Green, B. L. (2011). Treatment of complex PTSD: Results of the ISTSS expert clinician survey on best practices. *Journal of Traumatic Stress, 24,* 615–627.

Courtois, C. A. (1999). *Recollections of sexual abuse: Treatment principles and guidelines* New York, NY: W. W. Norton.

Foa, E., Davidson, J. R. T., & Frances, A. (1999). Treatment of posttraumatic stress disorder. *The Journal of Clinical Psychiatry, 60*(Suppl 16), 4–76.

Foa, E., Friedman, M., & Keane, T. (2000). *Effective treatment for PTSD: Guidelines from the International Society of Traumatic Stress Studies.* New York, NY: Guilford Press.

Foa, E., Keane, T., Friedman, M., & Cohen, J. (2008) *Effective treatment for PTSD: Guidelines from the International Society of Traumatic Stress Studies.* New York, NY: Guilford Press.

Institute of Medicine of the National Academies. (2006). *Posttraumatic stress disorder: Diagnosis and assessment.* Washington, DC: Author.

International Society for the Study of Dissociation. (2000). Guidelines for the evaluation and treatment of dissociative symptoms in children and adolescents. *Journal of Trauma & Dissociation, 1,* 109–134.

International Society for the Study of Dissociation. (2004). Guidelines for the evaluation and treatment of dissociative symptoms in children and adolescents. *Journal of Trauma & Dissociation, 5*(3), 119–150.

International Society for the Study of Dissociation. (2005). Guidelines for treating dissociative identity disorder in adults. *Journal of Trauma & Dissociation, 6*(4), 69–149.

International Society for the Study of Trauma and Dissociation. (2011). [Chu, J. A., Dell, P. F., Van der Hart, O., Cardeña, E., Barach, P. M., Somer, E., Loewenstein, R. J., Brand, B., Golston, J. C., Courtois, C. A., Bowman, E. S., Classen, C., Dorahy, M., Şar, V., Gelinas, D. J., Fine, C. G., Paulsen, S, Kluft, R.P., Dalenberg, C. J., Jacobson-Levy, M., Nijenhuis, E. R. S., Boon, S., Chefetz, R. A., Middleton, W., Ross, C. A., Howell, E., Goodwin, G., Coons, P.

M., Frankel, A. S., Steele, K., Gold, S. N., Gast, U., Young, L. M., & Twombly, J.]. *Guidelines for treating dissociative identity disorder in adults.* McLean, VA: Author.

Kezelman, C., & Stavropoulos, P. (2012). *The last frontier: Practice guidelines for treatment of complex trauma and trauma informed care and service delivery.* Kirribilli, Australia: Adults Surviving Child Abuse (ASCA). Retrieved from www.asca.org.au

National Institute for Clinical Excellence. (2005). *Post-traumatic stress disorder (PTSD): Themanagement of PTSD in adults and children in primary and secondary care.* London, England: Author.

Saakvitne, K. W., & Pearlman, L.A. (1996). *Transforming the pain: A workbook on vicarious traumatization.* New York, NY: W. W. Norton.

Shapiro, F. (2017). *Eye movement desensitization and reprocessing: Basic principles, protocols, and procedures* (3rd ed.). New York, NY: Guilford Press.

U.S. Department of Veterans' Affairs/Department of Defense. (2017). *PTSD: National Center for PTSD.* Retrieved from http://www/cpg.med.va.gov/PTSD

Child welfare supervision: Special issues related to trauma-informed care in a unique environment

Crystal Collins-Camargo and Becky Antle

ABSTRACT

The child welfare (CW) system must adopt a trauma-centered focus. Children served typically have experienced some form of trauma, and involvement with the system is, itself, traumatizing for children and their families. Frontline workers and supervisors also are influenced by their exposure to that trauma and work-related challenges. There is a need for clear articulation of a trauma-informed approach to supervision and for research as to its implementation and impact. The authors provide a rationale for why professionals in the CW system require trauma-informed supervision, reviewing relevant literature. Potential components of trauma-informed supervision are explored, with practical examples illustrating implementation.

Child welfare (CW) in the United States is designed to protect at-risk children, many of whom have been traumatized. This vulnerable population may experience trauma not only based on this maltreatment, but also in response to intervention by the CW system, as services are often involuntary and necessitate removal from the family. Although the concept of trauma is not new to the CW field, recent attention to the need for a trauma-informed approach has emerged (Kisiel, Fehrenbach, Small, & Lyons, 2009). More than one in 10 children served by the CW system is identified as demonstrating trauma symptomatology requiring clinical intervention (Caseneuva, Ringeisen, Wilson, Smith, & Dolan, 2011).

As CW services are provided through various forms of partnerships between the public and private sectors (McBeath, Collins-Camargo, & Chuang, 2012), the consideration of how the child welfare system can best meet the needs of these children and their families is relevant to a wide range of organizations seeking to serve these children and families. Families served by the CW system are typically multi-problem and in crisis, and the public and private agencies serving them often operate in a state of crisis, heightening the importance of supportive supervision (Collins-Camargo & Millar, 2012). The stress of the work and the impact of working with traumatized clients and in traumatizing situations may only be exacerbated by the pressures associated with media portrayals, public opinion, and the press for accountability (Chenot, 2011). Workers are often blamed for bad outcomes in child protection cases by the media, despite the complexities of this work and the facts of the case.

In this article, the authors will focus on trauma-informed (TI) supervision within the field of CW. For a number of reasons, CW supervision presents a variety of unique challenges underscoring the criticality of this role. Despite abundant research regarding CW, generally, a systematic review conducted by Carpenter, Webb, and Bostock (2013) found a weak evidence base regarding the impact of supervision in this field, specifically. Most studies were cross-sectional and reported the quality of supervision was associated with desired worker practice. The authors noted a lack of rigorous studies on the impact of supervision on clients. However, this observation should not minimize the value of studies on the influence of supervision on worker practice and outcomes, particularly when discussing trauma-informed supervision.

Kadushin classically distinguished educational, supportive, administrative, and, later, clinical supervision (Kadushin & Harkness, 2002). With educational supervision focused on teaching practice skills, and supportive supervision focused on assisting staff with managing the work and the stress associated with it, clinical supervision involves the critical examination of the intervention techniques and clients' response to them in order to promote service effectiveness. Public CW occurs within the context of a bureaucratic environment in which other forms of supervision may take a backseat to administrative activities. Since trauma is endemic to CW work, it is essential that CW supervision involve both clinical supervision to assist the worker in effectively working with the client as well as supportive supervision to help the worker deal with the response to serving traumatized clients and in potentially traumatizing situations.

Since there may be significant variance in educational preparation of CW workers (Zlotnik, 2003), the need for supervision to promote worker competence and enhance practice with traumatized clients becomes even more important. Based on a meta-analysis, Mor Barak, Travis, Pyun, and Xie (2009) found that effective supervision in child welfare, social work, and mental health settings promotes a positive work environment, contributing to worker effectiveness through task assistance, social/emotional support, and interpersonal interaction. In CW, effective supervision has been found to positively influence organizational culture, promoting evidence-informed practice and worker self-efficacy (Collins-Camargo & Royse, 2010), organizational climate (Mor Barak, Levin, Nissly, & Lane, 2006; Seibert, Silver, & Randolph, 2004), and perceived opportunities for life-work balance (Smith, 2005).

Another challenge inherent in CW supervision involves secondary traumatic stress (STS), vicarious traumatization, and compassion fatigue among frontline workers themselves. A notable proportion of CW workers experience threats of violence as well as indirect trauma (Goodard & Hunt, 2011). Conrad and Kellar-Guenther (2006) found that 50% of Colorado child protection workers scored high or extremely high on compassion fatigue, but only 7.7% were high or extremely high on burnout. Given the degree of trauma experienced by CW clients, staff experiencing emotional exhaustion is a concern. Research has suggested a relationship between emotional exhaustion and job satisfaction (Cahalane & Sites, 2008; Mena & Bailey, 2007). In one study (Mandell, Stalker, De Zeeuw Wright, Frensch, & Harvey, 2013), a key factor in those child welfare staff who had high emotional exhaustion but maintained job satisfaction was supportive and reflective supervision. We discuss the nature of reflective supervision later in this article.

Relatedly, researchers have examined factors related to CW worker retention, including supervision. Strolin-Goltzman (2008) did not find a difference between high and low turnover agencies based on supervisory factors, but did find differences based on organizational factors such as job clarity and coherence, and satisfaction with salary and benefits. Other researchers (Chen & Scannapieco, 2010) have found supervision is a factor in retention and/or turnover, and supervisor influence may occur through attending to emotional and psychological needs of staff. Kruzich, Mienko, and Courtney (2014) found that supervisory support was significantly and positively associated with worker psychological safety, which in turn was related to intent to remain employed. Supervision's effect may occur in part through work unit dynamics and individual attitudes and behavior, since workgroup psychological safety decreases turnover (Kruzich et al., 2014). Supervisor influence on organizational climate also may be at play, as Lee, Weaver, and Hrostowski (2011) found quality supervision served to mediate worker emotional exhaustion through psychological empowerment.

Trauma-informed care (TIC) in CW

There are a growing number of programs and initiatives designed to promote TIC in CW (Ko et al., 2008). Tools have been developed, such as *Creating Trauma-Informed Child Welfare Systems: A Guide for Administrators* (Chadwick Trauma-Informed Systems Project [CTISP], 2013a), *Guidelines for Applying a Trauma Lens to a Child Welfare Practice Model*(CTISP, 2013b), and the *CW Trauma Training Toolkit* (National Child Traumatic Stress Network [NCTSN], 2013).

Surprisingly, in the wave of attention to TIC in CW and in the literature (Kerns et al., 2016; Kramer, Sigel, Conners-Burrow, Savary, & Tempel, 2013), there is little mention of supervision. Bartlett and colleagues (2016) described use of trauma-informed leadership teams in CW offices in one state to help integrate trauma-informed care systems. However, they did not discuss the role of supervisors. In another statewide initiative to build capacity for TIC involving workforce development as well as implementation of revision of policy and practice guidelines, results indicated improvement in trauma-informed knowledge, practice, and collaboration; however, frontline staff reported greater improvement in worker practice capacity than did supervisors and managers, and ratings of trauma-informed supervision and support actually declined over time (Lang, Campbell, Shanley, Crusto, & Connell, 2016). These results suggest a possible lack of effective attention to trauma-informed supervision.

Simply stated, TIC is about professionals attending to the trauma experienced by clients and the facilitation of recovery without re-traumatization. We would suggest this is not new in CW, but perhaps packaged in a new way. Many child welfare practitioners may agree. Others have argued that, despite the awareness of the relevance of trauma in CW, implementation of trauma-informed practices has not always been successful (e.g., Kramer et al., 2013), and there is a need for public policy to drive this movement (e.g., Beyerlein & Bloch, 2014). A trauma-informed CW system is one in which

> ... all parties involved recognize and respond to the varying impact of traumatic stress on children, caregivers, families, and those who have contact with the system. Programs and organizations within the system infuse this knowledge, awareness, and skills into their organizational cultures, policies, and practices. They act in collaboration, using the best available science, to facilitate and support resiliency and recovery. (CTISP, 2013a, p. 11)

The elements of such a system include maximizing physical and psychological safety for children and families, identifying their trauma-related needs, enhancing child and family well-being and resilience as well as the well-being and resilience of professionals in the field, and partnering with youths and families, as well as other agencies serving them (NCTSN, 2013). Certainly, these elements require intentional action on the part of CW supervisors.

The Children's Bureau has funded three cohorts of discretionary grants targeting, in part, implementing TIC in CW. In preparation for statewide training and implementation of a trauma screening tool by CW workers and trauma assessment by behavioral health providers, the authors administered a survey to staff in one state's public agency to assess organizational readiness and capacity to implement trauma-informed care. Similar assessment was conducted in other states using a variety of instruments and methods as a part of this initiative (Strolin-Goltzman, Collins-Camargo, Akin, & McCrae, 2015). Surveys were administered online and by paper to assess readiness using standardized scales such as the Trauma Systems Readiness Tool

(Hendricks, Conradi, & Wilson, 2011). Surveys were completed by 171 CW workers, 44 supervisors, and 13 administrators in the CW agency. Comparisons were made in perceptions of readiness and capacity to provide trauma-informed care.

Preliminary data analysis showed no statistically significant differences between the three groups (workers, supervisors, and administrators) in CW. However, descriptive analysis indicated that, in comparing mean scores for many domains of trauma systems readiness, workers reported the lowest levels of readiness, followed by supervisors and administrators. This trend held true for the domains of training and education, psychological screening, trauma screening, understanding of trauma concepts, community connections to address trauma, parent-child trauma, vicarious trauma, and systems integration. (See Table 1 for descriptive statistics on these subscales.)

As indicated in Table 1, the most pronounced differences between workers and supervisors were in the areas of training/education and organizational

Table 1. Descriptive statistics comparing child welfare workers, supervisors, and administrators on subscales of the trauma systems readiness tool.

		N	Mean	Std. Deviation
Readiness training and education	Child welfare worker	169	19.4793	3.54073
	Child welfare supervisor	44	20.7045	2.86583
	Child welfare administrator/manager	13	20.5385	2.84650
	Total	226	19.7788	3.41040
Readiness psychological screening	Child welfare worker	170	8.3529	1.30276
	Child welfare supervisor	44	8.6364	1.08029
	Child welfare administrator/manager	13	8.1538	1.86396
	Total	227	8.3965	1.30064
Readiness screening	Child welfare worker	168	9.0952	4.16176
	Child welfare supervisor	44	9.3409	4.17603
	Child welfare administrator/manager	13	9.7692	4.30414
	Total	225	9.1822	4.15736
Readiness trauma concepts	Child welfare worker	169	11.6686	2.03751
	Child welfare supervisor	42	11.9286	3.07145
	Child welfare administrator/manager	13	13.2308	1.42325
	Total	224	11.8080	2.25975
Readiness connections	Child welfare worker	166	12.8193	2.01596
	Child welfare supervisor	44	12.8409	2.68452
	Child welfare administrator/manager	13	13.3077	2.09701
	Total	223	12.8520	2.16037
Readiness parent child trauma	Child welfare worker	167	36.2874	5.36286
	Child welfare supervisor	44	36.5000	6.81824
	Child welfare administrator/manager	13	36.3077	4.06990
	Total	224	36.3304	5.59210
Readiness vicarious trauma	Child welfare worker	167	16.5868	4.45492
	Child welfare supervisor	44	17.3636	4.66601
	Child welfare administrator/manager	13	18.0769	3.75192
	Total	224	16.8259	4.46321
Readiness systems integration	Child welfare worker	167	14.6168	2.69702
	Child welfare supervisor	44	14.3182	3.44912
	Child welfare administrator/manager	13	15.3077	1.49358
	Total	224	14.5982	2.80601

readiness to respond to vicarious trauma, with workers reporting lower levels of readiness or preparation in these domains than supervisors. This result suggests that workers may feel a greater need for training on trauma and attention to vicarious trauma than supervisors are aware of. Similarly, administrators reported higher levels of trauma systems readiness than supervisors in numerous areas, including screening, understanding of trauma concepts, community connections to address trauma, vicarious trauma, and systems integration. These data may indicate that administrators over-estimate the level of feelings of preparedness of their supervisors to handle trauma issues for clients and workers.

As a part of the same project, the authors also conducted focus groups with 12 CW workers and six supervisors following the pilot testing of the trauma screening procedures in this initiative. Key themes relevant to TIC in CW from these focus groups included the value of the trauma screening process, need for more training/preparation regarding how to handle emotions and disclosures of trauma during the screening process, and how to work with others, such as caregivers and behavioral health clinicians, around these trauma needs.

Additional themes relevant to supervision included the need to manage staff anxiety about change. Participants also reinforced the value of screening children for trauma and behavioral health needs amid concerns regarding staff workload, the need to incorporate trauma screening process questions and results into regular supervision discussions, and the need for supervisor advocacy with community partners to obtain necessary data such as comprehensive trauma assessments. These themes highlight the fact that trauma-informed care in CW builds upon and requires attention to existing issues and practices such as workload, and lack of procedures focused on trauma experienced by clients.

There is near silence in the literature on trauma-informed supervision in CW. There is a need to work to translate the elements of TIC outlined elsewhere (e.g., CTISP, 2013a, 2013b), which themselves need empirical support (Bartlett et al., 2016), into an approach to trauma-informed supervision. In addition, in light of research referenced earlier regarding secondary traumatic stress and compassion fatigue in this field, consideration needs to be given to TIC of workers and supervisors as well as their clients.

Proposed components of trauma-informed supervision in CW

The literature includes efforts to establish essential elements of CW supervision generally. Dill and Bogo (2009) purported models of supervision that integrate administrative, clinical, and educational components. One study conducted by the National Child Welfare Resource Center on Organizational Improvement (Hess, Kanak, & Atkins, 2009) involved interviews and surveys with workers, supervisors, managers, and experts in CW. Ultimately, 31 responsibilities were identified as "most important" for supervisors in this field that spanned administrative, clinical, and educational supervision. This study yielded a technical report, *Building a Model and Framework for Child Welfare Supervision*, that remains relevant as to the wide range of responsibilities of those in this field (Hess et al., 2009). A challenge that has not yet been surmounted is to establish if it is even possible to do 31 major things well. This no doubt contributes to the level of stress experienced by those in this role. Looking at this another way, a qualitative study of characteristics of an effective CW supervisor yielded five primary themes: mission/values, diversity, constant change, team identity, and community embeddedness (Hanna & Potters, 2012).

How would a TIC approach alter the elements of CW supervision? It would seem to be relatively straightforward, while understandably challenging in the fast-paced environment of CW work: attentiveness to the influence of trauma on clients, staff, and the supervisors themselves throughout the various roles and responsibilities of supervision. *Guidelines for Applying a Trauma Lens to a Child Welfare Practice Model* (CTISP, 2013b) offers some guidance regarding supervisory strategies in each stage of the intervention process, and, when considered in relation to the essential elements identified by the NCTSN (2013) for a trauma-informed system, as well as the broader supervision literature, some clear components emerge.

Maintain a trauma lens in practice

We argue that CW supervision in general already attends to issues of trauma in that it is not a revelation that our clients have typically been traumatized, and in fact this is typically the impetus for these children coming to the attention of the agency. However, more recent intervention strategies, such as universal screening for trauma and behavioral health needs and trauma-informed assessment and treatment, need to be reinforced through supervision. Workers can benefit from supervisors emphasizing the clinical relevance of these activities to CW goals of safety, permanency, and well-being. Coaching workers on interpretation of results generated by these tools, discussing them with clients, and applying findings to case planning is an important supervisory role. For example, a supervisor might say, "The assessment indicates the trauma this child experienced through emotional abuse by the father may be influencing his performance in school. How can we address this in the child's case plan?" NCTSN (2013) also emphasized considering cultural relevance when interpreting trauma history and selecting interventions, which supervisors can model with staff. For example, differing approaches to communication and interaction in some cultures may impact the sort of treatment recommended.

Supervisors can help workers identify protective factors as well as risk factors for use in case planning and decision making (CTISP, 2013b). This approach is critical in a system in which it is easy to focus on a deficit rather than strengths-based approach. Supervisors might ask workers, "Given these traumatic experiences of the child, how is he or she continuing to succeed in school? Who are the people or what are the internal strengths of the child that have made this possible? How can we build on these?"

Leadership in collaborating with partner agencies such as behavioral health providers is at times necessary to promote appropriate treatment from clinicians and support a TIC approach. As indicated by the data from the authors' (Strolin-Goltzman et al., 2015) statewide initiative described earlier, there is often a need for an advocacy role with partner agencies to support the best interest of CW clients. Supervisors may have more experience and/or confidence to advocate on behalf of clients with community partners. Behavioral health agencies are also in the process of becoming more trauma-informed, and they may need feedback regarding how their work impacts cases also served by the child welfare agency. For example, if it appears based on the child's report that therapy time is primarily spent discussing school activities rather than the impact of the trauma she experienced, the supervisor may request a meeting with the worker and therapist to model how to productively discuss implementing a more TI approach to treatment.

As such, supervisory influence can be provided through modeling when interacting with clients or others, as well as in supervisory meetings, as a way to help workers think through the implications of trauma history at each stage of intervention. *Guidelines for Applying a Trauma Lens to a Child Welfare Practice Model* (CTISP, 2013b) offers concrete examples of how supervisors can demonstrate trauma-informed practice at each stage in a case. For example, during the case planning process supervisors may review trauma screening results during supervision and assist workers in examining how a history of trauma may impact intervention and the family's response to it, so that this may be considered in the case plan developed with the family. When out-of-home placement is required, supervisors may discuss how the child's reaction to trauma may impact his or her response to placement, and how workers can support the child and foster family (CTISP, 2013b). This may play out at any stage of working with a child or family. For example:

- During investigation and initial assessment, the supervisor reviews the trauma screening results with the worker for thoroughness and helps him or her to determine how the results impact the need for and type of services.

- In meeting with the worker and parent, the supervisor provides examples of the child's behavior and responses in an effort to demonstrate how to help a parent understand how the trauma may be impacting it.
- When the worker indicates the foster parent is really struggling with caring for the child and that the placement may be in jeopardy, the supervisor brainstorms with the worker how to help the foster parent understand how the trauma of being placed in foster care may be influencing the child's behavior in order to guide the foster parents in responding supportively.
- In reviewing progress on meeting case plan objectives, the supervisor asks the CW worker to consider how prior trauma may be influencing how the client is responding in therapy, and subsequently helps develop a plan for exploring this with the client's therapist to improve the treatment process.
- In a case planning conference, the supervisor probes with the parent and worker to recognize the progress made in the resolution or management of issues related to their domestic violence victimization and extrapolate how that growth may positively impact their parenting.

Regardless of whether the trauma led to child welfare intervention or occurred as a result of it, TI supervision openly explores the role of it in what the client is experiencing, and helps the worker determine how this should influence treatment. In short, whenever supervisors ask workers to assess or analyze how the trauma history of a child or family being served may be impacting their responses or models how to intervene in light of identified trauma, this is promoting trauma-informed care.

Targeted reflective supervision

Reflective supervision is a skill that creates an opportunity for workers to think through the complex practice situations in which they have engaged, ways they approached interactions with clients, the effectiveness of the strategies used, and next steps in their work with families. In addition, supervision is a time to explore with workers their own emotional responses to these situations and interactions more directly (Harvey & Henderson, 2014). Unless supervisors intentionally guide workers through their own reactions to the heartbreaking and often volatile and dangerous circumstances they encounter with children and their families, these experiences will likely be left unsaid. When supervisors open this door and then respond empathetically, workers experience a safe environment in which self-reflection and processing of their own emotions can occur. Mills (2012) described how important this can be with respect to worker experiences with removing children from their homes. She described this as helping to support "emotional containment" (p. 301) and helping workers process the trauma experienced by their clients and prevent secondary traumatization.

Purposeful questioning can be used to guide workers to think through their interactions with clients and plan for future intervention. For example, "Why do you think Mrs. Smith may have reacted that way? Could it have been influenced by her own history of abuse?" Or, "What was that like to hear a five-year-old child describe these experiences?" Or, "When you meet with April next week, how might you approach this subject that would be mindful of her history and potentially yield a more productive response?" Or, "I can see that this experience had an impact on you. Can we talk about that?" The supervisor can then help workers plan, or even practice, how to approach a child or family in their next home visit. The following case example illustrates just one example of this, which, when considering that CW workers are confronting the effects of a wide array of trauma with nearly every child and family they interact with daily, requires substantial supervisory attention.

Jane, a 23-year-old worker, returns from an interview at school with Tammy, a five-year-old girl she placed in foster care after being physically abused by her mother. She is visibly upset as she recounts for Mary, her supervisor, that Tammy has disclosed that her teenage foster brother has been fondling her sexually. Before processing the interaction with the child, Mary acknowledges that Jane seems upset, and they discuss her response to what has happened. Specifics regarding how Mary would approach Jane's needs will be offered in the section on responding to indirect trauma. She helps Jane think through the interview with Tammy and the indicators of how the child is responding to what happened to her, verbally and non-verbally, by asking purposeful questions: "Talk me through how this came up, and what you noticed about Tammy's nonverbal cues when she was telling you this." They talk about the potential relationship between how Tammy is responding to this situation in relationship to what happened to her in her mother's home: "How do you think what happened to Tammy at home may relate to how she is feeling about what is happening to her now? What would be a good approach to exploring this with her, given what you know about her and her history?" They conduct an assessment of options for responding to the allegations as well as develop a plan for Tammy to receive a clinical and functional assessment by a mental health professional.

There may be no other social work setting in which reflective supervision is more important to promote effective intervention with clients who have experienced trauma than child welfare.

Action-oriented engagement with clients

A trauma-informed CW supervisor must be willing to get out into the field with workers as opposed to remaining in the office. Mor Barak and colleagues (2009) found task assistance had the greatest impact on positive worker outcomes. Task assistance may involve accompanying workers on difficult home visits or conducting challenging interviews jointly with them. Just being there and, when needed, actively engaging in dialogue with the client, is so important. This could also mean offering to take care of some tasks while the worker is attending to others, such as the myriad activities required when a child is placed in foster care, including petitioning the court, filling out necessary paperwork, arranging for school transportation, ensuring appropriate medical and behavioral health screening, and touching base with the foster parent on how the child is adjusting. Sharing the load during particularly intense times is a form of joining, and may help workers feel less overloaded. Such active engagement serves to protect and support workers as they face traumatic situations, as well as provide the opportunity for skill development and modeling.

Facilitating evidence-informed continuous quality improvement

Research has demonstrated the role of supervision in facilitating adoption of new practice approaches and manageable organizational change (e.g., Cooksey-Campbell, Folaron, & Sullenberger, 2013). Change is stressful, and this is a matter of organizational culture and climate. There is also evidence suggesting supervisors play an important role in promoting teamwork within CW units to support the use of evidence-informed practice (Collins-Camargo & Garstka, 2014). Promoting evidence-informed practice within the team requires creation of a safe environment, and the supervisor sets the tone. Supervisors can create the opportunity to discuss in team meetings how to use evidence from agency databases, client interaction, and published research to inform workers' practice. They may facilitate critical thinking in the work unit by actively discussing these topics in regular meetings, and rewarding workers for using evidence to improve their practice. This, in turn, can help workers feel greater self-efficacy in their work as well as expectancy valance, which represents the extent to which workers retain the belief they can make a difference in the lives of children and families. A continuous quality improvement approach grounded in evidence may, in fact, inoculate workers against secondary traumatic stress (Collins-Camargo, 2012).

When persons are struggling to perform challenging professional tasks that they feel less competent to do—not to mention question whether it is going to make a difference anyway—it is easy to understand how this can have a domino effect on individuals. When dealing daily with child maltreatment, domestic violence, and substance abuse within agencies that seem to demand more than is reasonable and overemphasize administrative tasks, it is easy to lose faith in the work. Sharing success stories in group supervision regarding clients with significant trauma histories who demonstrated resilience and achieved reunification with their children, for example, can also support a positive culture and inspire workers to persevere.

Supporting workers through preventing and responding to indirect trauma

There are three forms of indirect trauma: secondary traumatic stress (STS), vicarious traumatization, and compassion fatigue (Knight, 2013), all of which have application in the CW environment. As workers are regularly exposed to the horrifying details of the trauma experienced by abused children, they in turn may be traumatized, impacting their view of the world and the persons with whom they interact, in what is termed vicarious traumatization. When CW workers find thoughts of the trauma experienced by children on their caseload intruding in their personal life, entering into their dreams, and eliciting a trauma response of their own, this STS may seem very similar to posttraumatic stress disorder. Having an empathic response to working with an entire caseload of families experiencing various forms of trauma can take a cumulative toll on the worker in the form of compassion fatigue, changing the way they view the helping relationship from compassion to mistrust and resentfulness (Knight, 2013).

Supervisors should take a very intentional approach to prevention of and response to indirect trauma, and the literature provides some guidance in this regard. Bride and Jones (2006) found CW workers with lower levels of STS reported their supervisors used an action-oriented approach, offering help and providing visible support. Other research results support promoting compassion satisfaction (Conrad & Kellar-Guenther, 2006) and fulfillment (Radley & Figley, 2007), which require very purposeful efforts on the part of CW supervisors to find and acknowledge evidence that workers are having a positive impact on children and families. As noted earlier, it can be easy to focus on what is not going well in CW casework, which typically involves high caseloads and frequent crises. Supervisors might devote a portion of regular supervision meetings to celebrating successes, even if they are small steps of progress toward goals, as a way of reinforcing that workers are having a positive impact.

Regularly supporting and even requiring self-care activities goes a long way in preventing secondary trauma and compassion fatigue. In one study, workers with higher levels of trauma-informed self-care, of which supervision is an important part, experienced higher levels of compassion satisfaction and lower levels of burnout (Salloum, Kondrat, Johnco, & Olson, 2015). Given that supervisors often control caseload and workflow, they serve a critical role in adjusting for individuals in time of need, or even in a standard sort of way to provide periodic respite.

Supervisors should be trained to identify and respond to indirect trauma in their staff. Part of this is recognizing those who may be at higher risk, such as those who have their own trauma history (Figley, 1995) or underdeveloped emotional intelligence (Matthews & Zeidner, 2004). As supervisors watch for signs of STS or compassion fatigue among staff, they might step in and encourage a staff person to take a day off, leave early to engage in some form of self-care, or hand a case off to him or her (the supervisor) or another worker to assist temporarily if it is becoming too traumatic. Revisiting the case scenario described earlier, one can see how trauma-informed supervision requires the identification and response to high-risk situations when workers may be experiencing indirect trauma:

When talking with Jane about responding to Tammy's allegations of maltreatment in foster care, Mary also knows it is her responsibility to address potential indirect trauma associated with this situation. When appropriate, she acknowledges Jane's distress, probing for how she is responding, knowing she and Jane placed the child in this home: "I know it can be so hard to hear that this has happened to Tammy even though you couldn't have predicted it. How are you feeling? Can we talk about this some more this afternoon once you have taken steps to ensure Tammy's safety?" Mary may choose to share her own response to this situation: "Whenever something bad happens in a foster home where we have placed a child, I can't avoid feeling guilty and wondering if I should have done something differently. Have you ever experienced this?" Mary also considers what she knows about Jane's personal history as a potential childhood victim, or in her prior work at the agency. Maintaining appropriate boundaries and closely assessing and responding to Jane's response, Mary reminds Jane that often our memories of our own personal experiences can be triggered by talking with clients about the trauma they have experienced. She looks for signs in Jane's responses to suggest she may be unable to have a compassionate response, blaming or questioning the victim. After she leaves her office, Mary takes time to think through what Jane has had to endure in her casework recently and develops a plan for talking this through with her and assessing how she is handling the stress of the work to determine if compassion fatigue may be taking a toll. Within the next couple of days, Mary touches base with Jane to see how she is feeling about what happened, and the actions she has taken to protect Tammy since they talked.

Discussion of self-care and management of personal and professional stress should be a regular part of supervisory meetings to normalize conversations on these topics so that workers do not feel singled out. Building discussion of stress and self-care into regular supervision also allows the supervisor to continuously gather data to assess risk of STS and burnout, and then make adjustments in caseload or assignments as needed.

A component of trauma-informed supervision is application of this knowledge in the recruitment and selection of staff for CW work. Shackelford (2012) provided an extensive list of symptoms of both posttraumatic and secondary traumatic stress in CW workers, such as avoidance behaviors, memory lapses, emotional numbness, and irritability. Swift and appropriate response is essential in these circumstances, and the supervisor is responsible for responding quickly to get workers the help they may need. Trauma-informed supervisors know what resources are available to assist workers experiencing indirect trauma and how to access them, and are willing to advocate proactively and responsively on behalf of their staff with managers and service providers to alleviate workload volume and ensure intervention occurs.

Trauma-informed support of and for supervisors

The field often forgets the importance of supporting the supervisors themselves as they do this complex work (Collins-Camargo, 2012; Dill, 2007). Everything described in the prior section about workers applies in parallel to their supervisors in terms of what they need from middle managers. Regehr, Chau, Leslie, and Howe (2002) found high rates of exposure to critical events and a high amount of accountability contributed to nearly 50% of CW supervisors falling in the high or severe range for posttraumatic symptoms. Similar to research described regarding workers presented earlier, the literature offers strategies to address STS in supervisors, including self-care training and support groups (Dane, 2000), peer support and consultation through learning circles (Collins-Camargo, 2006), and middle manager supervision of supervisors to help clarify perceptions and process challenges (Figley, 1989). The aforementioned data from the authors' (Strolin-Goltzman et al., 2015) implementation of a TIC approach in CW suggest that there is a disconnect between perceptions of supervisors and administrators regarding trauma systems readiness and support needs. Middle managers/administrators must not assume that supervisors are impervious to the effects of STS. Managers also must not assume they are fully aware of or equipped to handle the complex trauma needs of the CW system, but instead should inquire about supervisors' needs and any gaps they may be experiencing in their important role.

More broadly, a trauma-informed approach to CW systems would clearly recognize the importance of the role of frontline supervisors in the agency. This includes operationalizing an organizational culture valuing supervision, recognizing high-quality supervisors, and addressing supervisor STS (Bell, Kulkarni, & Dalton, 2003). Supervisors are a conduit for TIC and supporting the work of the frontline. They are also a valued participant in organizational management, providing them with access to strategic information in the organization that helps them respond appropriately to organizational change and reinforce priorities (Choi, 2011). Ausbrooks (2011) studied why supervisors stay in CW and identified the following themes: a sense of mission, support systems, and coping skills.

From a trauma-informed perspective, this translates to understanding and embracing the reality that responding to trauma is a key part of this work, employing self-care strategies with not only their staff but themselves is critical, and relying on productive support systems within and outside the agency that understand the influence of trauma on the work being done is important.

Future directions

Obviously, while many of our assertions related to trauma-informed supervision are supported by related research, there is a need for the development of a fully articulated model and subsequent research related to its implementation and impact. In reviewing the 31 responsibilities of CW supervisors outlined by Hess and colleagues (2009), a trauma-informed approach to CW supervision would not likely add many additional responsibilities. For example, preventing and responding to indirect trauma is addressed directly in the list. A fully articulated model merely requires that in each of the activities in which a supervisor is engaged the influence of trauma is considered and addressed as appropriate.

The need for a trauma lens spans clinical supervision across the wide variety of human service settings in which it occurs. However, CW represents a practice arena in which it is critically important, for the range of reasons explored throughout this article: the trauma that brings clients to workers, the trauma that intervention sometimes inflicts, the bureaucratic and underfunded agencies in which the work occurs, and the susceptibility of the staff who are dedicated to working in this environment. A legend in the study and treatment of trauma, Charles Figley (2012), articulated this well: "Most CW workers care deeply about their clients and their families, and many may suffer from the inability to balance their own needs with those of their vulnerable clients" (p. 4). No one knows more about trauma in families and what happens in its wake than CW supervisors—the TIC movement is not a revelation to them. However, CW systems are typically moving too fast to stop and examine the implications of trauma in the work they do, or put practices and resources in place to respond most effectively to it. It is time we do just that, and enhance the evidence base on how we can most impactfully intervene.

Funding

The study referred to in this article was funded by the U.S. Department of Health and Human Services, Administration for Youth and Families, Children's Bureau through the Promoting Well-Being and Adoption After Trauma program.

References

Ausbrooks, A. R. (2011). Why child welfare supervisors stay. *Journal of Religion & Spirituality in Social Work, 30*, 358–384. doi:10.1080/15426432.2011.619901

Bartlett, J. D., Barto, B., Griffin, J. L., Fraser, J. G., Hodgdon, H., & Rodian, R. (2016). Trauma-informed care in the Massachusetts Child Trauma Project. *Child Maltreatment, 21*, 101–112. doi:10.1177/1077559515615700

Bell, H., Kulkarni, S., & Dalton, L. (2003). Organizational prevention of vicarious trauma. *Families in Society, 84*, 463–470. doi:10.1606/1044-3894.131

Beyerlein, B. A., & Bloch, E. (2014). Need for trauma-informed care within the foster care system: A policy issue. *Child Welfare, 93*(3), 7–21.

Bride, B. E., & Jones, J. L. (2006). Secondary traumatic stress in child welfare workers: Exploring the role of supervisory culture. *Professional Development: The International Journal of Continuing Social Work Education, 9*(2/3), 38–43.

Cahalane, H., & Sites, E. (2008). The climate of child welfare employee retention. *Child Welfare, 87*, 91–114.

Carpenter, J., Webb, C. M., & Bostock, L. (2013). The surprisingly weak evidence base for supervision: Findings from a systematic review of research in child welfare practice. *Children and Youth Services Review, 35*, 1843–1853. doi:10.1016/j.childyouth.2013.08.014

Caseneuva, C., Ringeisen, H., Wilson, E., Smith, K., & Dolan, M. (2011). *NSCAW II baseline report: Child well-being* (OPRE report #2011-27b). Washington, DC: Office of Planning, Research and Evaluation, Administration for Families, U.S. Department of Health and Human Services.

Chadwick Trauma-Informed Systems Project. (2013a). *Creating trauma-informed child welfare systems: A guide for administrators* (1st ed.). San Diego, CA: Chadwick Center for Children and Families.

Chadwick Trauma-Informed Systems Project. (2013b). *Guidelines for applying a trauma lens to a child welfare practice model* (1st ed.). San Diego, CA: Chadwick Center for Children and Families.

Chen, S., & Scannapieco, M. (2010). The influence of job satisfaction on child welfare workers' desire to stay: An examination of the interaction effect on self-efficacy and supportive supervision. *Children and Youth Services Review, 32*, 482–486. doi:10.1016/j.childyouth.2009.10.014

Chenot, D. (2011). The vicious cycle: Recurrent interactions among the media, politicians, the public, and child welfare services organizations. *Journal of Public Child Welfare, 5*, 167–184. doi:10.1080/15548732.2011.566752

Choi, G. (2011). Organizational impacts on the secondary traumatic stress of social workers assisting family violence or sexual assault survivors. *Administration in Social Work, 35*, 225–242. doi:10.1080/03643107.2011.575333

Collins-Camargo, C. (2006). Clinical supervision in public child welfare: Themes from a multi-site study. *Professional Development: Journal of Continuing Social Work Education, 9* (2/3), 102–112.

Collins-Camargo, C. (2012, spring). *Secondary traumatic stress and supervisors: The forgotten victims*. CW 360: A Comprehensive Look at a Prevalent Child Welfare Issue. Minneapolis, MN: Center for Advanced Studies in CW.

Collins-Camargo, C., & Garstka, T. (2014). Promoting outcome achievement in child welfare: Predictors of evidence-informed practice. *Journal of Evidence-Based Social Work, 11*, 423–436. doi:10.1080/15433714.2012.759465

Collins-Camargo, C., & Millar, K. (2012). Promoting supervisory practice change in public child welfare: Lessons learned from university/agency collaborative research in four states. *Child Welfare, 91,* 101–124.

Collins-Camargo, C., & Royse, D. (2010). A study of the relationships among supervision, organizational culture promoting evidence-based practice, and worker self-efficacy. *Journal of Public Child Welfare, 4,* 1–24. doi:10.1080/15548730903563053

Conrad, D., & Kellar-Guenther, Y. (2006). Compassion fatigue, burnout, and compassion satisfaction among Colorado child protection workers. *Child Abuse & Neglect, 30,* 1071–1080. doi:10.1016/j.chiabu.2006.03.009

Cooksey-Campbell, K., Folaron, G., & Sullenberger, S. W. (2013). Supervision during child welfare reform: Qualitative study of factors influencing case manager implementation of a new practice model. *Journal of Public Child Welfare, 7,* 123–141. doi:10.1080/15548732.2012.740441

Dane, B. (2000). Child welfare workers: An innovative approach for interacting with secondary trauma. *Journal of Social Work Education, 36,* 27–38.

Dill, K. (2007). Impact of stressors on front-line child welfare supervisors. *The Clinical Supervisor, 26*(1–2), 177–193. doi:10.1300/J001v26n01_12

Dill, K., & Bogo, M. (2009). Moving beyond the administrative: Supervisors' perspectives on clinical supervision in child welfare. *Journal of Public Child Welfare, 3,* 87–105. doi:10.1080/15548730802695105

Figley, C. R. (1989). *Helping traumatized families.* New York, NY: Brunner/Mazel.

Figley, C. R. (1995). Compassion fatigue as secondary traumatic stress disorder: An overview. In C. R.Figley (Ed.), *Compassion fatigue: Coping with secondary traumatic stress disorder in those who treat the traumatized* (pp. 1–20). New York, NY: Brunner/Mazel.

Figley, C. R. (2012, Spring). *Helping that hurts: Child welfare secondary traumatic stress reactions.* CW 360: A Comprehensive Look at a Prevalent Child Welfare Issue. Minneapolis, MN: Center for Advanced Studies in CW.

Goodard, C., & Hunt, S. (2011). The complexities of caring for child protection workers: The context of practice and supervision. *Journal of Social Work Practice, 25,* 413–431. doi:10.1080/02650533.2011.626644

Hanna, M. D., & Potters, C. C. (2012). The effective child welfare unit supervisor. *Administration in Social Work, 36,* 409–425. doi:10.1080/03643107.2011.604403

Harvey, A., & Henderson, F. (2014). Reflective supervision for child protection practice: Reaching beneath the surface. *Journal of Social Work Practice, 28,* 343–356. doi:10.1080/02650533.2014.925862

Hendricks, A., Conradi, L., & Wilson, C. (2011). Creating trauma-informed child welfare systems using a community assessment process. *Child Welfare, 90,* 187–205.

Hess, P., Kanak, S., & Atkins, J. (2009). *Building a model and framework for child welfare supervision.* New York, NY: National Resource Center for Family-Centered Practice and Permanency Planning and National CW Resource Center for Organizational Improvement.

Kadushin, A., & Harkness, D. (2002). *Supervision in social work* (4th ed.). New York, NY: Columbia University Press.

Kerns, S. E., Pullmann, M. D., Negrete, A., Uomoto, J. A., Berliner, L., Shogren, D.,... Putnam, B. (2016). Development and implementation of a child welfare workforce strategy to build a trauma-informed system of support for foster care. *Child Maltreatment, 21,* 135–146. doi:10.1177/1077559516633307

Kisiel, C., Fehrenbach, T., Small, L., & Lyons, J. S. (2009). Assessment of complex trauma exposure, responses, and service needs among children and adolescents in child welfare. *Journal of Child and Adolescent Trauma, 2*(3), 13–19. doi:10.1080/ 19361520903120467

Knight, C. (2013). Indirect trauma: Implications for self-care, supervision, the organization, and the academic institution. *The Clinical Supervisor, 32*, 224–243. doi:10.1080/ 07325223.2013.850139

Ko, S. J., Kassam-Adams, N., Wilson, C., Ford, J. D., Berkowitz, S. J., Wong, M., . . . Layne, C. M. (2008). Trauma-informed systems: Child welfare, education, first responders, health-care, juvenile justice. *Professional Psychology, Research and Practice, 39*, 396–404. doi:10.1037/0735-7028.39.4.396

Kramer, T. L., Sigel, B. A., Conners-Burrow, N. A., Savary, P. E., & Tempel, A. (2013). A statewide introduction of trauma-informed care in a child welfare system. *Children and Youth Services Review, 35*, 19–24. doi:10.1016/j.childyouth.2012.10.014

Kruzich, J. M., Mienko, J. A., & Courtney, M. E. (2014). Individual and work group influences on turnover intention among public child welfare workers: The effects of work group psychological safety. *Children and Youth Services Review, 42*, 20–27. doi:10.1016/j. childyouth.2014.03.005

Lang, J. M., Campbell, K., Shanley, P., Crusto, C. A., & Connell, C. M. (2016). Building capacity for trauma-informed care in the child welfare system. *Child Maltreatment, 21*, 113–124. doi:10.1177/1077559516635273

Lee, J., Weaver, C., & Hrostowski, S. (2011). Psychological empowerment and child welfare outcomes: A path analysis. *Child Youth Care Forum, 40*, 479–497. doi:10.1007/s10566-011-9145-7

Mandell, D., Stalker, C., De Zeeuw Wright, M., Frensch, K., & Harvey, C. (2013). Sinking, swimming and sailing: Experiences of job satisfaction and emotional exhaustion in child welfare employees. *Child & Family Social Work, 18*, 383–393. doi:10.1111/j.1365-2206.2012.00857.x

Matthews, G., & Zeidner, M. (2004). Traits, states and the trilogy of mind: An adaptive perspective on intellectual functioning. In D. Yun Dai & R. J. Sternberg (Eds.), *Motivation, emotion, and cognition* (pp. 143–174). New York, NY: Routledge.

McBeath, B., Collins-Camargo, C., & Chuang, E. (2012). The role of the private sector in the field of child welfare: Historical reflections, and a contemporary snapshot based on the National Survey of Private Child and Family Serving Agencies. *Journal of Public Child Welfare, 6*, 459–481. doi:10.1080/15548732.2012.701839

Mena, K. C., & Bailey, J. D. (2007). The effects of the supervisory working alliance on worker outcomes. *Journal of Social Service Research, 34*, 55–65. doi:10.1300/J079v34n01_05

Mills, S. M. (2012). Unconscious sequences in child protection work: Case studies of profes-sionals' experiences of child removal. *Journal of Social Work Practice, 26*, 301–313. doi:10.1080/02650533.2011.562603

Mor Barack, M. E., Travis, D., Pyun, H., & Xie, B. (2009). The impact of supervision on worker outcomes: A meta-analysis. *Social Services Review, 83*, 3–32. doi:10.1086/599028

Mor Barak, M. E., Levin, A., Nissly, J. A., & Lane, C. J. (2006). Why do they leave? Modeling child welfare workers' turnover intentions. *Children and Youth Services Review, 28*, 548–577. doi:10.1016/j.childyouth.2005.06.003

National Child Traumatic Stress Network. (2013). *Child welfare trauma training toolkit* (2nd Ed.). Retrieved from http://www.nctsn.org/nccts/nav.do?pid=ctr_cwtool

Radley, M., & Figley, C. R. (2007). The social psychology of compassion. *Clinical Social Work Journal, 35*, 207–214. doi:10.1007/s10615-007-0087-3

Regehr, C., Chau, S., Leslie, B., & Howe, P. (2002). An exploration of supervisors' and managers' responses to child welfare reform. *Administration in Social Work, 26*(3), 17–36. doi:10.1300/J147v26n03_02

Salloum, A., Kondrat, D. C., Johnco, C., & Olson, K. R. (2015). The role of self-care on compassion satisfaction, burnout and secondary trauma among child welfare workers. *Children and Youth Services Review, 49,* 54–61. doi:10.1016/j.childyouth.2014.12.023

Seibert, S. E., Silver, S. R., & Randolph, W. A. (2004). Taking empowerment to the next level: A multiple- level model of empowerment, performance, and satisfaction. *Academy of Management Journal, 47,* 332–349. doi:10.2307/20159585

Shackelford, K. K. (2012, Spring). *Occupational hazards of work in child welfare: Direct trauma, secondary trauma and burnout.* CW 360: A Comprehensive Look at a Prevalent Child Welfare Issue. Minneapolis, MN: Center for Advanced Studies in Child Welfare.

Smith, B. D. (2005). Job retention in child welfare: Effects of perceived organizational support, supervisor support, and intrinsic job value. *Children and Youth Services Review, 27,* 153–169. doi:10.1016/j.childyouth.2004.08.013

Strolin-Goltzman, J. (2008). Should I stay or should I go? A comparison study of intention to leave among public child welfare system high and low turnover rates. *Child Welfare, 87*(4), 125–143.

Strolin-Goltzman, J., Collins-Camargo, C., Akin, B., & McCrae, J. (2015, October). *Community assessment data and the development of trauma-informed, data-driven child welfare systems.* Paper presented at Council on Social Work Education Annual Program Meeting, Denver, CO.

Zlotnik, J. L. (2003). The use of title IV-E training funds for social work education: An historical perspective. *Journal of Human Behavior in the Social Environment, 7,* 5–20. doi:10.1300/J137v07n01_02

Trauma-informed supervision: Counselors in a Level I hospital trauma center

Laura J. Veach and Elizabeth Hodges Shilling

ABSTRACT

Trauma-informed counseling has increased in scope, including work in acute care hospital settings. In this article, we examine trauma-informed supervision, with particular attention to its implementation in a Level I hospital trauma setting involving specialized interventions at the bedside with severely injured trauma patients. Issues of supervision pertaining to substance use and post-traumatic stress response are emphasized. A case example is presented to demonstrate the unique needs of clinicians in an acute care hospital setting and the trauma-informed supervision practices we use with clinicians. Finally, we make recommendations for supervisors in acute care hospital settings and other similar settings.

Trauma, including psychological and physical trauma, has the potential to affect an individual in numerous important and long-lasting ways. It has been readily established that survivors of trauma demonstrate resilience, and yet may still struggle with various mental health or physical health concerns (Bonanno, Westphal, & Mancini, 2012; Dayton et al., 2016; Domhardt, Münzer, Fegert, & Goldbeck, 2015; McCleary & Figley, 2017; Munoz, Brady, & Brown, 2017). Importantly, with the sheer number of individuals exposed to trauma and the vast possibilities of experiences, clinicians are tasked with being appropriately sensitive to the impact of trauma. Trauma-informed care "brings to the forefront the belief that trauma can pervasively affect an individual's wellbeing, including physical and mental health" (Substance Abuse and Mental Health Services Administration, 2014, p. 8). Clinicians, including counselors, licensed clinical addiction specialists, social workers, and other mental health providers, tend to work in environments where psychological trauma is expected and is the primary focus. However, there are some settings, such as integrated care settings like acute trauma centers, where counselors may face clients with both psychological and physical trauma.

Acute trauma centers

Of the numerous types of trauma, physical injuries occur more frequently than all others do (SAMHSA, 2014). Globally, arguments have been made that injuries and deaths caused by traumatic injury are at an epidemic stage, with over 5 million deaths per year, far exceeding HIV, tuberculosis, and malaria-related deaths combined (Lawrence, 2017). According to the National Center for Injury Prevention and Control, Centers for Disease Control and Prevention (2016a), injury is the leading cause of death among persons aged 1–44 and, in 2014, traumatic injuries led to 2.5 million hospitalizations (CDC, 2016b). In the context of medical settings, the term trauma refers to "a bodily wound or shock produced by sudden physical injury, such as that from violence or an accident, including vehicle crashes, several falls, gunshots or knives, blunt forces, blasts and burns" (National Trauma Institute, 2017, para. 1). Trauma injuries represent a large portion of health care costs as well: in 2013, the medical and work loss costs of trauma were over $670 billion (Curtis, Thomas, Haegerich, Feijun, & Zhou, 2015).

In the United States, acute trauma centers are the primary location for treatment of traumatic injuries. Hospital acute care trauma centers involve a major hospital surgery team specializing in surgical care of severely injured individuals. A key component of hospital trauma centers is rapid response to injury as rapid response to trauma injuries can have a substantial impact on whether an individual lives or dies (Sangji & McDonald, 2014). The American College of Surgeons (ACS) created a system for recognizing the care ability at trauma centers (American College of Surgeons, Committee on Trauma, 2014). The ACS system identifies trauma centers at levels ranging from Level I (the most severely injured care) to a Level IV (optimally, the least severely injured care or preparation for transfer to a higher level of trauma care), with each level meeting a specific number of standards of care ("What is a Trauma Center?" 2016). These standards contribute to a greater chance of patients living after a trauma; in fact, the risk of death from severe trauma is 25% lower in patients who were treated at a Level I Trauma Center (Sangji & McDonald). Level I Trauma Centers have specialized trauma surgeons available 24/7 with immediate access to an operating room, resuscitation equipment, advanced diagnostic equipment, and blood products. In contrast, hospital emergency departments (ED) are separate entities entirely: ED physicians and staff treat a variety of illnesses and minor injuries, but do not provide the same level of intensive medical intervention for traumatic injury.

Trauma center patients can be hospitalized for traumatic injuries from a number of intentional and unintentional mechanisms of injury, including wheeled-vehicle crashes (e.g., cars, off-road all-terrain vehicles, motorcycles, bicycles, skateboards); violence-related assaults (e.g., gunshot wounds, stabbings, beatings, child abuse); falls from heights (e.g., roofs, tree-stands, hotel balconies, scoreboards, stairwells); self-inflicted injuries (e.g., suicide attempts by hanging, shootings, stabbings, poisoning, immolation, or other self-harm incidents); natural disasters (e.g., fires, lightning strikes, floods, hurricanes); or work-related accidents, such as crush or impalement injuries. Traumatic injuries are often quite serious and, as a result, physicians focus almost solely on the acute physical injuries during hospitalization (Phipps, Tittle, Zuhlke, & Bellanton, 2014). However, it is clear that trauma centers "are the first point of contact for injured trauma survivors at risk for the development of PTSD and related comorbid conditions" (Russo, Katon, & Zatzick, 2013, p. 489). Although outcomes like PTSD are common, several factors contribute to the total health impact of a trauma.

Mental health symptoms and diagnoses are critical components of trauma; preexisting mental health diagnoses are aspects of trauma patient care that are often overlooked and yet have a substantial influence on outcomes after a trauma (McQueen, 2016; Muscatelli et al., 2017; Phipps et al., 2014; Weinberg, Narayanan, Boden, Breslin, & Vallier, 2016). In a systematic review, 18–22% of patients had diagnosed psychiatric disorders prior to their ICU stay (Davydow, Gifford, Desai, Bienvenu, & Needham, 2009). Patients with prior histories of depression are more likely to experience poorer outcomes after numerous health events, including stroke, surgery, and trauma (Davydow et al., 2009); have a higher rate of morbidity after numerous types of surgery (Ghoneim & OHara, 2016); and are three times more likely to be noncompliant with medical treatment recommendations (DiMatteo, Lepper, & Croghan, 2000). In addition to depression, a history of anxiety appears to negatively affect outcomes for patients; anxiety symptoms prior to surgery were found to contribute to higher reported chronic pain post surgery (Theunissen, Peters, Bruce, Gramke, & Marcus, 2012); delayed wound healing (Gouin & Kiecolt-Glaser, 2011); and increased risk of postoperative respiratory failure (Zou et al., 2016). Finally, researchers have highlighted the increased risk of preexisting comorbid conditions, such as substance use disorders (SUDs) and post-traumatic stress disorders (PTSDs), in individuals admitted for traumatic injuries (Russo et al., 2013; Zatzick et al., 2006).

One of the primary foci of the standards for hospital trauma centers, outlined by the ACS, is prevention. An area of prevention highlighted by the ACS is alcohol and other drug use because of the important contributing factor substance use has on injuries. It is well established since Cherpitel's foundational work (1993) that, in more than any other hospitalized patient group, alcohol use disorders and misuse occur at higher rates in injured patients as compared to the general inpatient hospital population; continued research has verified that alcohol consumption, in terms of both volume and frequency, is causally linked to unintentional and intentional injuries (Cherpitel, 2013; Macdonald et al., 2013; Rehm et al., 2010); and heavy episodic drinking results in significantly increased risk of all types of injuries

(Rehm et al., 2010). As expected, alcohol consumption and risk of injury have a dose–response relationship (Taylor et al., 2010): that is to say, as alcohol consumption increases, the risk of injury increases.

Within trauma units, patients with positive blood alcohol levels on admission range from over one-third to nearly half (Afshar, Netzer, Salisbury-Afshar, Murthi, & Smith, 2016; Beydoun, Teel, Crowder, Khanal, & Lo, 2014; Field, Claassen, & O'Keefe, 2001) and reviews show 41% of readmissions for a subsequent trauma are alcohol-related injuries (Nunn, Erdogan, & Green, 2016). In order to address this widespread health issue, the ACS-COT developed a new quality standard in 2005 requiring all Level I U.S. Trauma Centers to provide screening for the most misused drug – alcohol – and intervene with problem drinkers (Zatzick et al., 2014). This intervention is most often referred to as alcohol screening, brief intervention, and referral to treatment (SBIRT).

Trauma-informed care in integrated care settings

Integrated care settings are medical settings that coordinate general medical and behavioral healthcare in an effort to optimize health outcomes (SAMHSA-HRSA, n.d.). Trauma-informed integrated care "refers to services that unite primary care, mental health, families, and communities while also integrating knowledge of the impact of trauma on all aspects of care" (Dayton et al., 2016, p. 392). Wissow (2016) noted that trauma-informed integrated care could be created by incorporating psychosocial-oriented counseling approaches with the physically oriented healthcare system. In fact, Wissow argued that an integrated trauma-informed care system is personalized and patient-centered, and coordinates healthcare beyond the traditional healthcare services "to include effective connections with services that address the so-called 'social determinants' of health and health-related behavior" (p. 389). The social determinants referred to by medical professionals are mental health factors and social factors that contribute to greater negative health, such as poverty. For example, a recent SAMHSA-funded project, Pediatric Integrated Care Collaborative, found that addressing social determinants of health can be accomplished by building collaborations with community mental health services and integrating mental health services into primary care offices (Dayton et al., 2016). Thus, integrated healthcare models addressing adverse health effects of trauma, both physical and emotional, have emerged as optimal in helping individuals achieve their fullest human potential.

One leading example of trauma-informed integrated care can be found in the US trauma hospital system of care. As described previously, acute trauma centers treat highly injured patients. Many of these patients present with current or previous mental health and substance use issues, and a significant number will experience PTSD or other related acute stress issues because of the trauma injuries. Therefore, acute trauma centers are optimal healthcare settings in which to integrate services that address the whole person, including counseling services. However, minimal research exists regarding trauma-informed clinical supervision related to substance use and traumatic disorders, such as PTSD, for those in an acute care medical setting (Darnell, Dunn, Atkins, Ingraham, & Zatzick, 2016; Field et al., 2001; Russo et al., 2013). To begin to address this gap, we will describe trauma-informed screening, counseling, and supervision in one acute trauma center.

Trauma-informed screening, intervention, and supervision in an acute trauma center

In our exemplary Level I Trauma Center, accredited since 1982 and located within a large southeastern academic medical center, over 3,500 trauma patients, ranging in age from infancy to centenarian, are admitted each year from urban and rural, multi-state geographic regions. The severely injured trauma patient may be in the hospital a few days to a number of months, and may have a strong support system at the bedside or be completely alone throughout their hospital stay. As a result of heightened recognition of the need for trauma-focused care, the Level I Trauma Center at Wake Forest School of Medicine is at the national forefront of trauma-informed counseling by being one of the only accredited trauma centers in the nation to employ specialized clinicians and supervisors solely dedicated to providing trauma-informed screening and intervention services. In addition, a robust training program provides opportunities for graduate students (master's and doctoral level) in helping professions to develop evidence-based, trauma-informed clinical skills.

Our model of trauma-informed care began with an alcohol SBIRT feasibility study in December 2006. Findings supported the provision of SBIRT in the adult trauma unit and services began with one faculty member, a PhD clinician with a background in mental health and SUD intensive interventional work, and one graduate intern. Over the past decade, more than 21,000 screenings (ranging from reviewing blood alcohol test results or specific nursing questions pertaining to substance use to individual screening sessions conducted at the bedside with a valid screening tool) have been provided by our clinical intervention team. Of those screened, a total of 10,500 patients over the past decade were considered to be drinking at risk; on average annually, approximately 1,100 screened positive for risky substance use or drinking; however, approximately 10% did not meet criteria for a brief intervention due to brain injury, surgical complications, death, or psychoses. One of our core values relates to excellence in patient care and, though we see individuals regarding highly sensitive and often stigmatized issues of substance use and mental illness, our team has not yet had a service complaint. Further, we have consistently maintained a less than 2% decline rate in offering substance use screening and intervention services to our hospitalized patients. Lastly, we have provided training to over 50 graduate students in our intervention models since 2007.

Over the years, expansion of SBIRT services led to additional staffing. Crisis intervention, acute stress, and PTSD screening and intervention services were also added within our trauma-focused care services. Since 2014, services expanded to the Pediatric Trauma Unit, the Intensive Care and Step-Down Burn Units, and, recently, two medical units under the Internal Medicine service. Currently, five full-time clinicians, licensed or provisionally licensed as both counselors and clinical addiction specialists, provide trauma-informed services to medically stabilized patients. During spring 2017, 10 clinical interns and practicum students were immersed in learning trauma-informed skills and represented four different counselor education preparation programs. In addition, over the past decade, we have provided services in accordance with our institutional mission to generate new knowledge in caring for individuals with substance use complications, acute stress, post-traumatic stress, crisis intervention, and other mental health complications by leading or participating in eight clinical and pragmatic research trials and feasibility studies (Doud et al., 2017; Ivers, Veach, Moro, Rogers, & O'Brien, 2015; Kazemi et al., 2017; Veach et al., in press; Zatzick et al., 2016).

Trauma-informed counseling in a Level 1 trauma center

The clinical team, both full-time clinicians and counselors-in-training, are tasked with providing trauma-informed SBIRT services and additional mental health services as needed. Our team's primary responsibilities within the hospital setting are twofold: (1) to provide screening and when applicable a brief intervention for risky or higher severity alcohol use issues (the most prevalent drug of abuse), and (2) to provide screening for acute stress and PTSD on our trauma and burn units. A secondary priority on all units is screening and intervening with other substance use issues. Additional services provided by our team include mental health support, crisis intervention, grief support, depression and anxiety screening, with intervention to patients, families of patients, and staff when our primary responsibilities have been attended to and team members are available.

The process of identifying patients who meet the criteria for screening is substantial and layered. When patients are admitted to any of our hospital services (i.e., adult trauma, pediatric trauma, adult burns, pediatric burns, and internal medicine), their information appears in a report that our team members receive at the beginning of each day. This report includes nurse prescreening questions related to alcohol and substance use, blood alcohol levels, gamma-glutamyl transferase [a test of liver enzymes that is used as a biomarker for heavy drinking (Peterson, 2004)], reasons for admission to the hospital and other basic information about the patients. Team members then review this report and electronic medical record information to gather the necessary information for categorizing. Patients are then categorized into six groups: (1) alcohol use concerns resulting in the need for screening and brief intervention; (2) not enough information available so follow-up with the patient is needed to discern need for screening and brief intervention; (3) other substance-use concerns are present resulting in need for screening and additional intervention; (4) patient does not meet criteria for substance use issue but presents with mental health concerns; (5) patient is currently not appropriate for services (i.e., injuries are too severe for intervention); and (6) patient does not meet any criteria so does not require services. Team members then prioritize patients to see based on the patient's category, physician and medical team updates during rounds, and discharge date, thus ensuring that the team meets the Level I Trauma Center requirements to screen all patients for alcohol use and follow-up with a brief intervention when applicable.

Importantly, patients do not sign up for these counseling sessions, and thus approaching and building rapport with clients are significant tasks for the counseling team. Additional factors that contribute to the nature of counseling in this environment include injury severity and level of sickness, presence of family and support persons for patients in their hospital rooms, and the stigma associated with SUDs – all of which add to the sensitivity and trauma-informed skill required from the intervention team. With this in mind, and if rapport is sufficiently built, counseling team members then can screen patients using, for example, the Alcohol Use Disorders Identification Test, a 10-item screening tool (Babor, de la Fuente, Saunders, & Grant, 1992). Counseling team members may then begin brief interventions with patients who screen positive for risky or higher levels of alcohol use. In this setting, these brief interventions are more accurately described as brief counseling interventions: the clinical team works diligently to be patient-centered, Rogerian, and respectful of the patient's expressed willingness to explore change.

An additional focus of counseling pertains to screening the individual for further complications with mental health comorbidity. For example, individuals with a previous diagnosis and treatment for a major depressive illness would receive more intensive intervention, such as a psychiatric consult to determine medication recommendations and further mental health treatment. Members of the trauma team would then provide additional counseling sessions to support the recommendations of the consult by offering supportive counseling, resources for medication information, and access to referral appointments and support groups. Finally, our trauma-informed counseling sessions may involve providing crisis intervention with someone who has experienced the death of a loved one in a motor vehicle crash, for example, or the recent prognosis of complete paralysis, amputation, or scarring disfigurement resulting from severe burns. The dynamic nature of the trauma center setting requires significant attention to trauma-informed supervision, detailed in the next paragraphs.

Trauma-informed supervision in a Level 1 trauma center

Trauma-informed clinical supervision can be described as "supervision that seeks to enhance the knowledge and skills of practitioners in understanding the complexity, dynamics, and potential behavioral manifestations of trauma" (Berger & Quiros, 2016, p. 145). For both the trauma-informed counselor and supervisor, it is important to become trauma-aware by enhancing knowledge about the impact and consequences of traumatic events related to individuals, families, and communities; obtain knowledge and skills with select trauma-related screening and assessment tools; and develop specialized skills conducting appropriate trauma-informed counseling interventions using collaborative, brief, solution-focus and strengths-based approaches that also foster the resilience of trauma survivors. In addition, key experiences of both the supervisee and supervisor need to be monitored and addressed as necessary. For supervisees, cultural orientation, training and skills, history in supervision, perceptions of support, personal trauma history, and vicarious trauma are important to consider in providing trauma-informed supervision (Berger & Quiros, 2016). For supervisors, training and practice experience, beliefs about trauma, knowledge and use of trauma-related practice models, and personal features (i.e., modesty, humility, and acknowledgment of limitations) are important. The nature of supervisory relationships, including "frequent and consistent supervisory meetings with a readily available supervisor" (Berger & Quiros, 2016, p. 147) and relational supervision approaches, are necessary for successful trauma-informed supervision. Supervisees and supervisors reported viewing several characteristics favorably, including focusing on empowerment of supervisees; emphasizing the importance of the supervisee–supervisor relationship and interactions; creating a safe and supportive environment for supervision; addressing the parallel process; encouraging supervisor and supervisee to continue to gain knowledge of trauma and trauma-informed care; and attending to and advocating for self-care (Berger & Quiros).

Clinicians working in the acute care trauma center environment often experience a parallel process with the patients, meaning that often clinicians' reactions to this work is similar to the patients' reactions to their trauma. The exposure to multiple and significant physical and mental traumas tends to result in a greater chance of secondary traumatic responses in our clinicians. Clinicians can experience secondary trauma responses including emotional, cognitive, behavioral, and existential symptomology (Substance Abuse and Mental Health Services Administration, 2014). Specifically, clinicians may experience emotions such as anger, fear, or helplessness. They may experience issues with boundary setting that result in rumination about clients or difficulty concentrating due to the emotional impact of this work. Finally, existential questions and concerns are especially common in this setting because of the frequency of facing death and dying.

Our trauma-informed supervisory approach is designed to meet the needs of clinicians-in-training and full-time clinicians in a dynamic and difficult setting with a high need for trauma-informed care. All of our supervision exceeds traditional weekly supervision meetings in order to meet the relevant clinician-centered needs when working within the trauma-informed approach, as underscored in a qualitative study on trauma-focused clinical supervision (Berger & Quiros, 2016). For first semester students and newly hired clinicians, substantial attention is paid to an intentionally slow process of exposure to the trauma patients and injury types. For example, students in their first semester of clinical experience and clinicians new to our setting spend a minimum of several weeks shadowing and observing trauma counseling without pressure to perform themselves. A consistent emphasis is given to processing student and full-time clinicians' experiences throughout their time, but for students and new clinicians this is especially true in the first few weeks. The first time a student sees a badly injured or burned patient can be particularly challenging, and trauma-informed supervision sessions can often optimize the processing of the experience.

Trauma-informed supervision is also provided for students and clinicians during weekly individual and triadic sessions, as well as in daily debriefing sessions, in response to clinician- or student-initiated supervision requests, or after clinicians or students experience particularly complicated sessions. It is a clear expectation that clinicians and students work as a team, which includes daily debriefing and opportunities to process thoughts and emotions. In addition, intentional brief supervision sessions, driven by both supervisors and supervisees, addressing relevant needs of clinicians and students, occur throughout each day in a dynamic fluid process aligned with Berger and Quiros' (2016) findings. Trauma-informed clinicians and student interns utilize audio recorded role-plays of client sessions during individual and triadic supervision to gain deeper awareness of trauma-informed practice and to increase self-awareness around skill strengths and areas for improvement. Students generally use role-plays during their first few weeks as a means to assess their readiness for clinical encounters with hospital patients. Live observation of students and clinicians is also utilized on a random basis to provide additional feedback. In addition, supervisors focus heavily on reflecting clinician experiences, especially as it relates to time-limited sessions with acutely injured patients. Attention is paid to the process of brief counseling and flexibility in the counseling approach due to the dynamic and changing nature of hospitalized patients. Supervisors will help clinicians reflect on their experiences with patients during interruptions from other medical staff as well and discuss strategies for managing sessions that are atypical, including in length, duration, and privacy.

Another integral part of our trauma-informed supervision involves ongoing training and feedback in substance use screening and brief counseling intervention approaches. Overall, substance use knowledge is important for trauma-informed counseling due to the frequent connections with substance use and trauma response and experiences. In addition, counseling students' limited instruction in substance abuse (e.g., Burrow-Sanchez & Lopez, 2009), combined with a prevalence of substance use and addiction issues in trauma survivors, contributes to a need for a greater focus on substance abuse training and feedback at our site. Supervisory sessions focus on developing awareness of substance use patterns, the hospitalized patient's response to the traumatic injury, and the precipitating event resulting in the current hospital admission.

A key focus within clinical supervision sessions is helping individual supervisees develop trauma-informed sensitivity. In this particular hospital setting, resources that are evidence-based and readily available, such as publications from the Substance Abuse and Mental Health Services Administration (SAMHSA), are key components of instruction. As noted in the *Treatment Improvement Practice (TIP) 57 Manual* (SAMHSA, 2014), it is important that the clinical team remains focused on recognizing patients' trauma-relevant symptoms, such as the following: hypervigilance; frequent reliving of the traumatizing experience (i.e., the precipitating event leading to the injury or past traumatic experiences triggered by the current hospitalization); safety issues for the hospitalized patient; opportunities for psychoeducation about traumatic injury and psychological responses; and options for referral to trauma-informed professionals post hospitalization. Another way of thinking about this is helping clinicians develop a trauma lens, as described by Berger and Quiros (2016). The trauma lens entails "approaching each client with awareness of possible traumatic experiences and their potential impact on client's perceptions, interpretations, emotional reactions, and behaviors" (Berger & Quiros, 2016, p. 147).

Viewing patients through a trauma-informed lens allows students to gain empathy for patients in new ways. For example, patients with trauma histories may present in a hospital environment, where they lack all control over their lives, as demanding or difficult. These behaviors can be frustrating for medical staff and difficult to understand. When a student or clinician is able to consider that these behaviors may be a direct result of traumatic experiences, they can then further empathize with the patient. As students gain additional mastery of basic clinical skills, the supervision focus shifts to include a greater emphasis on helping students demonstrate trauma-informed counseling interventions. For example, supervision sessions include discussions of ways to use collaborative, brief, solution-focused and strengths-based approaches in efforts to foster health, healing, and resilience.

As previously noted, it is expected that a number of traumatic events have occurred to trauma patients admitted to a Level I Trauma Center, so, uniquely, clinicians in our setting are managing consistent and frequent exposure to severe injury and death while providing clinical services. As a result, another substantial focus of supervision is secondary trauma. Much like SAMHSA (2014) recommends in the *TIP 57*, our supervisors work diligently to develop supervisory relationships that mitigate the experience of secondary trauma. Specifically, in line with SAMHSA's recommendations, supervisors take great care in developing strong supervisory relationships with an emphasis on safety and empowerment. At the onset of the supervisory relationships, supervisors provide supervisees with material on secondary and vicarious trauma and opportunities to discuss this. As the relationship continues, supervisors prompt supervisees to discuss potential feelings of secondary trauma, overwhelm, fatigue, grief, anxiety, and fear in a nonjudgmental way to normalize these for students. Additionally, supervisors monitor individual caseloads to balance these with clients who have and do not have trauma-related issues. An all-team member meeting at the beginning of the day gives the team an opportunity to review patients for the day and assign a mixed caseload to clinical staff and students. Through this process, supervisors are able to check-in daily with students and clinicians to gauge their level of fatigue or readiness for seeing patients and assign patients accordingly. In addition to individual supervisory relationships, the entire team has a strong emphasis on relationships and providing and accepting feedback. Modeling healthy professional relationships, feedback, and self-care are important parts of our trauma-informed supervision. The trauma-informed supervisor explains, for example, professional self-care activities with a work–life balance objective, such as setting aside a brief time each day to be mindful and make a brief gratitude list. Other supervision activities can include expressive arts activities, such as origami. The focus of using origami can be on increased awareness of a particularly difficult session or hospital experience, such as the unexpected death of a patient with whom the clinician had a recent session, and allows the supervisee to recognize the loss and its potential or realized impact on his or her developing well-being.

Additionally, the importance of intentional actions in support of counselor self-care cannot be overstressed. The trauma-informed supervisor's emphasis on addressing self-care is paramount. Research is lacking pertaining to trauma-informed clinical supervision's effect on supervisees or trainees, yet self-care appears to be an important predictor of effective trauma-informed counseling and compassion satisfaction (Butler, Carello, & Maguin, 2017). Finally, supervisors engage in, at minimum, biweekly supervision of supervision sessions that allow supervisors to receive similar learning and feedback opportunities as the supervisees.

Case example

This case involves a 22-year-old young single woman who suffered a severe burn (case is based on a representative composite, typifying issues with hospitalized individuals suffering from severe burns). Crystal was admitted to our Burn Intensive Care Unit with severe burns over 50% of her body due to a family violence assault. Her stepfather became enraged when he found her at their home in the act of injecting illegal drugs. In the ensuing altercation, the stepfather, Randy, became physically abusive and knocked Crystal into a gas fireplace in the home.

Upon admission to the trauma burn unit, our team identified Crystal as a patient meeting multiple criteria for intervention: she had a history of intravenous drug use, she was the victim of domestic assault, and she sustained substantial burns from the domestic assault. Of note, the burn injuries alone increased Crystal's risk for the development of acute stress and post-traumatic stress symptoms (Davydow et al., 2009). The first trauma-informed step taken with the care of Crystal involved our team clinician advocating for Crystal in medical treatment rounds. After consulting with her supervisor, our clinician recommended that the medical staff maintain sensitivity around dressing changes and medical interventions when involving touch since Crystal was physically assaulted and might have difficulty being touched while in the hospital.

Due to the severity of her burn injuries, Crystal was in the intensive care burn unit for 5 weeks, where she received multiple anesthesia-assisted procedures consisting of debridement, grafting, and re-grafting when several grafts failed. She was heavily sedated in the early weeks of her care but, as her grafts were showing signs of healing, she was increasingly more verbal. While Crystal was not able to communicate, the clinician continued to monitor her progress. During a debriefing session in week 2 of Crystal's hospitalization, the supervisor encouraged the clinician to consider additional aspects of Crystal's care while she was unable to communicate. Through a process of supervisor-guided brainstorming, the clinician was able to clarify that Crystal's family dynamics were a complicating factor and had the potential to provide additional stress for Crystal and the medical team during the entirety of her treatment. In an effort to ensure appropriate trauma-informed care, the clinician and supervisor brainstormed appropriate ways to monitor and intervene around this crucial factor. The clinician concluded that checking in regularly with the medical team and the family when present would allow opportunities to intervene early.

As Crystal became more verbal, the clinician and supervisor met to consider the likely first steps in supporting Crystal. The clinician and supervisor reviewed aspects of Crystal's history and things that had happened with family and friends during the recent weeks that were relevant to trauma-informed care. The supervisor made sure to illicit conversation about re-traumatization, encouraging the clinician to consider ways to minimize re-traumatization. The clinician decided that it would be important to describe her availability to Crystal, ensuring that Crystal would know during which hours the clinician could be contacted and the response time of the clinician to these contacts. Often patients are unaware that mental health and substance abuse clinicians are available during day time hours and providing clarity around this can ensure the client feels respected, heard, communicated with, and safe.

It was then that Crystal was seen for the first time by the team clinician, Lolly, a full-time licensed clinical addiction specialist associate and provisionally licensed professional counselor, to provide a brief trauma-informed session. In the beginning of her first session with Crystal, the clinician verified with Crystal first if she was in agreement with a session, was provided informed consent information, and, upon consent, intentionally began their relationship by giving Crystal the opportunity to demonstrate control and decision-making. Once Crystal agreed, she was offered a brief relaxation intervention, was introduced to a technique to help slow her breathing, and was shown how the relaxation technique could be used at her own initiative during difficult hospital treatment experiences. The clinician discussed her availability with Crystal and made a schedule of times when the clinician could stop by to see Crystal, thus respecting Crystal's need for autonomy, control, and decision-making.

Early on in the therapeutic relationship, Crystal discussed severe anxiety around her dressing changes and surgeries and issues sleeping at night because of night terrors and frequent awakenings by staff, thus providing additional information important to the screening process. The clinician was able to walk Crystal through ways to address her anxiety with the medical team. Despite empowering Crystal to advocate for herself, Crystal was not quite ready to take that step. The clinician asked Crystal's permission to intervene on her behalf and they decided collaboratively that meeting with the attending burn surgeon together would help. The clinician scheduled a time with the physician, brainstormed ways to approach the meeting with Crystal, and, at the behest of Crystal, led the meeting, checking in with Crystal at agreed upon intervals to allow her to comment. The meeting resulted in agreed upon changes in how dressing changes and preparation for surgery would occur, as well as shifts in how night staff responded to Crystal. This process helped Crystal gain more autonomy and increased her overall wellness during her hospital stay.

Crystal progressed over the course of the next 3 months and transitioned into a step-down unit where she received continued burn care by the surgical team, the occupational therapist, physical therapists, recreation therapist, a social worker, and the counselor for the burn unit. Her 16 sessions addressed goals related to her severe SUD involving a more intensive, multiple session intervention plan, including Crystal's goals of transfer to a specialized addiction treatment center when physically stable; her improved use of relaxation techniques; and her expression of a range of emotions as she continued her physical recovery while facing the residual scarring. Understanding the need for psychoeducation about acute stress and post-traumatic stress in burn survivors, the clinician discussed both with Crystal and helped her begin to develop coping skills for related symptomology.

The clinician was particularly challenged by the violent assault by the stepfather during her work with Crystal. After seeing Crystal screaming in pain one day, the counselor texted her supervisor, asking for a time to talk. The supervisor and clinician met later that afternoon to debrief about the session. The counselor shared that over the course of time working with Crystal she had become increasingly angry about the stepfather, his role in Crystal's injury, and their tenuous relationship. With severe burns, Crystal was in substantial pain for many of their sessions and the counselor was internally struggling with witnessing this trauma on a consistent basis. Additionally, the clinician shared that she was angry at Crystal's mother for not being there to support her and that, as a result, Crystal had very little social support. Lolly's supervisor normalized these feelings and opened a discussion about her awareness around where these feelings could be coming from. Lolly shared that she felt helpless at times with Crystal and the supervisor facilitated a discussion of ways Lolly could maintain boundaries and cope with the impact of her work with Crystal. Lolly shared that she had been over-identifying with Crystal and that she had not been sticking to her self-care plan; she agreed to intentionally center herself before beginning sessions with Crystal and start back with her self-care plan.

The trauma-informed supervision of the clinician, Lolly, included weekly individual or triadic sessions. The purpose of the supervision was to assist the counselor in enhancing her trauma awareness, explore goals to examine the client's change potential with substance use patterns in combination with specialized care for her SUD; give attention to effective relaxation techniques appropriate for burn patients; provide ongoing screening and intervention for PTSD and ASD; and introduce safety planning and screening for family violence risk factors. Lolly provided supportive counseling for Crystal to help her identify stressors and coping mechanisms pertaining to hospital-related medical procedures and to help her make arrangements for follow-up referral appointments for continued trauma-informed counseling. Supervision also included review of sessions with Crystal's family in accordance with the safety plan for any visitation by family. Lolly provided resources and recommendations to the family by phone and in person on a limited basis due to visiting restrictions of the stepfather, but was able to provide a referral to a family program for addiction and recovery. Trauma-informed supervision also included reviews of tapes of counseling sessions and live observation to monitor key awareness of vicarious trauma or over-identification with the particular issues present in the work with Crystal. Written self-care plans were also reviewed. Now, 3 years later, Crystal is an active peer support specialist with regular involvement in burn support group activities while maintaining a strong focus on her sustained substance-free recovery.

Suggestions for supervisors in acute care trauma settings

It is clear that there is a tremendous need for trauma-informed practice and trauma-informed supervision (SAMHSA, 2014) in acute trauma centers. In the case example we presented some of the typical responses from clinicians in our acute trauma center. Other responses common among clinicians in our setting include feeling overwhelmed by the pace and energy of the site, by the substantial physical trauma and illness experienced by patients and by the substantial learning curve associated with adjusting to a medical environment; and feeling anxiety about entering patient rooms, beginning brief counseling interventions, and interacting with medical professionals. While many new and seasoned clinicians experience similar feelings, students and clinicians at the hospital often face these feelings on a daily basis due to the ever-changing patient population and the uncontrolled environment within hospital patient rooms.

Little research exists on the specifics of how trauma-informed supervision looks in acute trauma centers or integrated care settings and yet a growing number of clinicians will find themselves working in settings like this as integrated care grows. Based on our experiences, we offer several suggestions to supervisors in acute care trauma settings that have the potential to be applied to other integrated care settings as well. Supervisors will benefit from the following:

- creating regular opportunities for supervision of supervision;
- seeking continuing education on trauma, injury, illness, and related mental health issues such as PTSD, SUDs, and depression;
- emphasizing self-care with their supervisees and taking additional care to model self-care for supervisees;
- focusing on the development of the supervisor-supervisee relationship with an emphasis on safety and empowerment;
- maintaining flexibility in how and when supervision is provided (i.e., checking in after tough clients early on in the student's development may be more beneficial and trauma-informed than weekly hour-long supervision meetings); and

- attending to secondary trauma experiences with supervisees through intentional, regular check-ins.

Conclusion

Although client responses to trauma vary substantially, certain clinical settings require special attention to and consideration of trauma. Trauma-informed clinical service and supervision are especially necessary for clinicians in hospital settings. In this article, we described physical traumas that result in hospitalization and an acute care hospital trauma setting where such traumas are treated, detailed the role of a team of clinicians providing trauma-informed substance abuse and mental health services, explored trauma-informed clinical supervision within this unique setting, and presented implications for other supervisors in similar settings. With substantial attention paid to trauma-informed supervision, clinicians with varying degrees of experience can be successful in dynamic and challenging environments like acute care hospital trauma centers.

References

Afshar, M., Netzer, G., Salisbury-Afshar, E., Murthi, S., & Smith, G. S. (2016). Injured patients with very high blood alcohol concentrations. *Injury*, *47*, 83–88. doi:10.1016/j.injury.2015.10.063

American College of Surgeons. Committee on Trauma. (2014). *Resources for optimal care of the injured patient.* Chicago, American College of Surgeons.

Babor, T.F., de la Fuente, J.R., Saunders, J., and Grant, M.. (1992). *AUDIT: The Alcohol Use Disorders Identification Test guidelines for use in primary care* (2nd ed.). Geneva: World Health Organization.

Berger, R., & Quiros, L. (2016). Best practices for training trauma-informed practitioners: Supervisors' voice. *Traumatology*, *22*, 145–154. doi:10.1037/trm0000076

Beydoun, H., Teel, A., Crowder, C., Khanal, S., & Lo, B. M. (2014). Past blood alcohol concentration and injury in trauma center: Propensity scoring. *The Journal of Emergency Medicine*, *47*, 387–394. doi:10.1016/j.jemermed.2014.06.024

Bonanno, G. A., Westphal, M., & Mancini, A. D. (2012). Loss, trauma, and resilience in adulthood. *Annual Review of Gerontology & Geriatrics; New York*, *32*, 189–210. doi:10.1891/0198-8794.32.189. Retrieved from https://www.cdc.gov/injury/wisqars/fatal_help/faq.html#citation.

Burrow-Sanchez, J. J. and Lopez, A. L. (2009), Identifying Substance Abuse Issues in High Schools: A National Survey of High School Counselors. *Journal of Counseling & Development*, *87*, 72–79. doi:10.1002/j.1556-6678.2009.tb00551.x

Butler, L. D., Carello, J., & Maguin, E. (2017). Trauma, stress, and self-care in clinical training: Predictors of burnout, decline in health status, secondary traumatic stress symptoms, and compassion satisfaction. *Psychological Trauma: Theory, Research, Practice, and Policy*, *9*(4), 416–424. doi:10.1037/tra0000187

Centers for Disease Control and Prevention, National Center for Injury Prevention and Control. (2016a). *Web-based Injury Statistics Query and Reporting System (WISQARS) Fatal Injury Data.* Retrieved from https://www.cdc.gov/injury/wisqars/fatal_help/faq.html#citation

Centers for Disease Control and Prevention, National Center for Injury Prevention and Control. (2016b). *Web-based Injury Statistics Query and Reporting System (WISQARS) nonfatal injury data.* Retrieved from https://www.cdc.gov/injury/wisqars

Cherpitel, C. J. (1993). Alcohol and injuries: a review of international emergency room studies. *Addiction, 88*(7), 923–937.

Cherpitel, C. J. (2013). Focus on: The burden of alcohol use - trauma and emergency outcomes. *Alcohol Research; Bethesda, 35,* 150–154.

Curtis, F., Thomas, S., Haegerich, T., Feijun, L., & Zhou, C. (2015). Estimated lifetime medical and work-loss costs of fatal injuries — United States, 2013 (Morbidity and Mortality Weekly Report (MMWR) No. 64 (38)) (pp. 1074–1077). Centers for Disease Control and Prevention. Retrieved from https://www.cdc.gov/mmwr/preview/mmwrhtml/mm6438a4.htm?s_cid=mm6438a4_w

Darnell, D., Dunn, C., Atkins, D., Ingraham, L., & Zatzick, D. (2016). A randomized evaluation of motivational interviewing training for mandated implementation of alcohol screening and brief intervention in trauma centers. *Special Issue on Studies on the Implementation of Integrated Models of Alcohol, Tobacco, And/Or Drug Use Interventions into Medical Care, 60*(SupplementC), 36–44. doi:10.1016/j.jsat.2015.05.010

Davydow, D. S., Gifford, J. M., Desai, S. V., Bienvenu, O. J., & Needham, D. M. (2009). Depression in general intensive care unit survivors: A systematic review. *Intensive Care Medicine, 35,* 796–809. doi:10.1007/s00134-009-1396-5

Dayton, L., Agosti, J., Bernard-Pearl, D., Earls, M., Farinholt, K., Groves, B. M., … Wissow, L. S. (2016). Integrating mental and physical health services using a socio-emotional trauma lens. *Current Problems in Pediatric and Adolescent Health Care, 46,* 391–401. doi:10.1016/j.cppeds.2016.11.004

DiMatteo, M. R., Lepper, H. S., & Croghan, T. W. (2000). Depression is a risk factor for noncompliance with medical treatment: Meta-analysis of the effects of anxiety and depression on patient adherence. *Archives of Internal Medicine, 160,* 2101–2107. doi:10.1001/archinte.160.14.2101

Domhardt, M., Münzer, A., Fegert, J. M., & Goldbeck, L. (2015). Resilience in survivors of child sexual abuse: A systematic review of the literature. *Trauma, Violence, & Abuse, 16*(4), 476–493. doi:10.1177/1524838014557288

Doud, A. N., Moro, R., Wallace, S. G., Smith, M. D., McCall, M., Veach, L. J., & Pranikoff, T. (2017). All-terrain vehicle injury in children and youth: Examining current knowledge and future needs. *The Journal of Emergency Medicine, 53,* 222–231. doi:10.1016/j.jemermed.2016.12.035

Field, C. A., Claassen, C. A., & O'Keefe, G. (2001). Association of alcohol use and other high-risk behaviors among trauma patients. *Journal of Trauma-Injury Infection, 50,* 13–19. doi:10.1097/00005373-200101000-00002

Ghoneim, M. M., & OHara, M. W. (2016). Depression and postoperative complications: An overview. *BMC Surgery; London, 16.* doi:10.1186/s12893-016-0120-y

Gouin, J.-P., & Kiecolt-Glaser, J. K. (2011). The impact of psychological stress on wound healing: Methods and mechanisms. *Immunology and Allergy Clinics of North America, 31,* 81–93. doi:10.1016/j.iac.2010.09.010

Ivers, N. N., Veach, L. J., Moro, R. R., Rogers, J. L., & O'Brien, M. C. (2015). Brief alcohol counseling intervention in a trauma setting with Latina/o clients (Special Issue). *Journal of Addictions and Offender Counseling: IAAOC Annual Review,* 107–124.

Kazemi, D. M., Jacobs, D. G., Portwood, S. G., Veach, L., Zhou, W., & Hurley, M. J. (2017). Trauma center youth violence screening and brief interventions: A multisite pilot feasibility study. *Violence and Victims, 32,* 251. doi:10.1891/0886-6708.VV-D-15-00141

Lawrence, R. (2017, November). *Tackling the Global Burden of Trauma: Perspectives of a Humanitarian NGO.* 4th Annual Meeting of the Pediatric Trauma Society, Charleston, SC.

Macdonald, S., Greer, A., Brubacher, J., Cherpitel, C., Stockwell, T., & Zeisser, C. (2013). Alcohol consumption and injury. In *Alcohol*. Oxford: Oxford University Press. doi:10.1093/acprof:oso/9780199655786.003.0019

McCleary, J., & Figley, C. (2017). Resilience and trauma: Expanding definitions, uses, and contexts. *Traumatology, 23*, 1–3. doi:10.1037/trm0000103

McQueen, M. (2016). Psychological distress and orthopedic trauma: Commentary on an article by Douglas S. Weinberg, MD, et al. *The Journal of Bone and Joint Surgery, 98*(5), e19. doi:10.2106/JBJS.15.01261

Munoz, R. T., Brady, S., & Brown, V. (2017). The psychology of resilience: A model of the relationship of locus of control to hope among survivors of intimate partner violence. *Traumatology, 23*, 102–111. doi:10.1037/trm0000102

Muscatelli, S., Spurr, H., O'Hara, N. N., O'Hara, L. M., Sprague, S. A., & Slobogean, G. P. (2017). Prevalence of depression and posttraumatic stress disorder after acute orthopaedic trauma: A systematic review and meta-analysis. *Journal of Orthopaedic Trauma, 31*, 47–55. doi:10.1097/BOT.0000000000000664

National Trauma Institute. (2017). *What is trauma*. Retrieved November 3, 2017, from https://www.nattrauma.org/what-is-trauma/

Nunn, J., Erdogan, M., & Green, R. S. (2016). The prevalence of alcohol-related trauma recidivism: A systematic review. *Injury, 47*, 551–558. doi:10.1016/j.injury.2016.01.008

Peterson, K. (2004). Biomarkers for alcohol use and abuse: A summary. *Alcohol Research and Health; Washington, 28*, 30–37.

Phipps, M., Tittle, M. B., Zuhlke, R., & Bellanton, B. (2014). Depression among trauma patients. *Dimensions of Critical Care Nursing, 33*, 136–141. doi:10.1097/DCC.0000000000000037

Rehm, J., Baliunas, D., Borges, G. L. G., Graham, K., Irving, H., Kehoe, T., … Taylor, B. (2010). The relation between different dimensions of alcohol consumption and burden of disease: An overview. *Addiction, 105*, 817–843. doi:10.1111/j.1360-0443.2010.02899.x

Russo, J., Katon, W., & Zatzick, D. (2013). The development of a population-based automated screening procedure for PTSD in acutely injured hospitalized trauma survivors. *General Hospital Psychiatry, 35*, 485–491. doi:10.1016/j.genhosppsych.2013.04.016

Sangji, N. F., & McDonald, K. (2014). Trauma and emergency care under the Affordable Care Act. *Bulletin of the American College of Surgeons, 99*(4), 20.

Substance Abuse and Mental Health Services Administration. (2014, March 1). *Trauma-informed care in behavioral health services*. Treatment Improvement Protocol (TIP) Series 57. Retrieved October 28, 2017, from https://store.samhsa.gov/product/TIP-57-Trauma-Informed-Care-in-Behavioral-Health-Services/SMA14-4816

Taylor, B., Irving, H. M., Kanteres, F., Room, R., Borges, G., Cherpitel, C., … Rehm, J. (2010). The more you drink, the harder you fall: A systematic review and meta-analysis of how acute alcohol consumption and injury or collision risk increase together. *Drug and Alcohol Dependence, 110*, 108–116. doi:10.1016/j.drugalcdep.2010.02.011

Theunissen, M., Peters, M. L., Bruce, J., Gramke, H. F., & Marcus, M. A. E. (2012). Preoperative anxiety and catastrophizing: A systematic review and meta-analysis of the association with chronic postsurgical pain. *Clinical Journal of Pain, 28*, 819–841. doi:10.1097/AJP.0b013e31824549d6

Veach, L., Moro, R., Miller, P., Reboussin, B., Ivers, N. N., Rogers, J. L., & O'Brien, M. C. (in press). Alcohol counseling in hospital trauma: Examining two brief interventions. *Journal of Counseling & Development*.

Weinberg, D. S., Narayanan, A. S., Boden, K. A., Breslin, M. A., & Vallier, H. A. (2016). Psychiatric illness is common among patients with orthopaedic polytrauma and is linked with poor outcomes. *The Journal of Bone and Joint Surgery, 98*, 341–348. doi:10.2106/JBJS.15.00751

What is a Trauma Center? ER or Trauma? (2016, May 26). Retrieved November 3, 2017, from http://share.upmc.com/2016/05/what-is-a-trauma-center/

Wissow, L. S. (2016). Introducing Psychosocial Trauma-Informed Integrated Care. *Current Problems in Pediatric and Adolescent Health Care, 46*(12), 389–390. https://doi.org/10.1016/j.cppeds.2016.11.003

Zatzick, D., Donovan, D. M., Jurkovich, G., Gentilello, L., Dunn, C., Russo, J., … Rivara, F. P. (2014). Disseminating alcohol screening and brief intervention at trauma centers: A policy-relevant cluster randomized effectiveness trial. *Addiction, 109*, 754–765. doi:10.1111/add.12492

Zatzick, D. F., Grossman, D. C., Russo, J., Pynoos, R., Berliner, L., Jurkovich, G., … Rivara, F. P. (2006). Predicting posttraumatic stress symptoms longitudinally in a representative sample of hospitalized injured adolescents. *Journal of the American Academy of Child & Adolescent Psychiatry, 45*, 1188–1195. doi:10.1097/01.chi.0000231975.21096.45

Zatzick, D. F., Russo, J., Darnell, D., Chambers, D. A., Palinkas, L., Eaton, E. V., … Jurkovich, G. (2016). An effectiveness-implementation hybrid trial study protocol targeting posttraumatic stress disorder and comorbidity. *Implementation Science; London, 11*. doi:10.1186/s13012-016-0424-4

Zou, J., Su, C., Lun, X., Liu, W., Yang, W., Zhong, B., … Chen, Z. (2016). Preoperative anxiety in patients with myasthenia gravis and risk for myasthenic crisis after extended transsternal thymectomy: A CONSORT Study. *Medicine, 95*(10), e2828. doi:10.1097/MD.0000000000002828

Trauma-informed supervision in deployed military settings

W. Brad Johnson, Matthew Johnson, and Kristin L. Landsinger

ABSTRACT

Uniformed mental health care providers often practice *in extremis*; that is, in difficult and dangerous contexts defined by deployment to combat theaters, isolated practice settings, and exposure —directly and indirectly—to traumatic experiences. Frequent exposure to client trauma heightens the risk of secondary traumatic stress and compassion fatigue among military health care providers. Supervision for military interns, residents, and junior practitioners must be competent, caring, and trauma-informed. In this article, we describe the unique characteristics of clinical practice in deployed military settings, including the unique professional and ethical quandaries for both practitioners and their clinical supervisors. We then offer a framework for trauma-informed supervision in deployed military settings, including several specific recommendations for supervisors in these contexts.

Clinical supervision is among the most frequent professional activities reported by mental health professionals (MHPs) across practice settings (Falender & Shafranske, 2007). There is broad consensus that effective supervision is a prerequisite for competent functioning on the part of trainees and early-career MHPs. Strong clinical supervision fosters a trainee's professional development, instilling and developing necessary knowledge, skills, and attitudes while monitoring and safeguarding client welfare and promoting ethical practice on the part of the trainee (Shallcross, Johnson, & Lincoln, 2010). Clinical supervision provides the structure and framework for learning how to apply knowledge, theory, and clinical procedures to solve human problems (Falender & Shafranske, 2007). Excellent supervision includes several integral components, including observation, feedback, evaluation, intentional modeling, facilitation of self-assessment, mutual problem solving, and professional gatekeeping.

Berger and Quiros (2014) recently observed that, ideally, supervision is a reflective process that offers a physical and emotional safe space and opportunity to examine the clinical work of the practitioner with the goals to enhance personal and professional growth, shape competence, and promote a high level of services. In essence, the supervisory relationship must become a safe space in which a supervisee can speak freely within the surrounds of a trusting environment. In addition, supervisors must attend to *both* the educative and supportive functions of supervision (Berger & Quiros, 2014). The *educative function* addresses teaching the supervisee about the relevant population, challenges typical of the specific setting and context, and strategies for successful and contextualized interventions. The *supportive function* refers to providing emotional support to help the supervisee cope with work-related challenges and stresses, identify personal issues that can impede the ability to provide competent services, and offer strategies to address them.

Above all, clinical supervision is fundamentally a relationship. Competent supervisors must be attentive to the relational dynamics that shape the formation, course, and outcomes of supervision (Johnson, Skinner, & Kaslow, 2014). Trainees have been known to gravitate toward supervising MHPs who have good interpersonal skills and can effectively demonstrate empathy, respect, genuineness, and support (Shallcross et al., 2010). Within the context of the supervision relationship, competent supervisors must balance sometimes competing roles (e.g., teacher, advocate, colleague, evaluator) with special attention to the best interests of the supervisee, the supervisee's clients, and the public at large. Recently, Johnson and colleagues reflected that the best supervisory relationships take on many of the characteristics of strong mentoring relationships (Johnson, Skinner, et al., 2014). As an assigned supervisory relationship moves along the mentoring relationship continuum from one end (formal, hierarchical, focused exclusively on skill development and assessment) to the other (a rich developmental relationship characterized by greater mutuality and relational mentoring), the supervisor begins to offer a range of both career and emotional or psychological functions, the relationship becomes increasingly reciprocal, and the supervisor becomes increasingly invested in the supervisee's professional development and success. Strong clinical supervision is an essential component of training and supporting military MHPs. In the following section, we introduce the distinctive contours of clinical practice in military settings with emphasis on the implications for clinical supervision.

Clinical supervision in military settings

Uniformed MHPs (at the present time, psychiatrists, psychologists, and social workers may be commissioned as health care service providers in the Air Force, Army, and Navy) face a host of unique challenges, stressors, and ethical tensions when compared to their civilian colleagues. For this reason, military medical training centers place a high priority on intensive training and deliberately challenging—yet well-supervised—training experiences for mental health care interns and residents (Johnson & Kennedy, 2010).

There are several factors that distinguish the military as a unique context for mental health care practice (Johnson, 2008, 2016). First, military MHPs are obligated to place the superordinate military mission before the interests of both self and individual service members. Supporting the overarching mission at hand is a legally binding duty for uniformed practitioners. This focus on the military mission (fighting and winning conflicts) is most apparent in time of war. Second, clinical work in the military context is often high-stakes in nature; the consequences of ineffective job assessments, clinical evaluations, and treatment are often more serious than in other contexts. For instance, clearing a psychiatrically impaired Special Forces member for a mission may place other service members in jeopardy. Conversely, declaring a team member with a critical skill set unfit to deploy may compromise the success of a key mission. Third, military MHPs have considerably more influence over the lives and careers of individual clients than may be true in civilian settings. A determination by an MHP that a client is psychologically unfit for deployment may reduce chances for promotion and continued military service. For example, a pilot who is diagnosed with major depression will not be allowed to fly until a course of treatment leads to a period of symptom-free functioning. If the depression doesn't abate quickly, the service member may be forced to move to a different job or medically retire from service.

Fourth, military MHPs have less ability than their civilian counterparts to decide whether to enter or exit clinical relationships with members of their military community. Although most professional ethics codes enjoin MHPs to provide services only within the boundaries of their competence, based on education, training, supervised experience, consultation, and professional experience, military MHPs often function in solo duty assignments, far from direct supervision or consultation, as the only mental health provider assigned to a military unit. Quite often, the culture of training in military settings teaches MHPs to take pride in their ability to effectively manage any client and clinical issue that walks through the door. Particularly when deployed as solo providers, uniformed MHPs may feel pressure to provide triage and even ongoing services to military personnel regardless of their established competence, presenting clinical and cultural variables, or specialized treatment requirements (Johnson, 2016; Moore & Reger, 2006). Fifth, many elements of military environments create unique ethical dilemmas for MHPs. Specifically, their roles as commissioned military officers (binding them to uphold federal statutes and military regulations) and their roles as licensed health care professionals (binding them to a code of professional ethics) can easily create tensions around issues such as confidentiality, multiple relationships, intrusions on privacy, and unintended disclosures.

In addition to these factors that distinguish health care service provision for military MHPs, many—if not most—uniformed MHPs will at one time or another occupy an embedded clinical duty assignment. By *embedded*, we mean that the MHP will be deployed as a member of a military unit, and obligated to place the unit's mission foremost. With the advent of the conflicts in Iraq and Afghanistan, more MHPs have been embedded with war-fighting units (ground units, air squadrons, aircraft carriers), and required to travel and live with the unit in active combat theaters (Moore & Reger, 2006). Deployed MHPs often report stressors—both for themselves and the clients they treat—specific to the deployment cycle. Linnerooth, Mrdjenovich, and Moore (2011) articulated stressors at each phase of the deployment cycle: *pre-deployment* (e.g., preparing their own family for deployment, understanding their role during deployment); *during a deployment* (e.g., understanding the line between therapy and "coffee talk" with colleagues, contemplating personal feelings about death); and *post-deployment* (e.g., readjusting to a normal day-to-day clinic routine and personal life); these three phases encompass the day-to-day realities for an active-duty MHP. All of these additional stressors may place uniformed MHPs at higher risk for secondary traumatic stress, compassion fatigue, and professional burnout. In fact, recent studies have suggested that the rates of burnout among military mental health service providers working in stateside clinics range from 21% to 28% (Ballenger-Browning et al., 2011; Kok, Herrell, Grossman, West, & Wilk, 2016).

Clinical supervisors in military contexts are licensed MHPs with at least three or four years more experience than a supervisee, often significantly more. A supervisor is also usually—but not always—of higher military rank. The vast majority of clinical supervision in military settings occurs within formal internship, residency, and postdoctoral training programs. Unlicensed MHPs must continue supervision until credentialed, even if they are deployed to a combat zone or stationed in a small or isolated duty station as the only uniformed MHP. Once a military MHP is licensed, often within the year following completion of an internship, supervision is no longer required. Clinical supervisors in the military are also busy practitioners in their own right. They see clients, conduct evaluations, and carry administrative military duties in addition to their supervisory work. In stateside military medical centers, the rhythm and routine of supervision is likely to be quite similar to that experienced by civilian supervisors. In deployed contexts, things are quite different. A supervisor may be required to travel to different locations to meet with supervisees stationed with different medical units. When this is not feasible, face-to-face supervision must be augmented by tele-supervision, both on the part of the assigned supervisor and training supervisors back in stateside medical centers. Most, but not all, clinical supervisors in the military have themselves been deployed at one time or another.

Supervisors of direct accession (post-training) military mental health care professionals, and of MHP trainees, have a unique opportunity to provide supervision related to self-awareness for signs and signals of distress and discussion of a tangible plan for what to do when signs and signals of distress occur.

In fact, because stress, emotional problems, and relationship turmoil can lead to diminished competence among supervisees (Elman & Forrest, 2007) and practicing MHPs (Sherman & Thelen, 1998), Johnson and Kennedy (2010) suggested that military supervisors "must emphasize trainee self-awareness and accurate self-assessment of competence" (p. 302).

For these reasons, supervisors in military settings must be attuned to the stressors linked to the cycle of deployment with particular attention to the unique stressors and vicissitudes of practice in embedded combat environments. They must prepare and support their supervisees accordingly. We propose that supervisors in military contexts own a heightened ethical/ professional obligation to ensure that supervisees are well-prepared for the challenges of military deployment and the high probability of working with severely traumatized military personnel.

In this article, we provide a framework and specific guidance for clinical supervisors in military settings. We specifically address the exigencies of supervision in those contexts characterized by military deployment and embedded work with combatant units. We first consider the unique risks and stressors associated with *in extremis* clinical work, defined as the provision of health care in environments characterized by physical danger, emotional distress, and exposure to trauma vicariously through work with active-duty military combatants. Next, we consider the specific phenomena of compassion fatigue and secondary traumatic stress and the associated risks to professional competence among military MHPs. We then discuss trauma-informed supervision as an essential framework for clinical supervision in military health care training and practice contexts, including the necessity of framing competence as a community obligation (Berger & Quiros, 2016). Finally, we conclude this article with several actionable recommendations for clinical supervisors working with military MHPs.

The deployed practitioner: *In extremis* clinical work

Thousands of military MHPs have deployed to combat zones in support of the global war on terror. These providers are often embedded within deployed military units and some of them have been routinely exposed—vicariously or directly—to traumatic events and disturbing images (Larner & Blow, 2011; Linnerooth et al., 2011). Deployment-related stressors for MHPs are ubiquitous and may include repeated and unpredictable deployments, extended absences from family, unpredictable living and work environments, stressful medical treatment decisions (e.g., making difficult triage and medical rationing decisions when casualties overwhelm available emergency services, providing health care to enemy combatants), exposure to seriously injured and psychologically traumatized service members, occasional exposure to direct threat, and nearly continuous exposure to traumatic client material (Gibbons, Barnett, Hickling,

Herbig-Wall, & Watts, 2012; Johnson, Bertshinger, Snell, & Wilson, 2014; McLean et al., 2011). For these reasons, it is often inevitable that some of these MHPs will become "wounded healers" (Daneault, 2008), uniformed healthcare professionals who have become so distressed—at least temporarily—that they have become impaired (Johnson, in press). Some of these MHPs have offered articulate and moving narratives of their personal struggles with trauma (Jadick, 2008; Kraft, 2007).

Accordingly, clinical work in deployed military settings has been described as *in extremis* health care practice (Johnson et al., 2011). *In extremis* was defined by Kolditz (2007) as "at the point of death" (p. 160). Like their colleagues in emergency medicine, refugee work, and disaster relief, uniformed MHPs face specific types and doses of stress less likely encountered by their civilian counterparts. Three primary types of risk in *in extremis* deployment contexts include risk of injury or death, risk of psychological trauma and emotional distress, and risk of ethical/professional distress (Johnson & Kennedy, 2010). Risk of injury or death is ubiquitous in combat theater clinical work. This risk is not only a consequence of enemy action, but also accidents and disease. In terms of risk for psychological trauma and emotional distress, there is now clear evidence that military deployment escalates the risk of psychological distress and impairment for all service members—including mental health professionals—when compared to non-deployed samples (Gibbons et al., 2012; Hoge, Auchterlonie, & Miliken, 2006; Jacobson et al., 2012; Sundin et al., 2014; Thomas et al., 2010). Finally, military deployment escalates the intensity and frequency of professional quandaries and occasional distress stemming from mixed-agency ethical dilemmas. These are dilemmas that occur when an MHP's ethical obligations to one party (e.g., an individual uniformed client) appear to directly compete or conflict with his or her obligations to another party (e.g., the immediate military commander or the broader military mission; Kennedy & Johnson, 2009). As one illustration of a mixed-agency ethical conflict, deployed MHPs have occasionally reported significant tension between efforts to safeguard the apparent best interests of an individual service member and the exigencies of the immediate military mission (Johnson, 2008). Some have questioned whether it is ever in the best interests of the individual service member to send him or her back into action when there is evidence of psychological impairment. In these situations, military supervisors must be particularly attuned to assist supervisees with working through their personal feelings, projections of their own trauma, and the potential for boundary erosion between supervisees and clients.

Trauma exposure and its consequences for deployed MHPs

Like all military personnel, military MHPs practicing *in extremis* and working daily with an often-traumatized population are considerably more likely than others in the population to suffer mood, anxiety, trauma, substance, and relational disorders

(Hoge et al., 2006). In addition, military MHPs are often quite junior and inexperienced, the very MHPs most vulnerable to work-related distress (Shapiro, Brown, & Biegel, 2007). Youth and inexperience translate to fewer inoculating experiences, both clinically (exposure to traumatized clients) and personally (exposure to the stresses of combat theater work). Unfortunately, the military often places advanced psychologists into the administrative and clinical supervisory realms, leaving the junior MHPs to perform the majority of the clinical work. Thus, clinical supervisors in military settings must be continuously alert to problems of professional competence in supervisees—as well as themselves—and must help supervisees to become vigilant to evidence of decrements in previous levels of competence as a function of distress (Johnson et al., 2011). Although uniformed MHPs do run the risk of direct exposure to traumatic events and subsequent trauma-related disturbances, evidence suggests that indirect exposure and cumulative emotional exhaustion pose greater threats to the deployed MHP's well-being and clinical competence (McLean et al., 2011).

Secondary traumatic stress and vicarious traumatization

Deployed health care providers may become secondarily traumatized by repeated and extended exposure to clients' traumatic disclosures (Figley, 2002; McLean et al., 2011). Regehr, Goldberg, and Hughes (2002) described the experience of *secondary traumatic stress* (STS) this way: "Through the process of hearing the graphic details of other people's horrifying experiences, the [MHP] can begin to experience symptoms that include intrusive imagery, generalized fears, [and] sleep disturbances" (p. 505).

Clinical supervisors must be attuned to the sometimes subtle shifts in supervisees caused by STS. In their theoretical model of STS, Bride and Figley (2009) articulated three elements that set the stage for STS. First, a provider is indirectly exposed to the traumatic experiences of clients. MHPs often share the emotional burden of clients' trauma, bear witness to the horrifying events, and, through their clients, themselves come face-to-face with trauma. Second, in the context of this exposure, the provider is being empathic, but this empathy comes with a price. Finally, the MHP is more likely to experience STS when specific risk factors are present. These include relative inexperience, degree of exposure to traumatic material, a high proportion of traumatized clients on one's caseload, and personal experience with combat-related or childhood trauma (Bride & Figley, 2009). Of course, military clinical supervisors must immediately recognize that each of these predisposing factors are likely to be in play for MHPs who deploy to combat zones, especially on multiple occasions.

In contrast, vicarious traumatization (VT) involves core changes in fundamental aspects of the therapist's self, including negative changes in cognitions, expectations, and relationship functioning as a long-term consequence of caring for others. In their seminal work on the topic, Pearlman and Saakvitne (1995) defined VT as the "negative effects of caring about and caring for others" (p. 31). According to the authors, VT is the "cumulative transformation in the inner experience of the therapist that comes about as a result of empathic engagement with the client's traumatic material" (p. 31). In a real way, empathy is the MHP's greatest asset and also possibly his or her greatest liability.

Compassion fatigue

In deployed military settings, MHPs working with seriously wounded or traumatized persons for an extended period, perhaps with little previous professional experience, are at greater risk of *compassion fatigue*, an emotional exhaustion syndrome resulting from excessive demands on one's own resources in empathizing with clients who are in serious pain (Figley, 2002). The compassion fatigue construct is closely aligned with VT. The more empathic the caregiver and the greater the experience of helplessness, inefficacy, and lack of support (Daneault, 2008; Shapiro et al., 2007), the greater the risk of compassion fatigue. Ongoing compassion fatigue may portend a corollary phenomenon, often termed *empathy failure* (Post, 1980). Empathy failure occurs when a previously competent MHP begins to process client experiences and feelings on a purely cognitive level, perhaps no longer capable of emotional processing and mirroring. In their research with ambulance workers, Regehr and colleagues (Regehr et al., 2002) found that those with empathy failure began to approach their work on purely technical levels, while remaining emotionally distanced from patients. Clinical supervisors must be carefully attuned to evidence of this sort of emotional numbing and disengagement in their supervisees. Over time, compassion fatigue is correlated with professional burnout in health care providers generally (Maslach & Leiter, 2008). Burnout evolves more slowly than compassion fatigue and describes a syndrome of emotional exhaustion, apathy, and, ultimately, feelings of hostility or aversion toward clients (Johnson, Bertschinger, et al., 2014; Linnerooth et al., 2011).

A case example

To illustrate the importance of trauma-informed supervision for uniformed supervisees in deployed military settings, we now offer a real case vignette from the experience of a uniformed clinical psychologist deployed to Iraq. Based on an earlier example from Johnson and colleagues (2011), we have updated the vignette to illustrate the effects of *in extremis* clinical work, secondary traumatic stress, and the corrosive effects of compassion fatigue, empathy failure, and burnout. We include the MHP's first-person experiential reflections, as well as reflections about her ongoing supervisory relationship.

> In a clinical session this morning, as my client sat across from me describing his difficult emotions and concerns, my brain went into lockdown. I stared at this

soldier, I saw his lips move and heard his voice, but my ability to take in what he was saying was lost. As he spoke, my mind was hijacked by an unwanted stream of disturbing images from the countless clients I had worked tirelessly to care for during the previous seven-month deployment. The mangled images included a young Marine burning to death inside his armored vehicle and a guard outside the dining facility having her head taken off by a rocket-propelled grenade. And then there was the intrusive image of one of my own long-term clients who was blown to pieces by an IED shortly before he was to return home to the States. Flooded by these memories, I lost all awareness of the soldier sitting in front of me. When my client finally asked, "Ma'am, are you okay?" I stared back blankly, feeling nothing. For the first time in seven months, I had absolutely nothing left to give, not compassion, not hope, not encouragement; some invisible boundary had been crossed and I was no longer able to relate to anyone else's sadness or process any more tragedy.

Two days following this experience, my spirits were lifted when my supervisor arrived for an impromptu visit. As a psychologist only two years post-internship and the only mental health professional assigned to my forward medical combat unit, I was fortunate to have a clinical supervisor located 20 miles away at a larger military medical unit. Mark was a psychiatrist and about 10 years my senior as an officer. Although we sometimes had short conversations via phone or e-mail, electronic communication was unpredictable and often impossible. To his credit, Mark made it a priority to make the dangerous trip via armored carrier or helicopter to my base at least once a month for face-to-face supervision sessions. As soon as he walked into the small tent that served as my "office," Mark could read my exhaustion. For the next half hour, he let me just talk. By then, I knew that Mark was unquestionably trustworthy and that our supervision sessions were genuinely safe territory. The flood gates opened and out poured a torrent of traumatic client stories, intrusive images, and my own experience of bone-deep depletion. Tears accompanied my words. To my surprise and profound relief, Mark refrained from focusing on any specific case, but merely mirrored back my sense of fatigue, shared some of his own struggles with symptoms of acute stress, and teared up when describing how he felt each time a member of his unit was lost. By meeting me where I was as a colleague and a friend, I found Mark's comments profoundly helpful and normalizing. Eventually, we discussed secondary traumatic stress and the risks this posed to "our," not just my own, competence. We agreed that both of us were struggling to preserve our competence in an extremely difficult context and we discussed strategies for doing so. Mark specifically encouraged me to turn to other health service providers, chaplains, and even a close friend or two in the unit to debrief more often and share hard experiences and concerns without compromising any client's confidentiality. When our time was up, my burden was lightened and I sensed that I could sustain good-enough clinical work for the remainder of the deployment.

The military clinician showcased in this case vignette is illustrative of thousands of health care providers who have deployed to combat zones in support of the global war on terror during the past decade and a half (Johnson, in press). In her experience, we see evidence of STS, compassion fatigue, empathy failure, and the inevitable decrements in professional competence so predictable in these circumstances. In addition, although this account does not examine the many possibilities for countertransference manifestations due to the provider's own individual history, it may also be playing an intricate part in the aforementioned decrements (Gelso & Hayes, 2007). Ironically, the more empathic this MHP may have been at the outset, the greater her risk of experiencing helplessness, inefficacy, and emotional detachment following extended periods of working empathically with traumatized clients (Shapiro et al., 2007). Were her STS and compassion fatigue to go unnoticed by a supervising MHP, it is likely that she would be at risk for a more general burnout characterized by apathy, exhaustion, and even persistent feelings of aversion and hostility toward her clients. This vignette illustrates, in a very real sense, how sustained competence in deployed military contexts may truly require a village. Closely knit and deliberately constructed communities of engaged and caring colleagues and supervisors might be the only way to ensure that individual practitioners are consistently functioning within competence standards. One strategy for deliberately constructing such a caring collegial "village" of colleagues is the *competence constellation* approach (Johnson, Barnett, Elman, Forrest, & Kaslow, 2013). Johnson and colleagues (2013) defined a competence constellation as "the cluster of relationships a professional has with people who take an active interest in and action to advance the individual's well-being and professional competence" (p. 347).

Trauma-informed supervision as an ethical obligation

Mental health professionals of all stripes are ethically obligated to actively prevent harm to those with whom they work. In the supervisory context, this ethical standard on avoiding harm means that supervisors must be vigilant to protect the public, especially consumers of supervisees' work (Amerian Psychological Association [APA], 2010). However, supervisors owe equal allegiance to supervisees. In military settings, clinical supervisors must provide training experiences that establish broad competence among military supervisees while inoculating them to the various stressors they may soon encounter. Yet, this intensity must be carefully controlled and attenuated so that supervisees are not overwhelmed or traumatized by the training itself (Johnson & Kennedy, 2010).

It may be tempting to place the burden for self-assessing competence levels in deployed environments exclusively at the feet of practitioners themselves. In fact, most professional ethical codes seem to reinforce this obligation on the part of the individual. For instance, the Ethics Code of the American Psychological Association (American Psychological Association, 2010) has codified the obligation this way:

> *Standard 2.06(b)*: When psychologists become aware of personal problems that may interfere with performing work-related duties adequately, they take

appropriate measures, such as obtaining professional consultation or assistance and determine whether they should limit, suspend, or terminate their work-related duties. (p. 5)

Unfortunately, there is considerable evidence that MHPs often are ineffective when it comes to accepting their own vulnerabilities and recognizing decrements in their own competence due to distress, and some continue to provide services when they are too distressed to do so effectively (Daneault, 2008). Moreover, research evidence from a range of health care disciplines reveals that most of us often are inaccurate in assessments of our own competence. Comprehensive reviews of social psychological and health care education research reveal that human self-assessments of any skill or professional competency are flawed systematically and consistently (e.g., Davis et al., 2006; Dunning, Heath, & Suls, 2004). Perhaps most concerning, MHPs whose competence is most compromised—by distress or burnout—often are among those least capable of effectively detecting problems with their own competence and responding appropriately (Davis et al., 2006). Of course, there are other reasons why supervisees may fail to share concerns about diminished competence with supervisors. In training contexts, military interns and residents may fear rejection or suffer shame if they do recognize their own ebbing performance. And some will employ narcissistic defenses to maintain the illusion of imperviousness to trauma and distress (Johnson et al., 2011).

Trauma-informed supervision

Recently, Berger and Quiros (2014, 2016) have articulated an evidence-based approach to *trauma-informed supervision*. Berger and Quiros noted that such supervision can help supervisees prevent, mitigate, and heal secondary traumatic stress and emotional exhaustion ubiquitous in contexts involving a significant caseload of trauma-exposed clients. Trauma-informed supervision should be mandatory rather than delivered "on an as needed basis" (Berger & Quiros, 2014, p. 298). It may include assessment of a supervisee's vulnerabilities and resilience relative to trauma, based on the supervisee's own life experiences. The military clinical supervisor may use assessment and discussion of supervisees' previous exposure to extreme stress or trauma and their strategies for resilience and adaptiveness to help supervisees address job-related stress and challenges, and exercise self-care. Depending upon the context for supervision, it may also be feasible to delegate a balanced trauma-related caseload to supervisees that are aligned with their experience and demonstrated competence. Such strategic assignment of traumatized clients might be far more attainable in formal training settings and more difficult in deployed contexts.

According to Berger and Quiros, there are five core elements of trauma-informed supervision:

(1) *Safety*: Environments that reflect acceptance and predictability in scheduling contribute to supervisees feeling comfortable to share work-related challenges and stresses and feel safe both physically and emotionally.

(2) *Trustworthiness*: When supervisees experience a strong working alliance and genuine care on the part of the supervisor, they are likely to feel safe sharing trauma-related reactions.

(3) *Choice*: Allowing supervisees to play an active role in the type of intervention used with a traumatized client is often critical.

(4) *Collaboration*: Supervisees benefit from experiencing the supervisory relationship as collegial and mutual in most respects, such that each member's realities are honored and each member's expertise brought to bear on the case at hand.

(5) *Empowerment*: Supervisees in trauma-rich contexts can feel empowered by validation, consistent feedback, and the opportunity to practice skills autonomously with monitoring by the supervisor.

Trauma-informed supervision emphasizes many of the virtues of communitarianism, in that supervisors endeavor to inculcate values of collegiality, community, and mutual interdependence in the supervisory relationship (Johnson, Barnett, Elman, Forrest, & Kaslow, 2012). In essence, the supervisory/training ethos is one best described as a learning community in which supervisors demonstrate egalitarian values, caring, reciprocity, and authenticity for those they supervise.

Finally, good trauma-informed supervision must also consider matters of *countertransference* and the parallel process playing out in the three-way relationship among client, supervisee, and supervisor. When a uniformed MHP works with a traumatized client, various emotional reactions can be triggered—by subtle or overt behaviors within the client—as a result of the MHP's own experiences with trauma (Gelso & Hayes, 2007). Countertransference reactions in the supervisee often originate in a very personal, perhaps unconscious area of the supervisee's experience; it is therefore crucial that the supervisor prioritizes the formation of a safe, therapeutic space wherein the supervisee can explore the countertransference material productively. As Gabbard (1996) reminded us, "the thoughts feelings, and behaviors that a therapist would most like to keep secret from the supervisor or consultant, are the most important issues to discuss with that supervisor or consultant" (p. 321). Trauma-related anxiety in the supervisee has proven to be a reliable predictor of countertransference manifestations in psychotherapists (Cohen, 1952; Hayes, Gelso, & Hummel, 2011), and it is likely that military MHPs with exposure—both direct and vicarious—to trauma, are at heightened risk for troublesome countertransference reactions to deployed and traumatized clients.

The skilled clinical supervisor is also attuned to the here-and-now psycho-dynamics between supervisor and supervisee (Freud, 1912; Sarnat, 2015), particularly owning the value of helping supervisees understand their bidirectional transference to supervisor and client (Schamess, 2006). In some respects, the relational dynamics in play between supervisees and their clients will be mirrored and repeated in the immediate relationship between supervisee and supervisor (Doehrman, 1976; Searles, 1955). Known as parallel process (Baudry, 1993), the competent supervisor in deployed settings will be thoughtful, gentle, but persistent, in helping the supervisee to become aware of trauma-related dynamics in the therapy relationship that are also evident in the supervisory relationship.

As an example, while many of the empirically supported trauma treatments require the client to repeatedly retell the traumatic narrative, MHPs might be required to retell the narrative to their supervisor in an effort to provide context for the therapeutic hour. This retelling can bring up feelings of anxiety, guilt, shame, disgust, and vulnerability in the therapist who is intimately associated with the narrative and the emotional difficulties it evokes. It would therefore serve the supervision hour well for the supervisor to explore the cognitive and emotional challenges within the narrative, as well as the parallel process occurring within the therapeutic and supervisory hours.

Recommendations for clinical supervisors in deployed military settings

We conclude this article with several practical recommendations for clinical supervisors of uniformed MHPs. These recommendations apply to both the training phase, as MHPs are prepared for deployments to combat zones, as well as to the deployment and post-deployment phases when an MHP is likely to be confronting and working through exposure to trauma.

Create a safe space in the supervisory relationship

Job one for the trauma-informed clinical supervisor is ensuring that the supervisee feels safe, supported, and cared for by the supervisor (Berger & Quiros, 2016). This requires that the supervisor tailor supervision to the individual needs of the supervisee so that he or she feels safe presenting authentically in the relationship. In their report of qualitative interviews with trauma-informed supervisors, Berger and Quiros (2016) wrote,

> In creating a safe space, which one interviewee described as "creating an oasis within the chaos," there was emphasis on balancing "being very attentive, gentle, supportive, and nurturing, while also nudging workers to challenge themselves, hold themselves accountable, and yet create a safe space to struggle toward professional growth." (p. 149)

One element of buttressing supervisees' defenses against trauma involves helping them to be as open as possible to—and even moved by—their own suffering, exhaustion, and compassion fatigue. For instance, supervisors might mirror supervisees' experience with genuine expressions of empathy or ask supervisees what they would say to a colleague—possibly employing the empty chair technique—who was suffering through a similar experience. The safe surround of the trauma-informed relationship should assist the supervisee in nurturing compassion toward the self. *Self-compassion* involves encouragement of feelings of caring and kindness toward oneself, and learning to harbor nonjudgmental attitudes toward one's own inadequacies, failures, and moments of diminished competence (Johnson, Bertschinger, et al. 2014). In a series of studies, Leary, Tate, Adams, Allen, and Hancock (2007) found that self-compassion effectively buffered people against powerfully negative life events. We propose that self-compassionate MHPs may subsequently be more accurate in their self-assessments of competence and more open to seeking consultation when secondary trauma and compassion fatigue occur.

Equip and inoculate supervisees for trauma exposure

Supervising MHPs in military training settings must be thoughtful about creating inoculating training experiences to ensure that supervisees are well-prepared for the exigencies of deployment and the very likely probability of repeated and prolonged exposure to secondary trauma in the context of their clinical work. Solid preparation for deployment must incorporate training in traumatology, battlefield triage, combat-related psychopathology, and some exposure to the varieties of client traumatic experiences they are likely to encounter (Johnson, Bertshinger, et al., 2014). Some examples of inoculating experiences include brief intensive military training schools for triaging combat wounds or surviving behind enemy lines and clinical rotations on rehabilitation units for service members recovering from both physical and psychiatric trauma. At the same time, the intensity of inoculation and training-based exposure must be carefully controlled and attenuated so that supervisees are not overwhelmed or traumatized by the training itself. In many respects, these efforts at preparation and inoculation will help supervisees grasp the personal, psychological, and professional risks associated with deployment (Johnson & Kennedy, 2010).

Beyond inoculation to traumatic client material, trauma-informed supervision must equip supervisees with a firm commitment to self-care and clear facility with self-care strategies. First, military MHPs must appreciate and accept the fluid, contextual, vulnerable nature of professional competence and accept their vulnerability to distress. Second, supervisors must help new MHPs hone self-awareness regarding their own signals of distress. Thus, a supervisor might engage in guided exploration with the MHP to identify concrete signs and symptoms of burnout, compassion fatigue, and secondary traumatic stress (Johnson, in press). Next, the supervisor can work with a supervisee to develop a vigorous and personalized plan for self-care in deployed settings (Bride & Figley, 2009; Linnerooth et al., 2011; Smith & Moss, 2009). Key elements of a self-care regimen may include physical fitness, nutrition, sleep, connection with colleagues, external consultation, and time for relaxation and creative pursuits.

Work toward a transformational (mentoring-oriented) supervisory relationship

A salient component of trauma-informed supervision is the creation of a sense of empowerment on the part of the supervisee (Berger & Quiros, 2016). Effective trauma-informed supervisors encourage supervisees to initiate and contribute to their own professional development plans while listening for their preferences, validating and supporting their unique clinical styles, and acknowledging their specific strengths. In military settings focused on preparation for and positive coping during deployment, supervisors must work to move the supervisory relationship along the mentoring continuum from primarily transactional (formal, hierarchical) to transformational (mutual, reciprocal, collegial, and empowering; Johnson, Skinner, et al., 2014). Transformational supervisory relationships are characterized by increasing reciprocity and collegiality, fluid expertise and complementarity, increasing vulnerability, and a holistic approach in which the supervisor becomes increasingly committed to both the supervisee's professional/ career and personal growth and development. Although the trust and social support common of more transformational/egalitarian supervisory relationships are likely to be vitally important for supervisees working with traumatized populations, supervisors must be sensitive to the fact that, at times, becoming more formal and directive can give secondarily traumatized MHPs the structure they require to effectively manage their own feelings and distress.

Remain attuned to transference dynamics

Supervisee countertransference reactions to traumatized clients can easily be triggered in uniformed MHPs who work largely with a combatant population. Supervisors must be diligent to form a safe supervisory space in which the supervisor can explore countertransferential material without reservation (Gelso & Hayes, 2007). Moreover, trauma-informed supervisors have underscored the importance of attending to a parallel process in their supervisory relationships; supervisees may reenact, in their interactions with the supervisor, the issues and emotions from their relationship with the client (Berger & Quiros, 2016). For instance, a supervisor may help a supervisee who becomes upset in supervision to discern how these feelings correspond with his or her client's expression of emotional distress during psychotherapy.

Help supervisees construct a viable competence constellation

In the context of secondary trauma exposure, military MHPs are always at risk of missing or minimizing evidence of compassion fatigue, secondary trauma, and diminished competence. The trauma-informed supervisor must collaborate with the supervisee—early in the supervisory relationship—to develop a competence constellation, framed by Johnson and colleagues (2012) as an MHP's network or consortium of individual colleagues, consulting groups, supervisors, and professional association affiliations that serve to provide both honest and frequent assessment of competence and ongoing collegial support. Beyond the individual supervisor, military training sites should provide numerous modalities for collegial support and competence maintenance, such as peer-to-peer consultation matches, psychotherapy opportunities external to the training program, support groups, continuing education gatherings, and, once deployed, ongoing consultation groups with MHPs in other locations. In the face of trauma, a well-constructed coalition of supportive professional relationships is essential for ensuring ongoing competence.

Deliberately model self-care, humility, and collegiality

One of the more powerful techniques available to the trauma-informed military supervisor is that of deliberate and intentional role-modeling for supervisees. Specifically, a supervisor with deployment and traumatic exposure experience can serve as a powerful exemplar regarding strategies for self-care, peer consultation, and steps taken to heal and regain equilibrium as a competent MHP (Berger & Quiros, 2016; Johnson, Bertshinger, et al., 2014). When a supervisor is authentic, humble, and willing to share personal and professional strategies for coping and thriving during and after deployment, then the supervisee's experiences with distress and fatigue are destigmatized and humanized.

Disclosure statement

The authors report no conflicts of interest. The authors alone are responsible for the content and writing of the article.

References

American Psychological Association. (2010). *Ethical principles of psychologists and code of conduct.* Retrieved from http://www.apa.org/ethics/code/index.aspx

Ballenger-Browning, K. K., Schmitz, K. J., Rothacker, J. A., Hammer, P. S., Webb-Murphy, J. A., & Johnson, D. C. (2011). Predictors of burnout among military mental health providers. *Military Medicine, 176*, 253–260. doi:10.7205/MILMED-D-10-00269

Baudry, F. D. (1993). The personal dimension and management of the supervisory situation with a special note on the parallel process. *The Psychoanalytic Quarterly, 62*, 588–614.

Berger, R., & Quiros, L. (2014). Supervision of trauma-informed practice. *Traumatology, 20*, 296–301. doi:10.1037/h0099835

Berger, R., & Quiros, L. (2016). Best practices for training trauma-informed practitioners: Supervisors' voice. *Traumatology, 22*, 145–154. doi:10.1037/trm0000076

Bride, B. E., & Figley, C. R. (2009). Secondary trauma and military veteran caregivers. *Smith College Studies in Social Work, 79*, 314–329. doi:10.1080/00377310903130357

Cohen, M. B. (1952). Countertransference and anxiety. *Psychiatry: Journal for the Study of Interpersonal Processes, 15*, 231–243. doi:10.1080/00332747.1952.11022877

Daneault, S. (2008). The wounded healer. *Canadian Family Physician, 54*, 1218–1219.

Davis, D. A., Mazmanian, P. E., Fordis, M., Harrison, R. V., Thorpe, K. E., & Perrier, L. (2006). Accuracy of physician self-assessment compared with observed measures of competence. *Journal of the American Medical Association, 296*, 1094–1102. doi:10.1001/jama.296.9.1094

Doehrman, M. J. (1976). Parallel processes in supervision and psychotherapy. *Bulletin of the Menninger Clinic, 40*, 1–104.

Dunning, D., Heath, C., & Suls, J. M. (2004). Flawed self-assessment: Implications for health, education, and the workplace. *Psychological Science in the Public Interest, 5*, 69–106. doi:10.1111/j.1529-1006.2004.00018.x

Elman, N. S., & Forrest, L. (2007). From trainee impairment to professional competence problems: Seeking new terminology that facilitates effective action. *Professional Psychology: Research and Practice, 38*, 501–509. doi:10.1037/0735-7028.38.5.501

Falender, C. A., & Shafranske, E. P. (2007). Competence in competency-based supervision practice: Construct and application. *Professional Psychology: Research and Practice, 38*, 232–240. doi:10.1037/0735-7028.38.3.232

Figley, C. R. (2002). Compassion fatigue and the psychotherapist's chronic lack of self-care. *Journal of Clinical Psychology, 58*, 1433–1441. doi:10.1002/jclp.10090

Freud, S. (1966). The dynamics of transference. In J. Strachey (Ed.), *The standard edition of the complete psychological works of Sigmund Freud* (vol. 12). London, UK: Hogarth Press. (Original work published 1912)

Gabbard, G. (1996). Lessons to be learned from the study of sexual boundary violations. *American Journal of Psychotherapy, 50*, 311–322.

Gelso, C. J., & Hayes, J. A. (2007). *Countertransference and the therapist's inner experience: Perils and possibilities*. Mahwah, NJ: Lawrence Erlbaum.

Gibbons, W. W., Barnett, S. D., Hickling, E. J., Herbig-Wall, P. L., & Watts, D. D. (2012). Stress, coping, and mental health-seeking behaviors: Gender differences in OEF/OIF health-care providers. *Journal of Traumatic Stress, 25*, 115–119. doi:10.1002/jts.21661

Hayes, J. A., Gelso, C. J., & Hummel, A. (2011). Managing countertransference. *Psychotherapy, 48*, 88–97. doi:10.1037/a0022182

Hoge, C. W., Auchterlonie, J. L., & Miliken, C. S. (2006). Mental health problems, use of mental health services, and attrition from military service after returning from deployment to Iraq or Afghanistan. *Journal of the American Medical Association, 295*, 1023–1032. doi:10.1001/jama.295.9.1023

Jacobson, I. G., Horton, J. L., LeardMann, C. A., Ryan, M. A. K., Boyko, E. J., Wells, T. S., & Smith, T. C. (2012). Posttraumatic stress disorder and depression among U.S. military health care professionals deployed in support of operations in Iraq and Afghanistan. *Journal of Traumatic Stress, 25,* 616–623. doi:10.1002/jts.21753

Jadick, R. (2008). *On call in hell: A doctor's Iraq war story.* New York, NY: NAL.

Johnson, W. B. (2008). Top ethical challenges for military clinical psychologists. *Military Psychology, 20,* 49–62. doi:10.1080/08995600701753185

Johnson, W. B. (2016). Military settings. In J. Norcross, G. R. VandenBos, & D. K. Freedheim (Eds.), *APA handbook of clinical psychology* (vol. 1, pp. 495–507). Washington, DC: American Psychological Association.

Johnson, W. B. (in press). Ethical considerations for working with military service personnel. In M. Leach & L.Welfel (Eds.), *Cambridge handbook of applied psychological ethics.* Cambridge, UK: Cambridge University Press.

Johnson, W. B., Barnett, J. E., Elman, N. S., Forrest, L., & Kaslow, N. J. (2012). The competent community: Toward a vital reformulation of professional ethics. *American Psychologist, 67,* 557–569. doi:10.1037/a0027206

Johnson, W. B., Barnett, J. E., Elman, N., Forrest, L., & Kaslow, N. (2013). The competence constellation: A developmental network model for psychologists. *Professional Psychology: Research and Practice, 44,* 343–354. doi:10.1037/a0033131

Johnson, W. B., Bertschinger, M., Snell, A. K., & Wilson, A. (2014). Secondary trauma and ethical obligations for military psychologists: Preserving compassion and competence in the crucible of combat. *Psychological Services, 11,* 68–74. doi:10.1037/a0033913

Johnson, W. B., Johnson, S. J., Sullivan, G. R., Bongar, B., Miller, L., & Sammons, M. T. (2011). Psychology in extremis: Preventing problems of professional competence in dangerous practice settings. *Professional Psychology: Research and Practice, 42,* 94–104. doi:10.1037/a0022365

Johnson, W. B., & Kennedy, C. H. (2010). Preparing psychologists for high-risk jobs: Key ethical considerations for military clinical supervisors. *Professional Psychology: Research and Practice, 41,* 298–304. doi:10.1037/a0019899

Johnson, W. B., Skinner, C. J., & Kaslow, N. J. (2014). Relational mentoring in clinical supervision: The transformational supervisor. *Journal of Clinical Psychology: In Session, 70,* 1073–1081. doi:10.1002/jclp.2014.70.issue-11

Kennedy, C. H., & Johnson, W. B. (2009). Mixed agency in military psychology: Applying the American Psychological Association ethics code. *Psychological Services, 6,* 22–31. doi:10.1037/a0014602

Kok, B. C., Herrell, R. K., Grossman, S. H., West, J. C., & Wilk, J. E. (2016). Prevalence of professional burnout among military mental health service providers. *Psychiatric Services, 67,* 137–140. doi:10.1176/appi.ps.201400430

Kolditz, T. A. (2007). Leading as if your life depended on it. In D. Crandall (Ed.), *Leadership lessons from West Point* (pp. 160–187). New York, NY: Wiley.

Kraft, H. S. (2007). *Rule number two: Lessons I learned in a combat hospital.* New York, NY: Little Brown.

Larner, B., & Blow, A. (2011). A model of meaning-making coping and growth in combat veterans. *Review of General Psychology, 15,* 187–197. doi:10.1037/a0024810

Leary, M. R., Tate, E. B., Adams, C. E., Allen, A. B., & Hancock, J. (2007). Self-compassion and reactions to unpleasant self-relevant events: The implications of treating oneself kindly. *Journal of Personality and Social Psychology, 92,* 887–904. doi:10.1037/0022-3514.92.5.887

Linnerooth, P. J., Mrdjenovich, A. J., & Moore, B. A. (2011). Professional burnout in clinical military psychologists: Recommendations before, during, and after deployment. *Professional Psychology: Research and Practice, 42,* 87–93. doi:10.1037/a0022295

Maslach, C., & Leiter, M. P. (2008). Early predictors of job burnout and engagement. *Journal of Applied Psychology, 93,* 498–512. doi:10.1037/0021-9010.93.3.498

McLean, C. P., Handa, S., Dickstein, B. D., Benson, T. A., Baker, M. T., Isler, W. C.,… Litz, B. T. (2011). Posttraumatic growth and posttraumatic stress among military medical personnel. *Psychological Trauma: Theory, Research, Practice, and Policy, 5,* 62–68. doi:10.1037/a0022949

Moore, B. A., & Reger, G. M. (2006). Clinician as frontline soldier: A look at the roles and challenges of Army clinical psychologists in Iraq. *Journal of Clinical Psychology, 62,* 395–403. doi:10.1002/jclp.20218

Pearlman, L. A., & Saakvitne, K. W. (1995). *Trauma and the therapist: Countertransference and vicarious traumatization in psychotherapy with incest survivors.* New York, NY: W. W. Norton.

Post, S. L. (1980). Origins, elements, and functions of therapeutic empathy. *The International Journal of Psychoanalysis, 61,* 277–293.

Regehr, C., Goldberg, G., & Hughes, J. (2002). Exposure to human tragedy, empathy, and trauma in ambulance paramedics. *American Journal of Orthopsychiatry, 72,* 505–513. doi:10.1037/0002-9432.72.4.505

Sarnat, J. E. (2015). *Supervision essentials for psychodynamic psychotherapies.* Washington, DC: American Psychological Association.

Schamess, G. (2006). Transference enactments in clinical supervision. *Clinical Social Work Journal, 34,* 407–425. doi:10.1007/s10615-005-0036-y

Searles, H. F. (1955). The informational value of the supervisor's emotional experience. *Psychiatry, 18,* 135–146. doi:10.1080/00332747.1955.11023001

Shallcross, R. L., Johnson, W. B., & Lincoln, S. H. (2010). Supervision. In J. Thomas & M. Herson (Eds.), *Handbook of clinical psychology competencies* (pp. 501–548). New York, NY: Springer-Verlag.

Shapiro, S. L., Brown, K. W., & Biegel, G. M. (2007). Teaching self-care to caregivers: Effects of mindfulness-based stress reduction on the mental health of therapists in training. *Training and Education in Professional Psychology, 1,* 105–115. doi:10.1037/1931-3918.1.2.105

Sherman, M. D., & Thelen, R. E. (1998). Distress and professional impairment among psychologists in clinical practice. *Professional Psychology: Research and Practice, 29,* 79–85. doi:10.1037/0735-7028.29.1.79

Smith, P. L., & Moss, S. B. (2009). Psychologist impairment: What is it, how can it be prevented, and what can be done to address it? *Clinical Psychology: Science and Practice, 16,* 1–15.

Sundin, J., Herrell, R. K., Hoge, C. W., Fear, N. T., Adler, A. B., Greenberg, N.,… Blies, P. D. (2014). Mental health outcomes in U.S. and U.K. military personnel returning from Iraq. *British Journal of Psychiatry, 113,* 1–8.

Thomas, J. L., Wilk, J. E., Riviere, L. A., McGurk, D., Castro, C. A., & Hoge, C. W. (2010). Prevalence of mental health problems and functional impairment among active component and national guard soldiers 3 and 12 months following combat in Iraq. *Archives of General Psychiatry, 67,* 614–623. doi:10.1001/archgenpsychiatry.2010.54

The intersection of identities in supervision for trauma-informed practice: Challenges and strategies

Roni Berger, Laura Quiros, and Jamie R. Benavidez-Hatzis, LCSW

ABSTRACT

This article discusses and illustrates the role and impact of the intersection of supervisors' and supervisees' social identities and the associated power and privilege within the context of supervision for trauma-informed practice. Based on current theoretical, empirical, and practice literature, challenges related to the supervisor's and supervisee's racial, ethnicity, gender, social class, and additional social affiliations are identified, as are strategies for addressing them within supervision for trauma-informed practice. A case example drawn from the authors' experiences illustrates the importance of attending to intersectionality in trauma-informed supervision Suggestions for future research efforts are offered.

In this article, we focus on the intersection of identities in the context of supervision for trauma-informed practice. The idea that one's identities impact one's professional relationships and functioning in general, and the supervisory relationship in particular, is not new. For example, Falender, Shafranske, and Falicov (2014) identified race-related attitudes, values, and awareness as critical in clinical supervision, and emphasized the importance of attending to interpersonal dynamics and the invisibility of guilt, shame, and internalized racism. It has been argued that supervision involves three individuals (supervisor, supervisee, and client) and that the inner worlds of each (i.e., their identities) shape the supervisory process and outcomes (Watkins, 2011; Werbart, 2007).

Although supervision for trauma-informed practice shares with all types and fields of supervision issues related to the intersection of the identities of supervisor and supervisee, it also presents challenges that are unique to its specific foci and content. To date, scholars have addressed individually diverse aspects of the intersection of identities (Hernandez & McDowell, 2010; Pfohl, 2004; Watts-Jones, 2010) and of supervision both in general and for trauma-informed practice in particular (Berger & Quiros, 2014, 2016). However, issues of this intersection within the unique context of supervision for trauma-informed practice have not been addressed.

This article is designed to attend to this gap in the literature. Based on the limited available knowledge and on our practice experience, we focus on trauma-informed supervision with attention to intersectionality. We begin with brief reviews of current knowledge about the intersection of identities and about supervision for trauma-informed practice, followed by a discussion and illustration via a case example of the nature, manifestation, and possible outcomes of intersection of the racial and ethnic, gender, sexual orientation, and other identities of the supervisor and supervisee in supervisory interactions for trauma-informed practice and strategies for effectively addressing identified issues. We conclude with directions for future research.

The intersection of identities

The intersection of identities is built on the view of identity as a complex, multifaceted, and fluid concept, and the understanding that one has simultaneously multiple identities based on one's affiliations with social groups according to gender, race, social class, ethnicity, nationality, sexual orientation, age, religion, and the like (Crenshaw, 1991). Each social identity carries with it labels and stereotypical views about the groups of which individuals perceive themselves as members (Phenice & Griffore, 2000). Through a comparison between the image of one's own and other groups, individuals become aware of the social perception of their own groups, are given labels and social attributes based on this membership, and internalize the social perceptions of these groups. These socially constructed identities mutually constitute, reinforce, and normalize one another. Depending on the power and privilege associated with them, one's identities can have both negative and positive effects, creating both oppression and opportunity for the individual (Warner & Shields, 2013).

The nature, dynamics, and outcomes of the intersection of one's identities have been studied in diverse cultural contexts. For example, Mensah (2014) studied the polymorphous, constructed, and fluid identity and its formation in African immigrants to Canada to develop a nuanced understanding of this population group that had been previously viewed through a homogenizing lens. Dancy and Jean-Marie (2014) studied the intersection of Blackness and smartness in African-American third-grade girls and the role it played in their learning mathematics. Burnes and Singh (2016) studied the intersection of gay, lesbian, bisexual, transgender, queer, and questioning (GLBTQ) identity and social class.

One's different identities are constructed and negotiated in the context of interpersonal relationships within the different sociocultural worlds with which one is affiliated (Jones, 2009). These identities may advantage or marginalize individuals and may be associated with inequality and limited access to economic, political, and social power (Phenice & Griffore, 2000). Each social interaction involves an encounter among the diverse identities of the "players" and the internalized social perception of their groups of membership (Galliher & Kerpelman, 2012; Warner & Shields, 2013).

As in all interpersonal exchanges, the intersection of the personal and professional identities of supervisor and supervisee plays a role in their interaction. Specifically, relevant to the intersection identities in supervision are differences in power and privilege associated with supervisor's and supervisee's *role* and *social affiliations.*

Role-related differences

Supervision is not egalitarian. Role-related structural power is intrinsic to the supervisory relationship, where disproportionate social power is accorded to the supervisor (Jernigan, Green, Helms, Perez-Gualdron, & Henze, 2010), who has the authority to put demands, allocate clients and tasks, and pass judgment on the supervisee's performance (Hewson, 1999). This power organizes and orchestrates social interactions, which in turn shape ideas, values, assumptions, and beliefs about the other (Beddoe, 2010; Kanter, 1993). Two types of structural power have been conceptualized (Nye, 2004). "Hard power" is coercive in nature and is the ability to influence behavior through physical, economic, and political force. It includes "carrots," such as a promise of economic gain through a possible job offer. "Soft power" operates through the creation of hierarchies within the professions. The presence of hard power reinforces these hierarchies by threat of loss of privilege, status, and economic gain, and by coercing actors back into predetermined behaviors, attitudes, and thought processes that reinforce privileged values and discourses. The use of power in supervision is reinforced through education, training, the media, social discourse, and consumerism. Exercising structural power in supervision may be manifested when the supervisee accepts without question the views, opinions, and ideas of the supervisor. In turn, this may be reflected in a parallel process whereby the client acquiesces to the views and observations of the supervisee in their work together (Deering, 1994).

Social affiliation-related differences

Supervisors' and supervisees' sociodemographic characteristics, including age, spiritual/religious affiliation, socioeconomic and immigration status, race, ethnicity, gender, and sexual orientation, affect their power. Supervision that involves supervisors with privileged identities and supervisees from traditionally marginalized social groups is particularly vulnerable to power dynamics that mirror power dominance in society at large, although power issues may also be apparent in supervisory dyads in which the individuals appear to be similar but hold different social identities (Jernigan et al., 2010).

The role and personal social affiliation positions may agree, such as when a supervisor enjoys power due to gender, race, and socioeconomic status. Thus, a Black female supervisee may be at the intersection of mutually exacerbating multiple marginalized social identities due to her gender and racial affiliation and her role in the supervisory relationship. However, role-related and personal identities of supervisor and supervisee may not be consistent with power relationships that exist in society, such as a female lesbian Latina supervisor supervising a straight older man. The importance of intersection of social identities in supervision was supported by a recent study that showed an association between an open discussion in supervision of supervisor's and supervisee's gender, race/ ethnicity, and sexual orientation and the quality of the working relationships, choice of interventions, and self-efficacy in trainees and interns in the helping professions (Phillips, Parent, Dozier, & Jackson, 2017).

Supervision for trauma-informed practice

As the number of clients who experience trauma following the exposure to natural or human-made stressors grows, so does the need for practitioners trained in trauma-informed practice. Trauma-informed practice means that practitioners working in settings which are likely to serve clients with histories of trauma, such as services related to addictions, mental health, child welfare, and corrections, remain sensitive to the possibility that, regardless of the presenting problem, their clients could have a history of trauma which may affect their current issues (Knight, 2015). Core principles of trauma-informed practice include understanding and recognition of trauma as both interpersonal and sociopolitical (Berger & Quiros, 2016) and "normalizing and validating clients' feelings and experiences; assisting them in understanding the past and its emotional impact; empowering survivors to better manage their current lives; and helping them understand current challenges in light of the past victimization" (Knight, 2015, p. 28).

To help supervisees become skilled at providing trauma-informed services, supervisors seek to enhance the supervisee's understanding of the complexity, dynamics, and potential behavioral manifestations of trauma and aptitudes in addressing them (Berger & Quiros, 2016). Specifically, practitioners should be trained in fostering trustworthiness, empowerment, choice, collaboration, and safety in their interactions with clients and in the culture of the agencies where they practice (Harris & Fallot, 2001). Researchers have found that supervision focusing on trauma was positively associated with better outcomes for clients and practitioners in various fields of practice (Bober & Regehr, 2006; Bussey, 2008; Hansel et al., 2011; Joubert, Hocking, & Hampson, 2013; Kitchiner, Phillips, Neil, & Bisson, 2007; Pack, 2014).

In addition to core elements and strategies of all supervision, supervision for trauma-informed practice also has unique aspects. Trauma-informed supervision combines knowledge about trauma and about supervision, focusing on the characteristics of the interrelationships among the trauma, the practitioner, the helping relationship, and the context in which the work is done (Etherington, 2009). Specifically, parallel to creating an environment that is safe and feels safe for clients, trauma-informed supervision requires creating a physical and interpersonal supervisory environment that feels safe for the supervisee, as this will enhance the outcomes for the supervisee and the client (Toren, 2008). Supervision should reflect a nonjudgmental, accepting, predictable strong working alliance between supervisor and supervisee built on trust and clear boundaries and expectations (Berger & Quiros, 2014, 2016). Although these elements are beneficial in all supervisory relationships, they are critical in supervision for trauma-informed practice because of their central role in providing trauma-informed services (Harris & Fallot, 2001). Supervision that emphasizes these elements enhances practitioners' skills for trauma-informed practice as it models to the practitioners, in the context of the supervisee-supervisor relationships, principles that can be emulated in the practitioner-client relationships in a parallel process. By participating in a supervisory process that emphasizes these elements, the supervisee learns experientially what their meaning and effects are and how they can be achieved.

To enhance the feeling of safety, it is critical that the supervisor foster a strong supervisory working alliance, assess the supervisees' vulnerabilities and resilience relative to trauma content, emphasize the importance of self-care, assign a trauma-related caseload that is balanced in severity, number, and types of clients' trauma, as well as take into account supervisees' length of professional experience and history of personal trauma. As issues of power (or lack thereof), independence, choice, trust, and control are key elements of trauma and trauma work, supervisees need to feel that their ideas matter, their preferences are honored, and power is shared, such that decisions are made collaboratively rather than dictated unilaterally.

In a recent study (Berger & Quiros, 2016), supervisors who provide trauma-informed supervision identified that effective trauma-informed supervision is shaped by *personal* and *professional* characteristics of the supervisor and of the supervisee, and characteristics of the *supervisory relationship. Personal* characteristics of the supervisee included cultural orientation and identity, training, history in the agency and in supervision, theoretical approach, perceptions of challenges and support, skills, personal traumatic experiences, indirect trauma, and clinical skills. Characteristics of supervisors identified as important were their formal training and practice experience in general and in trauma work in particular; commitment to an expansive definition of trauma, including sociopolitical trauma; familiarity with trauma-related practice models and advocating for the application of these models; willingness to challenge within the agency notions that were not trauma-informed; and personal characteristics of modesty, cultural humility, and acknowledgment of own limitations.

Supervisory relationships viewed as effective for trauma-informed supervision included frequent and consistent supervisory meetings and a strong emphasis on a compassionate, caring, and supportive supervisory style. On the organizational level, it was suggested that both clinical and administrative supervision encourage supervisees to feel comfortable to discuss their clinical issues and concerns, uninhibited by logistic considerations and fear of judgment, and models that emphasize relational aspects of the therapeutic alliance be used. Teamwork and supervision for all (clinical and other) staff involved in providing services to traumatized clients were recommended.

Challenges and strategies related to intersection of identities in supervision for trauma-informed practice

In supervision for trauma-informed practice, issues related to status, power, predictability, safety, vulnerability, and control that are at the essence of the experience of traumatized clients and trauma-informed practice correspond with the status and power aspects of the supervisory relationships. These issues impact how supervisors and supervisees define trauma, view its etiology, and assign meaning to it, particularly as it relates to social conditions of poverty, racism, homophobia, antisemitism, sexism, and ableism, what they see as appropriate manifestations of trauma reactions, coping strategies that they deem effective, and interventions that they endorse (Berger, 2015). Consequently, challenges to the supervisor and the supervisee exist requiring strategies to address them.

Challenges

Supervisors' and supervisees' racial, cultural, gender, sexual orientation, class, and other social affiliations may constrain authenticity in the supervisory relationship. Research has shown that non-White supervisees reported negative experiences when supervisors did not include a discussion of racial issues in supervision (Jernigan et al., 2010). Similarity and differences in social location in terms of gender, social class, immigration status, sexual orientation, race, and ethnicity of the parties in the supervisory dyad may impact how free the supervisee feels to ask questions and how free the supervisor feels to offer feedback. Will a Black supervisee feel safe asking a White supervisor questions without fear of being judged as unknowledgeable and thus confirming biases? Will a White supervisor hesitate to challenge a Black supervisee for fear of being viewed as politically incorrect or racist? Constantine and Sue (2007) found that Black clinicians supervised by White supervisors reported feeling invalidated in supervision due to a lack of awareness of racial and cultural issues. Manifestations of the absence of awareness were primarily focusing on supervisees' clinical weaknesses, blaming clients of color for problems that reflected oppression, offering culturally insensitive treatment recommendations, making stereotypical assumptions about Black clients and Black supervisees, and avoiding negative feedback for fear of being viewed as racist. The same may potentially apply to other social statuses such as gender, sexual orientation, disability, and social status.

Discrepancies may exist between one's own identity and society's perception of it and shape how individuals perceive and process discrimination. A dark-skinned, self-identified Latina may be treated as African-American and experience rejection from other Latinas because of her dark skin. A self-identified third-generation Holocaust survivor may be viewed by others primarily or solely as White. When this individual encounters an African-American supervisor whose self-identity reflects a history of lynching, slavery, and racial discrimination, unspoken content regarding trauma, which is shaped by these self-identities, may play out in subtle and not-so-subtle ways in their supervisory discussions.

Supervisees' social positions may affect their ability to contain, refrain from judgment, and listen to clients' painful stories for long periods and understand the complexity of the stories. They also may feel rejected and frustrated by clients' reluctance to share details of their experience, leading to losing confidence in their abilities. Consequently, supervisees may avoid discussing in supervision detailed reports about clients' traumatic experiences and their own reactions to these stories. The situation may become especially challenging for supervisees with unaddressed histories of personal trauma, in that the feeling of powerlessness in their role as practitioners may reactivate their sense of powerlessness when they were traumatized and compromise their professional competence.

Strategies

Effective strategies in addressing challenges that stem from the interplay of trauma work and intersectionality are those that empower supervisees, attend to relational components in supervisory interactions, create a feeling of emotional and physical safety and support, address parallel process, emphasize knowledge, and advocate self-care. Such strategies are *self-exploration, an ongoing open dialogue, flattening the power pyramid, creating relational safety,* and *sharing contemporary trauma knowledge.*

Self-exploration

Research and practice experience suggest that the dynamics and outcomes of the supervisory relationship are shaped by the social identities of the supervisor and the supervisee (Estrada, Frame, & Williams, 2004). Specifically, relative to trauma work, because social affiliations affect how practitioners view and approach trauma and traumatized clients (Berger, 2015; Quiros & Berger, 2015), it is of utmost importance to explore the supervisee's and supervisor's social identities and their related positions of privilege and oppression. For example, growing up in poverty may lead a practitioner to be less empathic to stress related to economic losses of a middle-class client. To help develop critical consciousness early on and throughout the supervisory relationship, it is useful to employ reflective questioning, in which both supervisee and supervisor search their own experience to recognize and challenge oppressive and dehumanizing political, economic, and social systems and their impact on their perspectives (Garcia, Kosutic, McDowell, & Anderson, 2009).

Contemporary American society privileges Whiteness, European-American culture, heterosexuality, middle- and upper-income status, maleness, U.S.-born citizenship, able-ness, and the English language. These identities enhance formal and implied opportunities in education, employment, and social organizations (Hernandez & McDowell, 2010). To create a context that respects diverse identities within the supervisory relationship, it is essential to examine if and how these privileged statuses and associated power or lack thereof are replicated in supervision. Such exploration of the supervisor's and supervisee's experiences with traumatized people of different social affiliations, preconceptions, beliefs, and values can clarify what the supervisee and supervisor bring to the supervisory relationships and how supervision may be affected. For example, do the supervisor and supervisee come from cultural groups with different legacies of trauma, such as the collective historical trauma of the Holocaust for a Jewish supervisee and the collective historical trauma of slavery for an African-American supervisor? Within same-race triads such as Black supervisor, supervisee, and client, do supervisor and supervisee share similar cultural identities (Jernigan et al., 2010)?

The examination of social identities helps in unveiling structural and relational power within the supervisory relationships as well as the supervisor's and supervisee's approach to clients' trauma, raising awareness of their own identity in interaction with the identities of others and enhancing the effectiveness of service to clients. The omission of discussing intersecting identities and the relationship to power may create problems both in the supervision and in practice (Mitchell, 2016). If intersecting identities of a supervisor and a supervisee and their relationship to power are not discussed in supervision, a supervisee who feels in a less powerful position may refrain from authentically conveying and employing with clients his or her own knowledge of and reaction to trauma, and substitute it by automatically adopting the supervisor's perspective. For example, how do references to the Holocaust by a Jewish supervisor and the legacy of slavery and current

Black Lives Matter ideology by a Black supervisee impact their perceptions of and approach to each other and to clients?

The discussion of intersection of identities becomes particularly relevant when supervisors' and supervisees' social identities differ and when clients share the supervisees' social affiliations. For example, a non-White female supervisor must question whether she views a White male supervisee as a representation of traditional oppressors and their current professional positions as a reversal of traditional gender- and race-based relationships, and if the supervisory process and outcomes for clients are affected. A White supervisor must examine if her assumptions about inferiority of non-Whites plays a role in the critique of the performance of a non-White supervisee. Such self-exploration can enhance the parties' ability to model meaningful relationships with people from all social groups and provide appropriate intervention strategies, as well as allow engagement in efforts to eradicate social and political manifestations of racism and oppression (Jernigan et al., 2010). Rather than a one-time event, a discussion of supervisor's and supervisee's social identities and their role in supervision must be part of an ongoing conversation. For example, a supervisor implementing routinely in discussions of clients a question how (not if) supervisee's and client's similarity or difference in social affiliation affects their interaction and how the supervisee intends to raise the question with the client, educates the supervisee of the importance of the issue.

Ongoing open dialogue

Self-exploration requires an open dialogue between supervisor and supervisee about effects on their trauma work of their respective identities, and associated structural power and social and cultural capital. Hernandez and Rankin (2008) advocated

> the co-construction of a dialogical context in which students and supervisees are able to raise questions, challenge points of view, ponder issues, confront opinions, articulate ideas, and express concerns. For those whose identities have been silenced by a lack of structural (material condition) or discursive (social discourses) privilege, this kind of dialogical context makes it possible to speak and consider the impact of what we do and say on others,(p. 33)

It is the responsibility of the supervisor to identify opportunities for this dialogue. To allow the dialogue, supervisors must attend to the relational aspect of the supervisory relationship by discussing issues that bother supervisees in their own life and their experience relative to sessions with clients, while refraining from being intrusive or turning supervision into therapy. Important in the dialogue is discussing countertransference content and parallel processes in the supervisor-supervisee and supervisee-client relationships.

Specific to trauma-informed supervision, the dialogue should adopt a sociopolitical lens to recognize supervisor's and supervisee's exposure to traumatic circumstances due to their social affiliations and the social identities associated with them, and examine how these play a role in their supervisory interaction. Supervisors should initiate an exploration of supervisees' trauma reactions to their own exposure to traumatic events, and to their indirect exposure by intensive work with traumatized clients, to allow the supervisee to gain in-depth understanding of what the client may feel. Supervisors' reactions to the report of supervisees' traumatic exposure may model for supervisees how to respond to their traumatized clients. For example, a supervisee with a trauma experience may report stress, nightmares, and diminished ability to enjoy activities he previously liked, symptoms suggesting the possibility of secondary traumatization. The supervisor can use principles of cognitive processing regarding the supervisee's experience (Berger, 2015) and discuss how the supervisee can apply the same to working with a client.

Flattening the power pyramid

Transparency, negotiation, and maximizing supervisee autonomy within the constraints of external requirements can minimize negative effects of structural power in supervision (Hewson, 1999). To facilitate growth for both and enhance supervisees' competence to establish an egalitarian, empowering relationship with clients, the supervisor should convey that none has exclusive ownership of knowledge, and create opportunities for supervisees to share their knowledge and experience, empowering supervisees to take the supervisor's knowledge as falsifiable and plausible. Rather than a unidirectional top-down approach, understanding of the client situation and developing an appropriate intervention plan should be conducted jointly and collaboratively between supervisor and supervisee. Structural and administrative conditions that augment supervisees' feelings of safety and triggers for feeling unsafe should be identified and minimized (Berger & Quiros, 2016). The mutuality of the process has special importance in the context of trauma-informed supervision because issues of power are central in trauma work (Afuape, 2012). A major element in traumatic experiences is the loss of control and being victim to external power, whether this is a result of interpersonal victimization or a human-induced or natural disaster (Foster & Hagedorn, 2014). Realizing one's own powerlessness can evoke fear, vulnerability, and anxiety. Participation in supervision where supervisees feel respected, validated, and empowered helps improve their ability to create the same with traumatized clients who are also struggling with the feeling of powerlessness. This is especially important when the supervisee is affiliated with minority groups affected by sociopolitical traumatic circumstances (e.g.,

GLBTQ, has a disability), as the power relationship in supervision may feel like a replication of power relationships in society (Quiros & Berger, 2015).

A collaborative process can be enhanced by encouraging supervisees to initiate agenda items and their self-identified preferences, acknowledging their ideas and knowledge, and supporting their professional development plan and working styles. Reflective supervision, a collaborative supervisory model arising largely from the field of early childhood mental health, offers a tool for flattening the power pyramid and has been advocated as effective in trauma-informed practice (Eggbeer, Shahmoon-Shanok, & Clark, 2010; Geller & Foley, 2009; Shahmoon-Shanok, 2006).

Efforts to understand and address issues of power in trauma-informed supervision is critical throughout the process, and needs to be adjusted with the shifting nature of power at different points. At the start of the supervisory relationship, experience and knowledge allow the supervisor to occupy a position of power. As the supervisee grows in knowledge and experience, this power differential shifts. Supervisors should be aware that they may feel discomfort as supervisees become more secure and may challenge the supervisory authority, and take deliberate actions to address their discomfort, such as discussing with the supervisee the impact of the changes in power differential and seeking peer consultation from other supervisors.

Creating relational safety

Supervisees who feel safe in the relationship with the supervisor are better equipped to identify their own trauma-related triggers, develop strategies for addressing their trauma reactions, and enhance their ability to provide effective services to traumatized clients (Berger & Quiros, 2016). A supervisee who shares a client's traumatic experience may try to avoid discussing the experience because it reignites painful memories and reactivates the practitioner's own trauma reactions. Practitioners might also assume that coping skills that helped them heal may be equally appropriate for a client. Safe space in supervision does not mean absence of conflict, nor is it a permanent state. Rather, allowing conflict to occur and be processed has the potential to enhance trust and openness (Beddoe, 2010), sharing, exploring, and attending to personal traumatic experiences of supervisees, as these affect their professional performance and approach to traumatized clients.

Sharing contemporary trauma knowledge

Both supervisor and supervisee bring to supervision their trauma-related knowledge. The supervisor typically brings familiarity with theories and empirical knowledge about trauma in diverse cultural contexts, and expertise in application of diverse practice models to serving traumatized clients. The supervisee may bring basic knowledge about trauma acquired in professional education, continuing education training, and possibly previous and current practice experiences. Both may also have access to tacit knowledge based on their personal affiliations and history. The supervisory relationship becomes an arena for the mutual sharing of expertise, knowledge, and experiences to enhance the provision of the best services to traumatized clients. It is the responsibility of the supervisor to seek ongoing training and remain informed about trauma research and practice. Sharing knowledge about social stress and trauma that are related to living circumstances such as residing in a poor neighborhood (Wadsworth et al., 2013) and understanding trauma from a sociopolitical lens (Quiros & Berger, 2015) are especially important when the client, supervisor, and/or supervisee are affiliated with groups that differ in their sociocultural background and status.

It is particularly important for supervisors to share with supervisees knowledge about symptoms of indirect trauma, including over-involvement with clients and excessive preoccupation with their issues, and withdrawal from the relationships with the client, with the supervisor, or from other interpersonal connections (Bledsoe, 2012; Pearlman & Saakvitne, 1995). It is also important to make supervisees aware of how their own social affiliations may impact on these symptoms and guide them in employing strategies for self-care. It is imperative that supervisors be deliberately aware of their own tendencies to become a rescuer of supervisees and develop a sense of grandiosity, just like the supervisee tries to do for the client.

Strategies for self-care advocated by supervisors may include managing workload by pacing and sequencing clients (e.g., avoid "crowding" all severely traumatized clients in one day), taking breaks for respite, and using cognitive strategies to separate work from personal life (not to "take home" one's clients and to "tune out" work-related thoughts). Researchers have found that even practitioners aware of the usefulness of evidence-supported strategies for self-care failed to engage in self-care activities (Bober & Regehr, 2006), suggesting the supervisors' critical role in enhancing the translation of knowledge about self-care into action.

Case illustration

The third author trained in an agency serving clients with traumatic experiences, concrete needs for housing, employment, and financial assistance, and often substance-related problems. Practitioners were social workers, psychologists, and mental health counselors, with a slightly larger number of males than females. The agency used a psychiatry-grounded biomedical trauma conceptualization, emphasized intrapsychic-focused interventions, and viewed exposure protocol as necessary for traumatized clients' recovery. An inherent unstated perception was that trainees in psychology were better suited for working with trauma survivors and the dominant view was that "good teaching cases," desired by all trainees, were individuals with a specific traumatic experience (e.g., accident, a death of a loved one, or a rape). Being assigned such clients offered the benefits of supervision by a renowned American White male trauma expert and better prospects for continued training, securing a full-time job, and gaining social and professional recognition. The view of a supervisor as "the best" reflects the dominant epistemology of power holders, often with limited input from supervisees and clients on whom structural power is exerted, and is a product of a socially constructed process of negotiating a hierarchical system of the stratification of the professional ladder.

The author, a novice Latina social worker, was assigned a 41-year-old Black/Latina client diagnosed with posttraumatic stress disorder (PTSD) following a history of multiple traumatic experiences. After 18 months of work with the client, focusing on creating safety and stabilization, she became the first client with whom the worker was to independently utilize an exposure protocol (Foa, Keane, Friedman, & Cohen, 2009). The worker began to self-doubt: Was the client ready for the exposure process or had she agreed to it to please the worker? Would the client go through the motions rather than experience a genuine therapeutic change? Was the worker projecting onto the client her own uncertainty about her readiness to effectively guide the client through an exposure treatment?

The worker took her concerns to the well-known supervisor, who responded by asking how long she intended to allow her own lack of confidence to cause the client to suffer from PTSD symptoms. While stunned by the supervisor's response (was she really hurting the client by "allowing her to suffer"?), it never occurred to the worker to question the supervisor's reaction. This interaction created a relational rupture between the supervisor and the worker, leaving her concerns about her own performance and feelings of responsibility for the client unexplored in supervision. Unlike previously, the client began to miss appointments, further delaying the opportunity to use the exposure protocol for addressing her trauma. The worker acknowledged to herself that she had been trying to avoid the supervisor (like the client avoided her). To preserve future training and employment opportunities, she decided to ignore the supervisor's attributing to her the responsibility for the client's suffering and discuss the "safer" topic of the client's missed appointments. The supervisor inquired if the worker had been avoiding him.

His question opened the door for an exploration of issues previously left unaddressed in supervision, such as whether the client's statement that "being Black, Latina, and a woman, hell, I am not even considered a human being," and her new behavior of missing appointments might be related to the worker's concern that the client was performing for her. Given her position on the intersection of being Latina, Black, and a woman, and her trauma history, the client experienced limited self-agency and diminished feelings of self-worth. These feelings were augmented by her family's expectation that, to avoid embarrassing them, she "be a good daughter," return to her assaultive husband, and be a "good wife," submitting to his sexual demands, irrespective of how degrading or painful to her.

The worker had discussed using exposure therapy with her client; however, she did not address with the client nor the supervisor the possibility that the discussion might induce in the client fear, a sense of loss of control, and worries about being retraumatized. The worker also worried that the client had agreed to the treatment protocol because she had to be a "good patient" like she was expected to be a "good wife." The worker's interpretation of her client's missing appointments as an attempt to restore agency and regain control was lauded by the supervisor, who inquired why it was not brought up previously. The worker related her hesitation and the accompanying feelings of a loss of control and anger to the supervisor's implying that she was responsible for the client's continued suffering, which led to her questioning her own competence. She further discussed feeling stuck by the supervisor's statement that women clinicians, more than their male counterparts, hesitate to implement exposure treatments and are more likely to "collude" with their clients, particularly around treatments pertaining to sexual assault. She questioned discussing her client's suspected superficial agreement with a supervisor who believed that women practitioners and clients colluded to avoid certain topics. Did her feeling of being stuck indeed indicate that she was colluding with her client?

To get herself unstuck and resolve the discrepancy between the supervisor's statements, fear of his disappointment in her, and her own beliefs and experience with the client, the worker chose to examine an alternate interpretation. Might the collusion represent a symbolic refusal both by the client (to treatment) and by herself (to learning what the supervisor tried to teach her)? Although both client and worker had been historically highly motivated, the client began to feel pressured by expectations to agree to the treatment; the worker began to feel the same about supervision. Consequently, each sought to regain control of their participation in the respective processes. These struggles were manifested in the client's ambivalence about the protocol and missed appointments, and in the worker's hesitation to follow the supervisor's explicit and the agency's implicit expectations that she begin the protocol. This situation illustrates the parallel process when worker and client are "trapped" in a powerless position in an encounter with an "other" whose social positioning renders authority and control.

The worker further questioned whether the supervisor's reaction attributing the client's suffering to the worker's hesitation may have been a response to her symbolic refusal of his authority. The supervisor expressed appreciation for the suggested interpretation, opening the road to a dialogue about the client's prior experiences leading her to treatment, the interaction between the client and the worker, the worker's potential ambivalence about the protocol, and her experience in supervision and in the agency's milieu. The worker and her supervisor discussed the opposite-sex dynamic between them and its potential contribution to their impasse. By incorporating the worker's input to understanding of the situation, the supervisor made a space that felt safer for her and reinforced her ability to choose how to proceed. This interaction illustrates how gender and role position may shape the supervisory relationships and its impact on the work with the traumatized client.

This case example illustrates how the identities of the individuals involved and the associated structural power shaped the dynamics of the supervisory process and its outcomes. Soft power was exercised by the supervisor and the agency through unilaterally imposing a biomedical conceptualization of trauma, creating a perception of what constituted a "good case." The supervisee internalized this perception of power, which led her to refrain from questioning the supervisor's authority and expertise, and forestalled a reasoned and thorough examination of the various factors impacting the client and her treatment. The supervisory relationships and the culture of the agency left no room for a critical discussion in supervision of the respective identities of supervisor and supervisee and of the assumption that the supervisor's assessments, which were reflected in the declarative nature of his statements, were not to be questioned because he occupied a privileged position due to his gender, race, experience, and reputation.

Consequently, a dissonance developed between the privileged epistemology represented by the supervisor and the supervisee's experience of herself and her client. The worker's resisting the supervisor and his supervision helped her assert some social power while simultaneously depriving her of getting the supervision she needed, potentially compromising the quality of her work with the client. Although the supervisee and her client shared a gender identity, though differed in race and professional standing, the supervisee and her supervisor differed in ethnicity, gender, professional authority, and organizational status in the agency, all of which impacted on the nature of the supervisory interaction. The case further illustrates a parallel process related to social positions. The supervisor's reactions reinforced the practitioner's self-doubt, anxiety, and feelings of loss of control. She, in turn, prompted these same reactions in her therapeutic encounters with her client, who complied with the supervisee's intent to utilize exposure therapy without questioning this decision.

Although the role of race was not readily apparent at the time of the interactions described in the case illustration, it became clear years later when the worker was in a supervisory role herself. She had a Black supervisee who was providing services to a Black teenager whose mother had kicked her out of her home numerous times and fled the country when she learned that Child Protective Services had been contacted. The client was placed temporarily in a foster home and expressed a desire to go back to live with her mother, who had since returned to the United States. In supervision, the supervisee advocated for an aftercare plan, involving returning the client to her mother's care, consistent with the young woman's wishes despite the concern of both the supervisor and supervisee that the client might be struggling with complex trauma resulting from chronic abuse and neglect. The supervisor realized that she and the supervisee disagreed about the meaning the mother held for the client and decided to address this directly. The conversation revealed a culturally ingrained difference between the meaning assigned to family by the Latina supervisor, who applied a Western-European perspective, and the Black supervisee, whose frame of reference was shaped by the legacy of disruption of Black families by White slave-holders. The supervisor acknowledged that she may have been unintentionally using her position of structural power to impose a "White" perspective of the mother as an abuser and betrayer.

Implications for future research

In this article, we discussed and illustrated challenges and strategies related to the intersection of social identities of the supervisor and supervisee in supervision for trauma-informed practice. Future researchers should examine the suggested strategies in the context of training for trauma-informed practice. Specifically, there is need for more nuanced empirical knowledge about differential processes and outcomes of supervision for trauma-informed practice in the context of diverse combinations of supervisor and supervisee in terms of their social positions and experience as they impact their approach to traumatized clients. For example, how do the dynamics of supervisory power play out in supervision for trauma-informed practice when the supervisor is non-White and the supervisee is White? When both are non-Whites? When the supervisor is a male and supervisee female and vice versa? When a supervisor from a modest socioeconomic background supervises a supervisee who comes from economic privilege? When the supervisor has a disability and the supervisee is able-bodied? When the supervisor is an immigrant and the supervisee U.S.-born? When the supervisor is GLBTQ and the supervisee is not? When the supervisee is significantly older than the supervisor?

Researchers to date have addressed these and similar questions relative to supervisory relationships and outcomes in general (e.g., Burkard, Knox, Schultz, & Hess, 2009; Kadan, Roer-Strier, & Bekerman, 2017). However, the same is not true for supervision for trauma-informed practice. The question remains as to the unique nature of supervisory relationships and outcomes in the context of supervision in the specific field of trauma practice, which is particularly vulnerable to issues of power. The following example illustrates the importance of such research. The first author was a recent immigrant from Israel while supervising a group of social workers comprised of U.S.-born and educated professionals and recent immigrants from the former Soviet Union, all of whom worked with adolescent immigrants and their families. Both clients and non-U.S.-born workers had considerable immigration-related traumatic experiences. On a certain occasion, one of the Russian supervisees turned to the supervisor and said with a mix of astonishment and appreciation in his voice, "It is amazing. You are newer in this country than I am. Your accent is heavier than mine. And yet, the Americans accept you as a knowledgeable authority figure and listen to you. This is so empowering." Researchers can help us deconstruct the power dynamics involved in supervision for trauma-informed practice and develop and test effective strategies to provide better supervision.

References

Afuape, T. (2012). *Power, resistance and liberation in therapy with survivors of trauma: To have our hearts broken*. London, United Kingdom: Routledge.

Beddoe, L. (2010). Surveillance or reflection: Professional supervision in "the Risk Society". *British Journal of Social Work, 40*, 1279–1296. doi:10.1093/bjsw/bcq018

Berger, R. (2015). *Stress, trauma and posttraumatic growth: Social context, environment and identities*. New York, NY: Routledge.

Berger, R., & Quiros, L. (2014). Supervision for trauma informed practice. *Traumatology, 20*, 296–301. doi:10.1037/h0099835

Berger, R., & Quiros, L. (2016). Best practices for training trauma informed practitioners: Supervisors' voice. *Traumatology, 22*, 145–154. doi:10.1037/trm0000076

Bledsoe, D. E. (2012). Trauma and supervision. In L. L. Levers, S. R. Seem, & K. M. Fallon (Eds.), *Trauma counseling: Theories and interventions* (pp. 569–578). New York, NY: Springer.

Bober, T., & Regehr, C. (2006). Strategies for reducing secondary or vicarious trauma: Do they work? *Brief Treatment and Crisis Intervention, 6*, 1–9. doi:10.1093/brief-treatment/mhj001

Burkard, A. W., Knox, S., Schultz, J., & Hess, S. A. (2009). Lesbian, gay, and bisexual supervisees' experiences of LGB-affirmative and nonaffirmative supervision. *Journal of Counseling Psychology, 56*, 176–188. doi:10.1037/0022-0167.56.1.176

Burnes, T. R., & Singh, A. A. (2016). Gay in the bank, queer in the streets: The intersection of LGBTQQ and social class identities. *Journal of LGBT Issues in Counseling, 10*(1), 55–71. doi:10.1080/15538605.2015.1138096

Bussey, M. C. (2008). Trauma response and recovery certificate program: Preparing students for effective practice. *Journal of Teaching in Social Work, 28*, 117–144. doi:10.1080/08841230802179118

Constantine, M. G., & Sue, D. W. (2007). Perceptions of racial microaggressions among Black supervisees in cross-racial dyads. *Journal of Counseling Psychology, 54*, 142–153. doi:10.1037/0022-0167.54.2.142

Crenshaw, K. W. (1991). Mapping the margins: Intersectionality, identity politics, and violence against women of color. *Stanford Law Review, 43*, 1241–1299. doi:10.2307/1229039

Dancy, T. E., & Jean-Marie, G. (2014). Faculty of color in higher education: Exploring the intersections of identity, impostorship, and internalized racism. *Mentoring & Tutoring: Partnership in Learning, 22*, 354–372. doi:10.1080/13611267.2014.945736

Deering, C. G. (1994). Parallel process in the supervision of child psychotherapy. *American Journal of Psychotherapy, 48*, 102–110.

Eggbeer, L., Shahmoon-Shanok, R., & Clark, R. (2010). Reaching toward an evidence base for reflective supervision. *Zero to Three, 31*(2), 39–45.

Estrada, D., Frame, M. W., & Williams, C. B. (2004). Cross-cultural supervision: Guiding the conversation toward race and ethnicity. *Journal of Multicultural Counseling & Development, 3*, 307–319.

Etherington, K. (2009). Supervising helpers who work with the trauma of sexual abuse. *British Journal of Guidance & Counselling, 37*, 179–194. doi:10.1080/03069880902728622

Falender, C. A., Shafranske, E. P., & Falicov, C. J. (2014). *Multiculturalism and diversity in clinical supervision: A competency based approach.* Washington, DC: American Psychological Association.

Foa, E. B., Keane, T. M., Friedman, M. J., & Cohen, J. A. (2009). *Effective treatments for PTSD: Practice guidelines from the International Society for Traumatic Stress Studies.* New York, NY: Guilford.

Foster, J. M., & Hagedorn, W. B. (2014). A qualitative exploration of fear and safety with child victims of sexual abuse. *Journal of Mental Health Counseling, 36*, 243–262. doi:10.17744/mehc.36.3.0160307501879217

Galliher, R. V., & Kerpelman, J. L. (2012). The intersection of identity development and peer relationship processes in adolescence and young adulthood: Contributions of the special issue. *Journal of Adolescence, 35*, 1409–1415. doi:10.1016/j.adolescence.2012.09.007

Garcia, M., Kosutic, I., McDowell, T., & Anderson, S. A. (2009). Raising critical consciousness in family therapy supervision. *Journal of Feminist Family Therapy, 21*(1), 18–38. doi:10.1080/08952830802683673

Geller, E., & Foley, G. M. (2009). Broadening the "ports of entry" for speech-language pathologists: A relational and reflective model for clinical supervision. *American Journal of Speech- Language Pathology, 18*(1), 22–41. doi:10.1044/1058-0360(2008/07-0053)

Hansel, T. C., Osofsky, H. J., Steinberg, A. M., Brymer, M. J., Landis, R., Riise, K. S.,... Speier, A. (2011). Louisiana spirit specialized crisis counseling: Counselor perceptions of training and services. *Psychological Trauma: Theory, Research, Practice, and Policy, 3*, 276–282. doi:10.1037/a0024644

Harris, M., & Fallot, R. (Eds.). (2001). *Using trauma theory to design service systems: New directions for mental health services.* San Francisco, CA: Jossey-Bass.

Hernandez, P., & McDowell, T. (2010). Intersectionality, power, and relational safety in context: Key concepts in clinical supervision. *Training and Education in Professional Psychology, 4*, 29–35. doi:10.1037/a0017064

Hernandez, P., & Rankin, P. (2008). Relational safety and liberating training spaces: An application with a focus on sexual orientation issues. Journal of marital and family therapy, *34*(2), 251–264.

Hewson, D. M. (1999). III. Empowerment in supervision. *Feminism & Psychology, 9*, 406–409. doi:10.1177/0959353599009004005

Jernigan, M. M., Green, C. E., Helms, J. E., Perez-Gualdron, L., & Henze, K. (2010). An examination of people of color supervision dyads: Racial identity matters as much as race. *Training and Education in Professional Psychology, 4*, 62–73. doi:10.1037/a0018110

Jones, S. R. (2009). Constructing identities at the intersections: An autoethnographic exploration of multiple dimensions of identity. *Journal of College Student Development, 50*, 287–304. doi:10.1353/csd.0.0070

Joubert, L., Hocking, A., & Hampson, R. (2013). Social work in oncology: Managing vicarious trauma—the positive impact of professional supervision. *Social Work in Health Care, 52*, 296–310. doi:10.1080/00981389.2012.737902

Kadan, S., Roer-Strier, D., & Bekerman, Z. (2017). Social workers from oppressed minority group treating majority group's clients: A case study of Palestinian social workers. *Social Work, 62*, 156–164. doi:10.1093/sw/swx008

Kanter, R. M. (1993). *Men and women of the corporation.* New York, NY: Basic Books.

Kitchiner, N. J., Phillips, B., Neil, R., & Bisson, J. I. (2007). Increasing access to trauma focused cognitive behavioural therapy for posttraumatic stress disorder through a pilot feasibility study of a group clinical supervision model. *Behavioural and Cognitive Psychotherapy, 35*, 251–254. doi:10.1017/S1352465806003201

Knight, C. (2015). Trauma-informed social work practice: Practice considerations and challenges. *Clinical Social Work Journal, 43*(1), 25–37. doi:10.1007/s10615-014-0481-6

Mensah, J. (2014). Black continental African identities in Canada: Exploring the intersections of identity formation and immigrant transnationalism. *Journal of Canadian Studies, 48*(3), 5–29. doi:10.3138/jcs.48.3.5

Mitchell, F. M. (2016). Creating space for the "uncomfortable": Discussions about race and police brutality in a BSW classroom. *Reflections, 21*(3), 4–9.

Nye, J. S. (2004). Power in the global information age: From realism to globalization. NY: Routledge.

Pack, M. (2014). Vicarious resilience: A multilayered model of stress and trauma. *Affilia: Journal of Women & Social Work, 29*, 18–29. doi:10.1177/0886109913510088

Pearlman, L. A., & Saakvitne, K. W. (1995). *Trauma and the therapist: Countertransference and vicarious traumatization in psychotherapy with incest survivors.* New York, NY: Norton.

Pfohl, A. H. (2004). The intersection of personal and professional identity: The heterosexual supervisor's role in fostering the development of sexual minority supervisees. *The Clinical Supervisor, 23*(1), 139–164. doi:10.1300/J001v23n01_09

Phenice, L. A., & Griffore, R. J. (2000). Social identity of ethnic minority families: An ecological approach for the new millennium. *Michigan Family Review, 5*(1), 29–39.

Phillips, J. C., Parent, M. C., Dozier, V. C., & Jackson, P. L. (2017). Depth of discussion of multicultural identities in supervision and supervisory outcomes. *Counselling Psychology Quarterly, 30,* 188–210. doi:10.1080/09515070.2016.1169995

Quiros, L., & Berger, R. (2015). Responding to the sociopolitical complexity of trauma: An integration of theory and practice. *Loss and Trauma, 20*(2), 149–159. doi:10.1080/15325024.2013.836353

Shahmoon-Shanok, R. (2006). Reflective supervision for an integrated model: What, why and how? In G. Foley & J. D. Hochman (Eds.), *Mental health in early intervention: A unity of principles and practice* (pp. 343–381). Baltimore, MD: Paul H. Brookes Publishing.

Toren, A. L. (2008). Supervision as a buffer to vicarious trauma among counselors-in-training (Doctoral dissertation). Available from ProQuest Dissertations and Theses database. (UMI No. 3314645)

Wadsworth, M. E., Rindlaub, L., Hurwich-Reiss, E., Rienks, S., Bianco, H., & Markman, H. J. (2013). A longitudinal examination of the adaptation to poverty-related stress model: Predicting child and adolescent adjustment over time. *Journal of Clinical Child & Adolescent Psychology, 42,* 713–725. doi:10.1080/15374416.2012.755926

Warner, L. R., & Shields, S. A. (2013). The intersections of sexuality, gender, and race: Identity research at the crossroads. *Sex Roles, 68,* 803–810. doi:10.1007/s11199-013-0281-4

Watkins, Jr., C. E. (2011). Toward a tripartite vision of supervision for psychoanalysis and psychoanalytic psychotherapies: Alliance, transference-countertransference configuration, and real relationship. *Psychoanalytic Review, 98,* 557–590. doi:10.1521/prev.2011.98.4.557

Watts-Jones, T. (2010). Location of self: Opening the door to dialogue on intersectionality in the therapy process. *Family Process, 49,* 405–420. doi:10.1111/j.1545-5300.2010.01330.x

Werbart, A. (2007). Utopic ideas of cure and joint exploration in psychoanalytic supervision. *International Journal of Psychoanalysis, 88,* 1391–1408. doi:10.1516/3374-N232-7582-7G10

A personal narrative on responding to the tragedy at Pulse in Orlando: A volunteer supervisor's perspective

John T. Super

ABSTRACT

In the aftermath of the massacre at Pulse in Orlando, Florida, the helping professions united to help meet the counseling needs created by the traumatic event. This article is a first-person account of a supervisor working with more than 600 volunteer professional helpers who helped the victims, families, friends, and others impacted by the massacre. An event like this elicits both personal and professional responses and, in working with the helpers, the two responses both impacted the work that was done by the supervisor. This account provides a better understanding of skills and dispositions helpful in responding to a community trauma and the personal impact on the supervisor.

Around 2:00 a.m. on June 12, 2016, an event occurred in Orlando, Florida, that captured the world's attention. A single gunman entered the Pulse nightclub armed with rounds of ammunition and proceeded to methodically shoot club patrons, ultimately injuring 53 and killing 49 people. Although this story was told through the media, this narrative is my account as one of the first to respond to the cognitive and emotional needs of those affected or impacted by the trauma.

As a responder, I was aware of my distinct roles as a helping professional and as a gay man who lived in Orlando. I worked with victims' families, patrons, local residents, and helping professionals after one of the deadliest mass shootings in the United States and, while helping others, I was internally negotiating through feelings of fear, anger, sadness, pride, and vulnerability. Professionally, during that time the most pressing cognitive needs were educating those I came into contact with (e.g., helping professionals, agency volunteers, potential clients) about the grieving process, focusing on trauma responses, addressing irrational thoughts, helping them understand how and why the shooting occurred, and, ultimately, finding meaning in the tragedy. Meanwhile, personally, I was experiencing some of the same issues as those seeking trauma counseling and was much less certain on how to deal with my own feelings. Our clients included victims, patrons of Pulse, and those in the community affected by the shooting whose emotional needs varied greatly, but commonly included processing the residual fear and feeling unsafe in their daily lives, understanding the worry their loved ones could be hurt, and beginning the process of the grief cycle.

In this narrative, I examine the tragedy from the personal and professional perspectives of an individual instrumental in organizing the response of the helping professions. While striving to provide the details to help readers who may face a crisis response, having experienced this trauma made writing this narrative difficult. As an academic, I learned to lessen internal and external distractions and focus on writing. This narrative goes beyond those typical situations because, as I sat down to write, I was reliving each of those days and moments. I often stepped away to examine my reignited emotions of sadness, fear, and exhaustion that I experienced the first few days after the massacre. During the first year after the attack, my focus was helping others understand their reactions and, to do this, I bracketed my own thoughts and feelings about what happened. Although this bracketing may be noble and even possibly needed, shelving my response limited me doing exactly what I was trying to help others do: process their thoughts and emotional reactions to the largest mass shooting in U.S. history, and one that happened in a city I called home.

Personal

In June 2016, we moved our main home from Orlando to Gainesville, Florida, to be closer to a teaching position I accepted at the University of Florida. We have aging family in Orlando, requiring my husband and I to be in Orlando regularly to manage their needs, so we also moved into a small home in Orlando the week before the shooting occurred. Around 5 a.m. on Sunday, June 12, I woke from a deep sleep to a text from a friend traveling out of state, both checking on my safety and worried about the news he was seeing. With my grogginess and the unusual safety check, I was confused by his message and why he was worried about my safety. To better understand the context, I turned to the local news and heard the first reports of a shooting at a club. Initially, the local news reported shots were fired and several were dead. As the minutes turned into hours that morning, the details of the shooting became clearer and the number of fatalities grew. With a rapidly developing situation, social media provided unfiltered information faster than broadcast news, so I turned to social media to learn more. I read a post from a fellow counselor who felt helpless and suggested that those in the counseling community might be useful at The Center. The Center is an Orlando-based, not-for-profit agency providing programs and services to the gay, lesbian, bisexual, and transgender+ (GLBT+) community, including mental health care services and counseling. (For the purposes of this article, the term GLBT+ will be used. The population is known by several acronyms and the term LGBT+ is generally inclusive of those who identify as gay, lesbian, bisexual, transgender, queer, questioning, intersex, asexual, and Allies.)

Until that Sunday morning, our exhausting weekend had been filled with moving, unpacking, and setting up the house in Orlando. In fact, I planned to spend that day unpacking dozens of moving boxes and settling in. However, as I read the posts on social media, I realized my weekend plans might change since there were ways I could help. For years, I had worked as a volunteer counselor at The Center, providing counseling to those in the Orlando GLBT+ community. During my work there, I learned The Center provides programs and services to meet the social, emotional, physical, intellectual, and spiritual needs of the Orlando GLBT+ community, and has an ongoing need for volunteers. I also knew those The Center helped often felt vulnerable, and this tragedy would only compound those feelings.

I began my counseling career by helping couples in the Orlando GLBT+ community but, after years in private practice, I decided to continue my studies, receiving a terminal degree in counselor education. As an academic, I had worked with universities in both Central Florida (the Orlando area) and North Central Florida. That morning, reading through social media, I recognized I could choose to help or to continue settling into our new home, and sat with that choice for a while before making the decision to help. Prior to joining the faculty at the University of Florida, I had taught in a counseling program at a university in Orlando. My decision was impacted by knowing those affected or impacted by the shooting could be (a) previous students, (b) previous supervisees, (c) previous colleagues, and/or (d) previous clients. In those moments as I weighed the choice of volunteering, I considered the training I had received as a Red Cross disaster mental health care responder, and decided to help.

On the morning of June 12, that very distinct moment stood out—the moment in which I considered maintaining the plans for my day or choosing to be involved in the response. Looking back, the decision should have been easy, but I weighed both options and debated over the answer. In weighing my options, I imagined that many helping professionals would respond and my choosing to stay home and unpack boxes would have little impact on the overall efforts. I also knew volunteering for a not-for-profit could be time-consuming and require a great deal of my energy. However, I was personally aware that something significant was happening in the city I lived in and in the GLBT+ community of which I was a part. Realizing this, I was compelled to respond. Ultimately, I realized I both wanted and *needed* to help.

During the drive to The Center, I prepared for what I might find, and imagined two possible scenarios. The first scenario was that The Center would be in a state of bedlam and the second was that The Center would be calm with little or no activity taking place. Even as I was anticipating these conditions, I was also struggling to understand the attack and worrying about my personal safety. The identity of the gunman was still unknown, the motive was only speculation, and the extent of the attack was still emerging. The unknown details were unsettling, and I worried about the city. I was afraid of learning that I knew some of the victims, and I experienced survivor's guilt. The guilt stemmed from doing what many do in response to collective trauma, realizing the possibility of my being at Pulse and feeling guilty that I was safe while others were hurt. On several occasions, I had gone to Pulse with friends on similar Saturday evenings, and I imagined my experiences there with what was emerging in the news. This was overwhelming and I did what many helpers do in similar situations: compartmentalized my personal thoughts and feelings to be present for those who needed help.

Arriving at The Center, I found the reality there was somewhere in the middle of calm and bedlam. There was a feeling of shock comingled with people jumping into action. Many of those already at The Center, which was the immediate epicenter for the GLBT+ community's response, were trying to better understand the shooting and how to appropriately respond.

Navigating through the building, I found the counselor spearheading the mental health response, and I followed the Red Cross' training protocol. I identified my qualifications and my professional experience as a counselor, supervisor, and educator in offering to help. This identification process gives the leader an understanding of how volunteers can best be used. Even though I was knowledgeable in counseling and trained in disaster response, I was surprised when he asked another counselor educator and I to join in leading the volunteer helping professionals, as he knew the response would be sizable and several leaders were needed. In a short period of time, there were three of us working together to organize the grassroots response, with him leading the efforts. In those first few minutes we realized the following: (a) we were in a period where the scope of the tragedy was developing and the helping response needed to be flexible (i.e., it could grow or constrict as we better understood the attack and what would be needed to help Central Florida heal), but had a growing awareness of the magnitude; (b) there were more and more helping professionals arriving, eager to work with those affected and impacted by the shootings to help them process what happened; (c) there was limited space for providing crisis counseling at The Center; and (d) the response efforts would need to be immediate, short term, and ongoing.

In those first few hectic hours, I recognized the blending of my personal and professional lives as a stream of volunteer helping professionals flooded into The Center and, in those volunteers, I recognized people from both of my lives. I recognized some from previously working as one of The Center's counselors, friends I'd known from living in Orlando, former students, and counseling colleagues who joined the response. Although these aspects of my life were distinct, they blended together in the days that followed the shooting, leaving me with a sense of pride and wholeness as I watched these people I knew—personally and professionally—unite to help so many.

Professional

The volunteer helping professionals

After the initial leadership meeting, I studied the environment before we met with the volunteer helping professionals. I appreciated watching colleagues reunite after their professional lives had gone in different directions, and I noticed the sadness, anger, and fear around the event that brought them together. I also noted that the volunteers were eager to start and looking for direction. With this understanding, I felt responsible to lead, yet I was still unsure of what was needed from the volunteer helping professionals. In those first few minutes of organizing the response, leadership was emerging to meet both the physical and emotional needs of the city and the GLBT+ community. At that time, there were many who wanted to help, but few who wanted to lead. Leadership during a crisis requires committing intellect, emotion, energy, and time. People with the requisite leadership skills and the willingness to commit were understandably rare during a time where most of the helpers were still processing their own reactions to the shootings.

That day, there were some shared traits among the volunteer helping professionals who responded after the shooting. All were struggling to understand the emerging news, to make sense of the increasing number of fatalities, and to set aside their worry for loved ones so that they could help. Amid the hectic environment, a sense of structure emerged; some of our volunteers began organizing the arriving helping professionals, some started talking to the many gathering for a sense of community at The Center about their thoughts and feelings, and others began gathering the resources needed for those directly affected.

While all of this was happening, many of the helping professionals were also processing their own range of shared emotions, including shock, anger, sadness, concern, grief, fear, and love. I often found myself talking to them as they worked, helping them find shared experiences and emotions to strengthen the growing sense of community. Also, the helping professionals were personally connecting to the trauma. Many times, they recognized their own vulnerability with statements such as, "I've been to Pulse before and that could have been me." As they processed these thoughts and feelings, many were also learning how they were personally linked to the shootings. Some learned of friends who were at Pulse that evening or neighbors mourning the loss of a victim, while others learned of coworkers connected to the victims. These moments of vulnerability and personal connection were significant and monumental to the professional helpers, and they often needed time to process with peers or supervisors.

During those first few hours, an unbelievable number of helping professionals marched through the door in response to a social media post asking for those willing to volunteer their professional services to help. Often those volunteering reported they needed to do something to help and could not stay home and do nothing. We quickly realized using an online spreadsheet to create the registry of the volunteers was needed. It included their contact information, their availability, and how they could help. To help place the volunteers in the positions in which they could be the most useful, volunteers also listed any special skills, training, or talents. We, as the leaders, discussed the cognitive and emotional needs of potential clients, and drew from personal knowledge and experience to identify the crucially needed characteristics in the helping professionals: (a) experience working with trauma; (b) experience working with the GLBT+ or Latin communities; (c) training in Eye Movement Desensitization and Reprocessing (EMDR), a modality for treating trauma; (d) bilingual ability, most importantly speaking Spanish; (e) experience in casework and connecting people to local resources; and (f) license to prescribe medications.

In the days that followed the tragedy, we were thankful and surprised that the registry grew to more than 600 helping professionals. I was proud of the number who responded from our collective professions, surprised at the large number, and also felt a greater sense of responsibility as I knew those volunteers were relying on me to help lead them. They included a wide range of professions, including counselors, social workers, educators, psychologists, psychiatrists, pet-assisted therapists, aroma therapists, counselors using expressive arts for healing, and clergy. The helping professionals were flexible and ready to go anywhere and do anything they could to provide assistance. In counseling, a common phrase is "meet the clients where they are," meaning to emotionally and cognitively match the client's levels of readiness and emotionality without judgment. Following the massacre, the professional helpers physically and literally met the clients where they were (e.g., civic centers, blood donation lines, nightclubs). The helpers responded to the tragedy for various reasons. Some were currently working with GLBT+ or Latin clients, some were parents and recognized the trauma to the families, and some worked with trauma or grief and knew their professional experience would be valuable. Regardless of their motivation to respond, I witnessed a genuine and enthusiastic desire in the helpers to do something, often combined with a feeling of not knowing what to do.

On that first day, the helping professionals were committed to helping others make it through the tragedy and began assisting almost immediately. In the first few hours, they helped Orlando residents at The Center understand their thoughts and emotions while watching the news reports. Also, the helping professionals focused on The Center's staff and, by early afternoon, were talking with those waiting in the long lines to donate blood. During this process, it was important for me as a supervisor to focus on the parallel processes the helpers and the clients were experiencing: as the clients worried about their friends and families, the helpers also worried about their loved ones. When the clients talked to counselors about their fears, shock, or anger, many of the helping professionals felt the same way. Although helpers regularly experience similar thoughts and feelings as their clients, the magnitude of these shared emotions were much greater for those working in the aftermath of the shootings. During those first few days, there were many shared thoughts and emotions with those who volunteered their professional services. But as they worked together to help others, their actions contributed to their own healing process.

Leadership and supervision

Leadership

Our early leadership meeting set the stage for the next few hours, days, and weeks. We created a leadership structure that identified the immediate needs of those seeking help, the necessary tasks to meet the needs, and the resources needed to help. Those volunteer helping professionals with advanced organizational skills were asked to create the registry, manage contacting and scheduling volunteers, and categorize the needs into (a) immediate needs, (b) short-term needs, (c) long-term needs, and (d) multifaceted needs. We initially envisioned the immediate need was to have helping professionals available the day of the shootings and for the first few days after for anyone in the area who wanted to talk about the tragedy, and for our grassroots efforts to provide grief counseling until the Red Cross mental health care team arrived to take over. We discussed that the area would be healing from the tragedy for months, if not years, and identified this as a long-term need. The multifaceted needs were categorized as needs for the clients, for the helping professionals, and for the overall operation to meet the comprehensive needs of a shocked city. Although this was sound logic, the reality of what the community was facing was startling and overwhelming to everyone involved. In those moments, I found it helpful to rely on my clinical training of focusing on clients' immediate needs as a way to quiet my thoughts and feelings.

Some unique leadership characteristics accompany unexpected traumatic events like the massacre at Pulse. In the first few hours after the shootings, the Orlando news outlets broadcasted that anyone wanting to talk could visit with our helping professionals to receive free grief and trauma counseling, triggering us to prepare for potentially many clients. In those first few hours and days, estimating the number of needed helping professionals was difficult since there were no established client patterns, often giving us more helpers than clients. As a result, we were challenged to keep the helping professionals engaged and motivated, which required me to be an involved and creative leader. That first morning, there was an immediate peak in clients at The Center, but the numbers waned over the next few hours and days. In looking back, it is evident that those in Central Florida were experiencing shock from the event and were continuing to process what occurred, and thus were not seeking out immediate help.

During that first week, flexibility and adaptability were necessary leadership skills for responding to the quickly changing environment. In traditional clinical settings, clients come to counseling seeking help. However, because of collective shock, few clients came to The Center. As supervisors, we knew the lack of clients did not diminish the need for help. We knew we had to be creative in connecting helping professionals to those in need of help. We asked the helpers to leave the counseling rooms and meet the clients in various ways, including circulating through The Center looking for individuals in distress and talking to them, visiting blood donation centers and talking to the lines of donors about their feelings related to the shooting, attending vigils to provide support to those having strong emotional reactions, and circulating among the patrons in Latin and GLBT+ nightclubs to help those who might be using alcohol as a coping mechanism.

Another leadership skill was challenging my belief of how counseling should occur for the amplified emotional circumstances we were operating in. During non-crisis events, those considering counseling report that seeking out counseling creates anxiety (Young, 2012). The loss of personal safety amplified the non-crisis anxiety to greater levels and, to accommodate the amplified feelings, we used pet-assisted therapists to lessen the discomfort. For example, on the second day two clients came for trauma counseling and one of the clients reported her roommate (the other client) had not left his bedroom since the attack; as a result, she had persuaded him to speak with a helping professional. His face displayed much worry, fear, and anxiety as he walked in, and using a pet to lessen these negative emotions was very helpful for him. As he was met by the pet-assisted therapist, he focused on petting the dog while reluctantly explaining why he was there. The interaction with the pet, the pet-assisted therapist, and the helping professional overcame his defense mechanisms and he agreed to a private counseling session. After nearly 90 minutes talking to a professional helper, he managed a smile while thanking the counselor as he left. In looking back, the multidisciplinary approach contributed to lessening the client's anxiety in accepting help and broadened my view of how the process should occur.

Leadership required many roles. The first was managing and organizing the needs at off-site locations as we began sending volunteers into public locations. On the day after the shootings, we started sending helping professionals to places where we knew counseling would be needed (e.g., workplaces, media outlets, hospitals, nightclubs, and civic organizations). Each site required different helping skills and characteristics, and as leaders we needed to quickly adapt and organize the localized response. Examples of the varied requirements were multilingual abilities, comfort working into a nightclub that catered to GLBT+ patrons with a leather fetish, and knowledge of and experience with trauma. The professional helpers came with a high level of motivation, but at times the motivation needed to be focused. For example, one helping professional worked on creating sign-in sheets for clients, yet the environment was dynamic and signing in was a low priority. So, that volunteer shifted her efforts to answering calls on a hotline broadcast on the local news for those who were emotionally distressed.

Another needed leadership role was mediating between and connecting the helping professions. The helping professionals were from various disciplines and each one's expertise needed to be honored. I soon realized that they came with varying knowledge about trauma. Educating them on how to work with trauma was important and ensured that all clients received competent assistance. Also, as a leader it was important to advocate for each profession to transcend professional differences. For example, someone trained with a medical model might advocate for prescribing medication for anxiety, while someone trained with a wellness model might advocate for talk therapy to address the same issue. As a supervisor, I often approached the difference of opinion as facilitating both professionals to find shared solutions to benefit the client. This advocacy created an understanding between the professionals that multiple disciplinary responses existed and, ultimately, everyone shared the same goal of helping the clients.

The final role was surprising and one I was not prepared for: working with the media. With a tragedy like this, a strong media presence was a reality and, as supervisors, we managed the reporters. The reporters were interested in speaking with those helping the people affected or impacted by the shootings, and myself or another supervisor would handle the media, allowing the helping professionals to focus on the counseling response to the tragedy. On the first day, as details of the shooting and numbers of casualties grew, the attention of reporters also grew. The local news reported our location provided grief counseling, resulting in a rapid increase in the number of reporters at The Center. The reporters sought information from anyone directly related to the tragedy, which included some of our clients. An initial goal for the supervisors was to protect the clients and helping professionals from the media to avoid retraumatizing or scaring them away from seeking help. It was natural that we were protective of those affected by the attack and lacked trust in the reporters.

Nevertheless, that protective goal changed on the first afternoon when I realized that some who were connected to the massacre at Pulse needed to talk to the media to externally process their thoughts and emotions. This became clear when I was asked to stand beside and support a young man who was giving an interview to an international news agency about his experiences in the nightclub. During the shootings, he carried friends out and returned for those who needed medical care. After leaving the hospital, he went home, showered, checked in with his loved ones, and came to The Center to connect with others who had had similar experiences. As I stood beside him, ever ready to interrupt the reporters' questioning at the first sign of emotional distress, I watched this young man answer the questions and share his experiences. I realized his emotional responses weren't the fear or distress I thought it would be, but one of growing resolve and resilience. Because of him, I realized the telling of a story could help in the healing process, and so developed more of a narrative theoretical approach in my work with clients. The experience also affected supervision, as I initiated conversations with the helpers, focused on various client processing styles, and encouraged the helpers to share their own stories as a method of processing their emotional reactions.

Supervision

During the aftermath of the shootings and working in a trauma response mode, supervision had many similarities with standard supervision, and also required making some adaptations. During non-crises, many helping professionals default to using a brief therapy model (Triantafillou, 1997; Zhang, Yan, Du, & Liu, 2014) that often extends into multiple sessions. In those first few hours and days after the shootings, one supervisory adaptation was reminding them to focus on a one-session model instead of thinking from a multi-session approach. Also, in trauma counseling, a vital aspect of supervision is assisting the helping professionals in debriefing some of the trauma they worked with (Sommer & Cox, 2005). Supervision styles vary, and my style of debriefing includes exploring thoughts, feelings, perceptions, memories, and anything associated with the events. This process gives the supervisee an opportunity to examine lingering thoughts and emotions, and the space to express residual feelings to hopefully move through the moment and reduce the potential for compassion fatigue. In a tragedy response such as this one, the ratio of supervisors to supervisees was much larger than would meet standard ratios. I began accommodating the unbalanced ratio by encouraging counselors to debrief with one another and praising those who I saw listening to and validating the emotions of their colleagues. Also, the supervisees included many practitioners working with trauma for the first time and, to prepare them, I adapted a technique in training marriage and family therapists of encouraging them to hypothesize what working with trauma could look like (Rivett & Street, 2009). Hypothesizing helps those new to working with trauma prepare for what is typically experienced in counseling sessions and thinking through the process of identifying appropriate interventions to use with commonly presented issues.

Professionally, for me, June 12, 2016, was a day of constant motion and response to emerging needs. Looking back, it was necessary to fill all the supervisory duties and roles without preparation or forethought. In the first few days, the crisis required some standard clinical supervisory skills and some additional ones that developed in the moment. In a traditional academic setting of training helping professionals, supervisors regularly focus on the trainees' wellness as the trainees focus on the clients, and, to an extent, this remained true. However, during this crisis response, as a supervisor it was important for me to recognize that helping professionals were also dealing with their personal emotions as they helped others process the aftermath of the shooting. For example, on the second day the volunteers talked to one another as they waited for clients to come to The Center. To switch the focus to supervision, I would gather the helping professionals into a circle and ask them to talk about their thoughts on the developing news and how the news might personally and emotionally affect their sessions. To focus on their well-being, I encouraged them to identify the emotion they were feeling in the moment and process their experiences to help them be emotionally available to their future clients. Also, teaching those unfamiliar with crisis counseling to work in a triage mode and shifting helpers' thinking from multi-session counseling models to what could most help the client in one session were additional supervisory skills. For example, in those first few days, the sounds of media helicopters hovering over the city were common and this sound triggered negative emotions in many helpers and clients. One mode of long-term treatment is to gradually expose clients to sounds to desensitize their reactions. In this case, the counselors often had only one session and, instead of exposure to the sounds, the helping professionals might restructure irrational beliefs (e.g., imminent danger, gunfire) attached to the sound to make a quick change. Finally, during the first few weeks, many of the helpers worked long hours and focused their energies on clients' needs. Because of this, another important skill was focusing the helping professionals on their own personal wellness and normalizing their emotional reactions.

During this time, I realized my supervision training and experience had not prepared me for the magnitude of this crisis response. As a result, I approached supervision much more organically and I made several changes that were helpful, based on the helping professionals' responses to my actions. Clinical supervision often occurs with individuals or small groups (Borders & Brown, 2005). The first change occurred as the trauma response required us to work with large supervision groups. In more traditional clinical supervision, confidentiality is paramount (Bernard & Goodyear, 2014) and, to ensure confidentiality, private spaces are often used and the supervisor meets with one or a few helpers. The second change in the days immediately following the massacre was that supervision often occurred in public spaces and we avoided discussing confidential information. Also, most supervision was spontaneous and in response to a supervisee's immediate needs. Finally, supervision changed to reflect a more logistical and practical focus (e.g., preparing the helping professionals to provide counseling and answer questions of emotionally distraught callers on the crisis lines), or involved announcements of upcoming events (e.g., supervision groups, volunteers needed to provide counseling at the vigil) and specific needs (e.g., bilingual support materials for clients).

Often, supervision was as dynamic as the environment we were working in. Supervision ranged on a continuum from a more traditional supervisory experience to a dynamic and spontaneous supervision response. Taking advantages of pauses between clients to focus on the helping professionals' development and well-being was meaningful. If one or more of them were eating, this became a moment for a supervisor to check in on their thoughts and emotions. Supervision also happened in motion, when we were walking between sites or clients. Individual supervision occurred rarely and only as needed, most often when a supervisee was experiencing a strong emotional reaction and needed individual attention. For example, I was asked to help a helping professional who struggled in a session when she realized a personal connection to the shootings mirrored the fears her client was experiencing. When the helping professional and I talked, she explained her worries that friends may have been hurt in the club and couldn't set those thoughts aside in the moment. She and I discussed the options of temporarily pausing her thoughts while with the client or pausing her volunteering to help others to confirm her friends were safe. Ultimately, she realized the worries were more a reaction to the collective trauma than realistic fears.

Just as there were situational considerations for the professional helpers, I also learned how important the considerations for supervisors were. As a supervisor, the act of supervising became more situational than traditional. Traditional clinical supervision is more intentional, such as structuring an activity or supervisory intervention toward a purpose (Bernard & Goodyear, 2014), but in this situation supervision became more creative. For example, at the end of the first day a group of professional helpers gathered around a conference table and began coloring in a donated coloring book. I asked them to identify how the images created were affected by the day's work. Those within the group connected their creations to their cognitive and emotional responses to helping clients working with the trauma. They explained their color choices, relating the choices to their feelings of shock, fear, and even optimism. The coloring became a vehicle for processing their reactions in a way that was comfortable and conversational for them. Their stories were rich with introspection and full of emotion. The impromptu supervision in a nontraditional format taught me a great deal about supervision, and moving forward I determined to remind myself to be creative and present when supervising. To remind me of this lesson, some of the images they colored that day are framed in my office.

Operating in this crisis required me to examine personally held beliefs and biases, then adapt functional beliefs and abandon any that were not useful. This process was somewhat surprising to me, as the beliefs and biases were ones I weren't expecting. For example, when I asked a young female adult from a higher income background to go into a GLBT+ leather and bondage paraphilia club, I felt uncomfortable. I thought she might be offended and, after asking her, I was surprised with her comfort and willingness to go. This example represents multiple shifts I had as a supervisor during this experience, the first in giving up beliefs about the professional helpers' comfort in uncomfortable situations. The second altered belief was changing the expectation of clients coming to us, to the professional helpers leaving the grief counseling center to find counseling opportunities for those who needed it.

Helping professionals and supervisors who respond to a crisis like the shootings at Pulse must rely on their education and experience, but also be willing to adapt for unpredictable circumstances. Although supervision in this crisis had many similarities with standard supervision, I benefited from challenging my supervisory beliefs, adjusting for changes to a less-traditional professional helping environment, and gaining a greater awareness of the professional helpers' increased stress and emotional responses from the collective trauma experienced by all those who responded. Personally, after working in this trauma response mode, I better understood some of my biases, I challenged my views of supervision, and I learned how to better supervise during a crisis.

Conclusion

Responding to an event like the one that happened at Pulse must be immediate; it cannot be planned. During those first few hours and days, as a leader and a supervisor, my work included a great deal of assessing the overall needs, understanding who needed help, and organizing an appropriate response. Such a dynamic and changing crisis environment requires many supervisory roles. In situations such as this, the roles a supervisor should be prepared to fill are many: educator, counselor, clinical supervisor, manager, ambassador, and spokesperson for the helping professions, while assisting those living in the area to understand how the healing process begins.

In the months following the shooting, it was helpful for many to identify what was learned from the experience, and, as a supervisor, it was important for me to focus on what I learned about supervision in a dynamic and emotional time. First, supervisors must consider the needs of supervisees differently during a response to trauma. There will be those who have a strong desire to help and participate, and there also will be those who recognize the time isn't right for them to help; both perspectives can be honored. In addition, supervisors must remain aware that working across disciplines requires recognizing the value and strengths of the academic and professional training of one's own discipline, but not limiting expectations of a discipline based on perceptions and beliefs. Finally, supervisors can and should encourage all helpers, including those in training programs, to participate in the Red Cross training as preparation for responding to a crisis.

Responding to the tragedy at Pulse provided opportunities to grow both professionally and personally. In reflecting on the tragedy's short-term personal effect on me, I recognize several moments of growth. Initially, I experienced guilt from leading and supervising the helping efforts and not directly counseling. I learned that, much like education, leadership is a vital role that supports those helping the clients. In addition, I learned more about a city and the people among which I lived. I recognized my pride in fellow citizens for their varied responses, from donating to help the efforts to reaching out to those who had the potential to be marginalized (e.g., GLBT +, Latins, Muslims) and standing in solidarity with those persons. Also, I felt an enormous pride in the helping professions from the large-scale response and the initial work.

In the months after, and in writing this narrative, I am still recognizing the long-term effects, both cognitively and emotionally, from being involved in the response. Acting as a supervisor during the crisis, I was focused on helping the clients and the helping professionals without taking the time to focus on myself and the emotions I experienced during this process. Friends and colleagues would remind me to take care of my cognitive and emotional needs, which I did, as needed, to navigate through our collective efforts, but I spent much more effort focusing on others. Also, the other leaders were in constant motion and the time to collectively process our own reactions as leaders was nonexistent. In class, I often remind students that we must attend to our emotions or they will get our attention in other ways; this was certainly true for me as a result of my being involved in the response. The vicarious trauma began surfacing in the weeks that followed in the form of extreme emotional reactions, emotional disengagement, and cognitively avoiding the topic at a personal level. This method proved to be unsuccessful and forced me to focus internally to begin the healing process. Interestingly, writing this narrative ignited underlying thoughts and emotions, allowing for a delayed grieving and sadness that the constant activity following the tragedy prohibited. The writing allowed the opportunity to create a personal narrative examining those ignored thoughts and emotions.

My personal involvement with the direct grief counseling efforts ended at the end of the second week, when I needed to focus on teaching and heading the clinical experiences for our counseling program. As the Red Cross became more involved in the area, the initial plan was to merge our efforts into the Red Cross' efforts. In a leadership discussion, we decided not to merge with the Red Cross and instead to indefinitely continue the grassroots response. When this decision was made, it became apparent that my personal and professional commitments needed to be a priority and I needed to step out of the response to the shootings. Although I left the daily operations, I remained involved in the counseling efforts.

This narrative can best be concluded by thinking back to June 12, 2016. At the end of that day, I drove home physically, mentally, and emotionally exhausted. During the drive, I inventoried my feelings and realized I was feeling sad for what I saw, shocked at the anger and hatred of one man, stunned that this could happen in a city I call home, and curious about how and why the shooting occurred. But I also experienced pride as I saw rainbow flags hung outside homes, businesses, and public spaces to display solidarity. I pulled into my driveway that evening to see my new neighbor hanging a rainbow flag in front of his home. I thanked him for the support and shared how meaningful it was for me after working at The Center all day. He said he felt helpless and it was the only thing he knew to do to support a city that was in shock and hurting. To finish the day, I watched an awards show for self-care, to help me focus on anything not related to the tragedy. Watching the show, I saw the ribbons celebrities wore in support of Orlando and heard the speeches memorializing the attack. I found the focus of those on national television to be surprising and almost surreal, in that they were talking about a city I thought of as home. And, even as I knew the tragedy had affected the world in momentous ways, I also knew, collectively, the world was beginning to heal.

Disclosure statement

No potential conflict of interest was reported by the authors.

References

Bernard, J. M., & Goodyear, R. K. (2014). *Fundamentals of clinical supervision* (5th ed.). Upper Saddle River, NJ: Pearson, Prentice Hall.

Borders, L. D., & Brown, L. L. (2005). *The new handbook of counseling supervision.* New York, NY: Taylor & Francis.

Rivett, M., & Street, E. (2009). *Family therapy: 100 key points and techniques* (1st ed.). New York, NY: Routledge.

Sommer, C. A., & Cox, J. A. (2005). Elements of supervision in sexual violence counselors' narratives: A qualitative analysis. *Counselor Education & Supervision, 45,* 119–134. doi:10.1002/ceas.2005.45.issue-2

Triantafillou, N. (1997). A solution-focused approach to mental health supervision. *Jounal of Systemic Therapies, 16,* 305–328. doi:10.1521/jsyt.1997.16.4.305

Young, M. E. (2012). *Learning the art of helping: Building blocks and techniques* (5th ed.). Upper Saddle River, NJ: Pearson.

Zhang, W., Yan, T. T., Du, Y. S., & Liu, X. H. (2014). Brief report: Effects of solution-focused brief therapy group-work on promoting post-traumatic growth of mothers who have a child with ASD. *Journal of Autism and Developmental Disorders, 44,* 2052–2056. doi:10.1007/s10803-014-2051-8

Trauma-informed intercultural group supervision

Anthony Haans and Nora Balke

ABSTRACT
Trauma-informed group supervision is a novel way of providing much-needed supervision to trauma helpers. We describe a structured group supervision method originally developed for Western trauma supervisors. Core features of the method are two identification rounds: first, identification with the client as a person and, second, identification with the position of the case presenter. We explain why we designed this structured identification approach and elaborate its main features. This method has been applied in many intercultural contexts and post-conflict regions of the world. Finally, we formulate some basics of intercultural application and contracting for group supervision.

Background and context

At the end of the 20th century, the first author (clinical psychologist-psychotherapist), together with colleague Johan Lansen (psychiatrist-psychotherapist), discussed experiences of trauma supervision in the Netherlands. We had worked with survivors of political violence for more than two decades and supervised trauma helpers for several years. Lansen had made an inventory of challenges of trauma supervision in the Netherlands, and we designed a training course on case supervision for experienced general supervisors and inexperienced trauma supervisors (Lansen & Haans, 2004). Our intent was to prepare supervisors to engage in trauma-informed supervision with therapists working with survivors of torture and war and refugees.

In 2003, this training course was employed at the Treatment Centre for Survivors of Torture (BZfO (BehandlungsZentrum für Folteropfer; Berlin)) in Berlin, Germany, an international center for the support of refugees (Balke, 2015). For more than a decade this training has attracted experienced professionals from the fields of trauma, personality disorders, addiction, and juvenile mental health. These professionals use their experience to support less experienced or novice trauma helpers. As a result of participation in this course, participants developed an identity as trauma-informed supervisors and acquired the necessary core supervisory skills.

The supervision course consists of several basic modules that have one shared characteristic: to offer a frame of reference and actions for supervisors, helping them to encounter trauma-related impediments in their work. These modules include the following: individual supervision, group supervision, team supervision, team dynamics, and organizational coaching. Attention is devoted to negotiation and contracting, intercultural supervision, trauma-related supervision, and specific supervision methods, such as psychodrama, art, and music, in response to the specific needs of supervisees. The course takes place for 31 days across a year and a half. Back home, participants must conduct at least 30 supervisory sessions in their professional field, using individual, group, or team modalities. These supervision sessions are individually supervised in 15 so-called learning supervision sessions, by an experienced, independent supervisor who is familiar with the content of the course. At the conclusion of the course, trainees are required to write a short essay on supervision in their field or specialty.

The need for a structured approach to trauma-informed group supervision

Group supervision is a well-known format in the mental health professions and its possibilities have been widely researched (e.g., Enyedy et al., 2003; Kaduvettoor, O'Shaughnessy, Clyde, & Weatherford, 2009; Ray & Altekruse, 2000). Recently, more theoretical and empirical inquiry has been devoted to trauma-informed supervision (TIS; Bergerand & Quiros, 2014), but literature on specific trauma-informed *group* supervision (TIGS) has remained rare since our original publication in 2004. Since there is, unfortunately, no research material available, we will first provide an extensive vignette describing specific features and challenges of TIGS in a cross-cultural context. This vignette reflects the challenging phenomena that occur in most trauma-related supervision groups. In reality, the combination and intensity can vary according to the specific context of the group. For sake of clarity and readability, we have combined these different situations into one, composite group example: the examples are real; the combination is constructed. In this example, we focus on two trauma-related pitfalls: countertransference, and a related group dynamic, unproductive roles that result from social and intercultural contexts. These processes are not unique to trauma treatments; they often occur in many other therapeutic contexts. In trauma work, these processes often are more complex and challenging (Smith, 2009).

First, we give a short description of this composite supervision group. An international supervision group in Berlin includes participants who primarily work with refugees and politically traumatized individuals. They are working in different organizations supporting refugees in the capital and province. There are eight participants: five males, three females, which include three social workers, three psychologists, one art therapist, and one psychiatrist. In this vignette, the following group members play a key role and we provide a short description of them. (For sake of privacy these names are changed, and ages are estimated.)

Tammo (45) is a Kurdish PhD psychologist who was born in Kurdistan who has lived and studied in Germany since he was in his twenties. He has much experience in intercultural trauma support and therapies. He works in an institution engaged in trauma therapy. He plays an active role in the Kurdish community in Germany and at home.

Bernd (40) is a German social worker. He has worked in different settings like drug addiction and street-corner work, and for the last seven years in a sheltered home for refugees.

Heidi (30) is a social worker connected to a Charitas Beratungsstelle für Flüchtlinge (a Christian church related counselling sevice for refugees) that supports asylum seekers during the registration process. This is her first assignment providing trauma-related support to refugees.

Ibrahim (55) is a psychologist from Iraq who fled from the Saddam Hussein regime about 30 years ago after his graduation. He has specialized in community support and works in a community center.

Gerhard (40) is a German psychiatrist. He has worked internationally in refugee support and works in a region east of Berlin in a psychiatric hospital with people from the former German Democratic Republic.

Aisha (32) is an art therapist with a Tunisian/French background who has been living in Germany for 10 years. She took several refresher courses in art therapy and trauma assistance, and works in a community center with children and adults from different cultures, many of whom have experienced trauma. She also is a rather well-known sculptor in Berlin.

The group has been meeting for more than a year, every three to four weeks. They met at previous trainings they all had attended. They also interact with one another professionally. During one of these trainings they decided to start a trauma-oriented supervision group and found a supervisor, a highly regarded expert in the field of clinical supervision. He does not have experience as either a trauma therapist or supervisor of trauma therapists. He has come to the second author for incidental consultative supervision (Holloway, 1995). The group operates in a format originally developed by Balin (Salinsky, 2009). Sessions loosely proceed along the following format:

(1) One of the members introduces a case.
(2) Other group members then ask questions, and freely discuss the case, while the case presenter listens.
(3) At the end of the discussion, the presenter reflects on what she or he has heard.

Trauma-related challengers to TIGS: Countertransference

Vignette 1

Six months ago, a distinctive feature of TIS occurred in the supervision group. Heidi, the social worker of German origin, introduced a male client from Chechnya. In her work in a charity organization that assists refugees, one of her tasks is to collect information about clients' history of torture and trauma. The client was a former policeman who was arrested several times by his former colleagues because he had criticized his superior and expressed dissatisfaction with his transfer to another region. The transfer resulted in a separation from his wife and children. After his third arrest, he flew to Germany alone. He is waiting for asylum status and wants to be reunited with his family. Heidi was in support of his goal and asked for advice from the group members for the next steps to be taken.

The session opened quite productively. Based upon their different professional backgrounds, the other members asked relevant questions about this man and his life. Then the climate changed when Tammo, the German/Kurdish psychologist, asked more details about the client's experiences in the years before imprisonment. Heidi reported that it was her impression that he was an honest policeman in his small hometown. When he was transferred to a bigger city, the problems began. She stated that his new superiors and colleagues were cruel, and they engaged in the torturing and battering of prisoners. Heidi's client refused to participate in these activities. He was then imprisoned by his former colleagues, and was beaten and tortured (he still has the scars), and reported being very depressed from that time on.

Ibrahim, the therapist originally from Iraq, said he believed that Heidi's client must, perhaps reluctantly, have participated in these cruelties and that his imprisonment might have been for other reasons. Heidi became angry, stating that Ibrahim was "always suspicious," assuming everyone was a perpetrator. She asserted that she had no evidence that her client had any involvement with the mistreatment of prisoners. Bernd described one of his experiences where a refugee client reported how so-called comrades forced junior colleagues to participate in beating and torture as a kind of "initiation ritual." Heidi calmed down and agreed to consider this point and to inquire about this possibility with her client. Then the group continued discussing how to support her client with his request for asylum and reunification with his family. Heidi felt relieved and had a clear idea on how to proceed.

In the next group supervision session, Heidi once again brought up this case. She reported that she asked the client for more details about his actions. He reluctantly acknowledged that he had participated in the torture of others. He gave few details, but what he did tell Heidi was very shocking for her. She knew such things happened, but had never heard a person who had committed these deeds describe them. Although he claimed he was forced to torture prisoners by his superiors and colleagues, she saw this as cowardice. She also believed his actions regarding his family were cowardly. With the only explanation being "they were after me," he left his family alone in their dangerous hometown and did not bring them with him. Although her client expressed great remorse, Heidi no longer wanted to work with him.

At this point the group was stuck and did not know how to proceed. Some accused Heidi of being too condemnatory, and others argued she should not work with perpetrators. The supervisor himself was ambivalent, shifting from one position to the other. The group ended with the members dissatisfied.

Theoretical background of the vignette

Counselors who work with trauma survivors experience strong emotional reactions (Knight, 2013; Smith, 2009). All too frequently, they ignore these reactions, focusing instead on their client, professional methods, and techniques. The lack of attention to counselors' personal reactions is reinforced by the organizations that employ them. Opportunities for staff to discuss and therefore manage their reactions are mostly rare. When therapists are unable to give voice to their feelings, they are even more susceptible to disappointment, mental exhaustion, disillusionment, and indirect traumatization (Gurris, 2005; Strohmeier & Scholte, 2015).

Heidi's and the group members' reactions to her client may be viewed as manifestations of countertransference. In this case, the practitioners' reactions stem from their reactions to Heidi's client (Knight, 2013). We use this concept in a more general sense, as described by Kiessler (2001). He distinguished a continuum, with therapist-connected countertransference that stems from the therapists' own unresolved conflicts at one end. At the other end is client-induced countertransference (subjective countertransference), which stems from the client and is experienced by all involved caregivers. The strong emotional responses caused by the victim-perpetrator conflict of Heidi's client are an example of the latter. Wilson and Lindy (1994) considered trauma countertransference reactions mainly as the therapist's reactions, in individual or group settings, to the life and the behavior of their patients (to the right of the continuum). They distinguished two main forms of countertransference. The first is an exaggerated retention of distance (Type I: over-distancing) and the second is losing adequate proximity (Type II: over-involvement).

Heidi's actions reflected both manifestations in, respectively, sessions 1 and 2. In supervision, when supervisees present a difficult case, they often adopt one of the two stances identified by Wilson and Lindy (1994). No matter which position they take, their understanding of the case remains limited and restricted. They can only view the client from an either/or perspective; for example, the client is either "all good" and therefore truly a victim, or "all bad" and unworthy of the clinician's empathy. Group supervision can be very helpful because peer feedback helps the presenter develop a more differentiated, balanced, and complete understanding of the client. To minimize the negative effect of these countertransference reactions on both the therapist and the therapeutic relationship with the client, supervisors must encourage their supervisees to openly and honestly discuss their emotional responses from the start of the supervisory relationship. This must be done without pathologizing the supervisee. When the supervisor encourages open discussion in a group format, this normalizes and validates supervisees' reactions.

When Heidi was in the "good or bad" countertransference mode, she distorted her image of the client, a person with many contradictory characteristics, and stereotyped him as either a perpetrator or a victim. Even with continued help from the supervisor and her peers, Heidi still could not develop a more accurate and realistic perspective of him by the end of session 1, to recognize that the client could be both victim and perpetrator. It is for this reason that the Balint method of group supervision is insufficient in trauma-informed supervision. In session 2, Heidi rejected the client. Because of the unrecognized countertransference, her internal split is acted out by the group that separates into two "either/or" camps. The supervisor becomes aware of this split but is unable to share his inner experience in the supervision group, due to his own countertransference reactions, which he later disclosed to the second author. To overcome these difficulties, our group supervision model includes an identification round with the *client as a person*. We describe this later in this article.

Group dynamic challenges in TIGS: Unproductive roles of group members

The composition of a supervision group often is multidisciplinary. A variety of helping professions are present. Other social components are important like gender distribution, differences in experience, and so on. Although professionals intend to be helpful, they often get stuck in fixed roles, positions, and communication styles (Lansen & Haans, 2004). The next vignettes provide an example of this.

Vignette 2

In this group, Bernd is a very compassionate social worker and Aisha is a gifted art therapist. Both respond with much empathy when supervisees present their clients to the group. Gerhard, a German psychiatrist, and Tammo, the Kurdish PhD psychologist, are much more clinical in their approach. Although nearly all studied in Germany, they differ with respect to their level of education. If Bernd, Aisha, or someone else without an advanced degree presents a case, Gerhard and Tammo (the most highly educated and most experienced) often ally with each other and adopt a condescending attitude toward the others. They have firm ideas and can explain eloquently what is wrong with the client and which approach should be used based upon the literature, and always have suggestions about what other group members should do. Tammo, and to an even lesser extent Gerhard, does not present many cases for supervision. When they do, they maintain the discussion at a very clinical/technical level, neglecting their emotional responses. They focus on professional boundaries and skills. In response to unexpected complications in their relationships with clients, Tammo and Gerhard typically express anger with them, because they "did not respond properly."

Although all want to avoid top-down communication in favor of discussions among equals, communication in this group actually reflects stereotyped bureaucratic roles that members encounter at their work. In a supervision group that is comprised of individuals from various cultural backgrounds, fixed roles and alliances develop based upon the values and traditions of Western and non-Western group members (Gupta & Kumar, 2007). This is illustrated in the next vignette.

Vignette 3

About two months ago, Tammo introduced a female Kurdish client for discussion. He described this woman, her difficulties with her husband and children, and how she managed to survive in a southern neighborhood of Berlin. His supervision question was quite clear: Should he refer her to the community social worker or start supportive counseling by himself? After the case presentation, the question round that followed was appropriate. All were interested and asked many questions, such as "Where is she living?"; "What is her contact with the neighbors?"; "What school do her children go to and how are they doing?"; and "What kind of services have you delivered?"

The following case analysis emerged. This patient had severe posttraumatic stress disorder (PTSD) complaints that were very intrusive, but eye movement desensitization and reprocessing (EMDR) therapy had not been helpful. The intrusive symptoms had diminished somewhat, but the client still was quite isolated, relying on a few female Kurdish friends, and had hardly any contact with other people. She had done some cleaning work in Berlin households but stopped a few months ago. She sent her husband to school for meetings with the children's teachers, but never went there herself. In the third discussion round, the confusion started. Aisha and Ibrahim accused Tammo of being too rigid in his trauma method, and ignoring the social context of the patient. They believed he should have initially directed his attention to her social circumstances and waited to introduce the EMDR until he had a good relationship with her. Members quickly started a discussion about how appropriate it was to start supportive counseling, believing it might be too late. Tammo felt accused and, instead of listening, became defensive. The discussion became very emotional, with members condemning one another or trivializing the disagreement. The German participants initially were silent, trying to defuse the heated atmosphere, as did the supervisor. But their suggestions were largely ignored or only briefly adhered to by the other three. The group achieved no consensus, nor could Tammo decide upon an appropriate course of action. The group ended quite tensely and members were dissatisfied.

Theoretical background of the vignettes

Aisha and Ibrahim attacked Tammo. Aisha has no formal trauma therapeutic training and Ibrahim was educated a long time ago. Both had been largely educated through their practice and learned to pay attention to their clients' social context. Tammo is a postgraduate-educated trauma therapist with much experience in directive trauma treatment like EMDR. These treatments are often considered by non-Western professionals as "disease-oriented, Western treatment methods" that attach too little importance to social and mental health aspects of clients' lives (Tay & Silove, 2017).

At first glance, divisions seem to be the result of cultural differences, but they also are the result of professional disagreements. Both dynamics challenge the "myth of sameness" (Bernard & Goodyear, 1992). Groups often begin with what members have in common. For example, in this group, originally intercultural trauma work was the common factor. But numerous divisions became clear. If this group is going to be productive, these dynamics must be addressed. Intercultural groups readily reveal divisions related to majority and minority cultures. Minority group members often view themselves, and are viewed, as a unified front. In this example, the myth of sameness of the "Middle Eastern subgroup" is challenged. Aisha and Tammo were both born and socialized in Germany, while Ibrahim was not. However, Aisha and Ibrahim allied with each other in the dispute, reflecting their professional perspectives.

During this intense subgroup discussion, the German-born group members were silent. This was related to their position as members of the majority culture (Rudolph, 2005). Although they wanted to be helpful, they did not know how to deal with the conflict in "the minority culture." Therefore, the German subgroup retreated to a safe position by not getting involved, except to offer "outsider" opinions about calming down. They would not get involved with the substance of the disagreement. The supervisor did not address these fixed and defensive communications.

In supervision groups, the dynamic of "being different" must be dealt with through dialogue based upon "acceptance, appreciation, and respect towards the other" (Rudolph, 2005, p. 41). Thus, it becomes necessary to develop an "inter-subjectivity between individuals and groups" (Rudolph, 2005, p. 41; translation by authors). To encourage this type of discussion, we introduce a second identification round in our model: identification of the *task* and *position* of the supervisee. In this round, group members are gently confronted with one another's social, cultural, and ethnic differences, and develop understanding and empathy.

Trauma-informed group supervision

These vignettes illustrate why we designed this Trauma-Informed Group Supervision (TIGS) Method in our field of psychological trauma (Lansen & Haans, 2004). We found that trauma supervisors were confused in their approach because of the complexity of the clients' problems and the emotional reactions of the supervisees. We also observed that in group (and team) supervision the professional and social position of the trauma helpers resulted in isolation, feelings of powerlessness, and status fixations, which hampered an open fraternal dialogue. We designed a group supervision session of seven rounds, including two rounds to overcome these difficulties: identification with the client and identification with the position of the case supervisee. TIGS is based on common case group supervision and peer supervision principles (Hawkins & Shohet, 2000). Structuring was and is very important to increase benefits from supervision (Valentino, LeBlanc, & Sellers, 2016).

Table 1 presents the resulting group supervision sequence.

A supervision session takes between 60 and 90 minutes, depending on the complexity of the case and supervisees' experience with this method. The length of the rounds depends on the dynamics of the session.

Round 1: Selection of case and case presenter

Each group starts with an inventory of those members who want to present a case. These cases are briefly mentioned and the presenters briefly explain why they want assistance with the case, formulate a preliminary supervision question, explain if it is urgent or not, and provide basic relevant information. Then the group selects by consensus which case to take. During this round, the supervisor engages in the following actions: she or he ascertains whether there is clear agreement, ensures that everyone has an equal chance to present a case, and encourages democratic decision making and case introduction.

Table 1. Group Supervision Sequence.

Round	Action
Round 1	Selection of case and case presenter
Round 2	Presentation of the case
Round 3	Questions for clarification
Round 4	Identification with the client as a person
Round 5	Identification with the task and position of the case presenter
Round 6	Supervision *with* the group
Round 7	Conclusion

Round 2: Presentation of the case

The case presenter provides a short summary of the case. In the initial stages of the supervision group, the case often is an individual client. As the group develops, a family case or a therapy group may be presented. If a multi-person case is brought up, the model needs small adaptations, especially in Rounds 3 and 4, where more identification with different clients involved may be required (e.g., in a case involving a family with mother, father, and child, all three identifications can be carried out). In all cases, pseudonyms are used to protect clients' identities. The case presentation is as brief as possible. Mainly, it provides the name, age, and a little of the background of the client. Also, the length and frequency of contacts is provided. Audio or video tapes are not used in this format for practical reasons we discuss later.

At the end of the presentation, the case presenter reformulates his or her preliminary supervision question as specifically as possible: "What is the issue I have with this case, and what do I want to achieve?" This question must be clear to the presenter and the group members. The supervisor and the group members can help the supervisee accurately formulate a supervision question. They may offer alternative perspectives to make sure the question thoroughly addresses the issue (Lansen & Haans, 2004).

Such a process may go like this: At first, the presenter starts with the question "What is going on?," which is vague and lacks an acting subject. With help, she or he refines the question in different stages:

(1) I want to understand what is going on. (Supervisee identifies herself as actor, but the question remains too vague.)
(2) I want to know why this patient confuses me all the time. (Supervisee is an active subject, client is in the question, but "all the time" is too broad.)
(3) I want to know when and why this patient confuses me during our talks. (Specific subject, situation, and interpersonal dynamics are clear.)

In the next scenario, the presenter begins with the question "What do I do about it?" This question also is too vague and lacks a direct object. With help, she or he modifies the question to provide more direction to the supervision work:

(1) I respond with anger. How can I change this? (The subject and his or her feelings are clear, but the reasons for this anger, and the direction of change is still unclear.)
(2) I respond with anger when he tells me how he treats his wife and children. How can I be more empathic? (The subject, the situation, and the direction of change are clarified.)

This clarity is necessary to begin the discussion. However, during the supervision session the supervisee may become aware of other, previously unknown aspects of the case and his or her response, and appreciates new perspectives on the case. This requires the supervisor to regularly ask if the supervision question is still valid and reflects the concerns of the presenter. If necessary, the supervisee may be helped to reformulate the question with help from the supervisor and other group members.

It is critical that the supervisor devotes sufficient time to this round, as the supervision question guides the rest of the supervision sequence. It is the rail along which the supervision proceeds. The length of the case presentation may vary. What really matters is that the group and case presenter have a clear idea of the supervision question.

Round 3: Questions for clarification

After the presentation, the other supervisees are invited to ask questions about the case. Their instruction is clear: They are only to ask questions that help them better understand the case. These questions are then answered by the case presenter. This round ends when the supervisees have asked enough questions to be able to identify with the client. At regular intervals, the supervisor monitors this by asking, "Do you have sufficient information to identify with the client?" If not, supervisees continue to ask their questions. Once they believe they have the necessary information, the session moves on to the next round.

During Round 3, the supervisor ensures that only questions that require factual answers are asked. Supervisees' questions often contain their interpretations. For example, a member makes an assumption and asks, "What kind of psychiatric disorders exist in the family?" instead of "Are there any kind of psychiatric disorders in the family?" Group members also often ask questions that actually are suggestions. For example, the question "Should he not go into couples therapy instead of individual therapy?" could be reformulated as "What kind of support is being given to him?" or "Has the appropriateness of the current intervention been evaluated?"

The importance of reformulating questions cannot be overstated. A supervisee might ask of the presenter, "Why have you not considered calling in the child welfare social worker?" Although this question may at first glance appear neutral, it reveals condemnation of the case presenter. With the supervisor's encouragement, the supervisee rephrases the question as, "Has there been any contact between the client and other services?" If a member is unable to formulate a factual question, other group members are invited to offer suggestions to her or him.

Stage 4: Identification with the client

During this round, all group members identify with the client *as a person* while the case presenter attentively listens. The supervisor encourages group members to take time to reflect. She or he then encourages members to frame their responses as follows: "I am [name given to client], and I feel_____." Every participant expresses feelings evoked by the case presentation and questions. No comments are given at this point. When a group member finishes, another group member can start. He or she concentrates on feelings and is not allowed to discuss or complete another's answers since the complexities of the case mean that members may be hesitant and uncertain. When all group members have had a chance to express their feelings, the case presenter is invited to reflect on the question "What has struck you in these sequences?" The presenter explains to the group what she or he has learned from their reactions. The supervisor then asks the case presenter if the original supervision question remains valid or should be changed. This identification round can be very powerful, since strong feelings are evoked as members put themselves in the shoes of the client. Group members often get quite emotional. We often use techniques that help de-escalate tension and intense affect, such as changing chairs, walking around, or using an energizer like walking around and then freezing when the supervisor claps his or her hands.

During this round, the supervisor monitors the emotions that are being expressed. She or he attends to whether a full range of feelings is reflected and whether there are similarities and dissimilarities in the supervisees' responses. She or he also notes if there are any manifestations of collective countertransference. This happens if critical aspects of the case that are too emotionally laden are ignored by most or all of the supervisees. This was reflected in the collective countertransference described earlier in the second and third vignettes.

Round 5: Identification with the task and position of the case presenter

In this round, all participants identify with the role of the case presenter. The focus is not on her or him as a person, but rather on the position she or he is in and the task she or he has with respect to the client. The group members follow the same procedure as in the preceding round. For example, if the case presenter is a social worker, they start with the phrase "I am the social worker with [name patient] and I feel ___." With each profession, the statement changes accordingly.

In this round, the supervisor again pays attention to the diversity of feelings and encourages members to be honest with themselves and one another. The primary rationale for this round is that it minimizes the rifts that may develop in groups based upon professional status and the perceived hierarchy that often results. Supervisees can look beyond their own discipline, their culture, and professional positions. They learn to empathize and recognize their underlying similarities and differences.

This also is a difficult round, since supervisees are more comfortable providing solutions and suggestions—often under the guise of feelings—rather than expressing the feelings themselves. The supervisor must be prepared to intervene, helping members refocus their attention on feelings and reminding them that in the next round their attention will be directed toward identifying solutions. She or he can do this by providing a friendly reminder such as, "This is more a suggestion or solution; please save this for the next round."

In response, participants often reply with a comment like, "I feel stuck." However, this is not a feeling but a description of a situation. The supervisor can then ask, "How do you feel when you get stuck?" Hidden messages of disapproval also can emerge. One group member might say, "I feel I should have used EMDR," which is implicitly stating the case presenter should have used this method. The supervisor might then ask, "What do you feel in this position if you notice you have not used a potentially useful method?"

If group members focus on *feelings* in the position of the case presenter, group members generally demonstrate much empathy and understanding of the presenter's situation. Group members also realize they have been in the same position themselves and have experienced the same feelings. At the conclusion of this round, the case presenter reflects on the most significant elements of the case, based upon the discussion so far.

Often the case presenter reports feeling helpless, powerless, confusion, and alone or isolated in the first three rounds. After this round, they are surprised by the amount and quality of understanding and support they have received from their peers. All group members become more conscious of and more willing to acknowledge that they, too, have had moments of distress in their own professional careers. This empathic awareness produces a sense of equality and sets the stage for the next round, which depends on members feeling neither inferior nor superior to others.

Round 6: Supervision *with* the group

In this round, the group engages in a joint reflection of possible solutions based on the discussions generated in preceding rounds. The supervisor first verifies with the case presenter if the supervision question is still valid. If so, they engage in Round 6. If not, the supervision question is reformulated by the case presenter. Most of the time group members, having a more complete understanding through the preceding sequences, can assist with this, if needed. After this new formulation, they start with Round 6, a discussion in which all are free to offer their opinions about solutions. The case presenter actively participates as well. At the close of this discussion, the case presenter selects solutions relevant to him or her based on the supervision question.

In this round, the supervisor conducts the group in a manner referred to as "supervision with the group". Proctor distinguishes three forms of group supervision authoritative, participative and cooperative. (Proctor, 2008, p.32; Proctor 2000). *Authoritative* group supervision (in a group) is really nothing more than individual supervision by the supervisor in the context of a group. Group members sit and observe. In *participative* group supervision (with the group), the supervisor is "responsible for supervising and managing the group; also for inducing and facilitating supervisees as co-supervisors" (Proctor, 2000, p. 38). In *cooperative* group supervision, the supervisor "is a group facilitator and supervision monitor; supervisees also contract to actively co-supervise" (Proctor, 2000, p. 38).

In a newly formed group, the supervisor may rely upon participative group supervision with the group. As the group matures, with the assistance of the supervisor, she or he can rely more upon the solution-finding capacities of the members and gradually make a transition from supervision *with* the group to cooperative supervision *by* the group. In times of crises or when restructuring the group, she or he may need to return to the participative form of group supervision. The supervisor must be clear about which approach she or he selects. Authoritative group supervision is never advisable, since it is not empowering to members, nor does it promote peer learning. But when the group deviates from the agreed upon procedure, she or he can take authoritative action and correct in a non-intrusive way. The same applies if the group crosses boundaries of integrity and confidence.

The two identification rounds, Rounds 4 and 5, typically result in a more detailed and comprehensive and empathic understanding of the client and the case presenter. Furthermore, hierarchical and individual professional positions that can disrupt discussion and understanding are diminished, resulting in more egalitarian relations between members. During the sixth solution round, the supervisor monitors the discussion to ensure that these achievements are maintained. If she or he notices that supervisees' understanding of the case is compromised or the old unproductive positions reemerge, she or he redirects the group's attention to outcomes of the previous rounds.

The supervisor must believe in and promote the self-help capacities of her or his supervisees. After all the dialogue and reflections that have preceded this round, group members provide valuable insights. The case presenter ultimately decides what course of action she or he will take based upon the feedback received. There are times when the case presenter believes at the outset of this round that she or he has a solution, even before the discussion starts. This may result in a much shorter round, particularly when other supervisees express their agreement with the resolution. However, the supervisor should assess whether the presenter has come up with a realistic solution or has circumvented further reflection. If the supervisor believes the latter is the case, she or he encourages the group to suggest other options and invites the case presenter to reflect on these and consider them in addition to the strategy she or he developed.

The supervisor initially refrains from offering her or his own solutions. Our "first golden rule" is as follows: "Wait until you have heard all solutions of the group members; only add a solution of your own if this one has not been mentioned." Most of the time the supervisor's insights will have already been expressed by group members. Sometimes, the supervisor may think that the mutually agreed upon solution is unlikely to be successful. We do not interfere unless there is a threat of harm to the client; this is our "second golden rule." If our assumptions are incorrect, the supervisee will let us know this in the next session. However, if the agreed upon solution did not work, the case presenter will come back to the case and again reflect on why it went wrong and how to proceed.

Round 7: Conclusion

All participants share what the supervision session has meant for their own practice. This round tends to be brief, although group members usually report that they gained new insights relevant for their own practice. This discussion points out to all participants how much they have in common, regardless of discipline, title, position, cultural background, and work setting.

Frequently asked questions

We designed this identification round model to overcome frequently occurring difficulties in TIGS, such as professional confusion and strong emotional and countertransference reactions in Round 4. Round 5 aims at sharing feelings of helplessness and relieving feelings of isolation. It also facilitates a fraternal dialogue in the solution round. During our trainings students often ask the same questions about this method. Since our readers might have these questions as well, we answer the most common of these.

(1) Why identification rounds?

   It is important to help supervisees move beyond a focus on method and technique and appreciate the emotional aspects of the case for both the presenter and the client.

(2) Why factual questions?

   It is important for all supervisees to have a solid and comprehensive understanding of the case before they offer insights and suggestions.

(3) Why do you need one supervision question?

The supervisor assists the group in settling upon one question that serves as a guide and directs the ensuing conversation. The question also provides supervisees with a frame of reference and provides direction and structure to the discussion.

(4) Can the case presenter change the supervision question?

Yes, she or he can. This typically occurs during the questioning and identification rounds. These discussions assist the presenter in seeing the case in a new and different light, which, in turn, can lead to a refinement in the supervision question.

(5) Why identification with the client?

Typically, the presenter has only a limited insight into the client. In an earlier case scenario, the presenter, Heidi, demonstrated a restricted understanding of her client, which led her first to over-identify with him and later to distance herself from him. The presenter's ability to develop an appropriate intervention strategy—and other members' ability to learn from the case—depends upon acquiring a complete understanding of the client's emotional reactions and lived experiences.

(6) Why identification with the role and position of the case presenter?

The case presenter's feelings and reactions impact her or his work with the client. Until these reactions are discussed, she or he often feels alone, which undermines her or his work with the client. When members discuss these feelings, they appreciate their common experiences. It also helps the other team members remember similar feelings they may have had in their own practice. These shared emotions provide a necessary foundation for the solution round.

(7) Can other supervisees say anything?

Yes, they are encouraged to ask any questions and share any concern or insight that is relevant to the case, particularly during Round 3 (questioning), Round 4 (identification with the client), and Round 5 (identification with the case presenter). This ensures that, by the time the group moves into the solution round, all supervisees have the information they need to offer informed suggestions and solutions.

(8) Who decides on the applicability of the solutions?

The case presenter is the only one responsible for deciding upon a solution that she or he believes is appropriate for the case. There may be times when the supervisor offers additional insights, as noted previously. Typically, however, the presenter makes the decision and then follows through with it.

Intercultural trauma-informed supervision

Originally, we designed our supervision course for Dutch supervisors working with trauma helpers, counselors, and therapists working with Dutch clients who shared a similar cultural background with one another and with their clients. But when we transferred our supervision method to Berlin, it became clear that many of the supervisees worked in cross-cultural contexts where clients and supporters, but also mutual colleagues, had culturally different backgrounds, as described in our vignettes. A second reason to focus on the intercultural aspects was the result of the international application of this method. Over the past decade, the group and individual supervision models were implemented in many post-war and natural disaster areas like the Middle East, Iraq, Sri Lanka, India, the Democratic Republic of Congo, and Algeria. The full training was implemented as a postgraduate training in Georgia by the second author, and will be implemented in Iraq, Kurdistan, and Ukraine in the near future. Thus, an important new perspective was developed: *intercultural* trauma-informed supervision (Haans, Lansen, & Brummelhuis, 2007). We have expanded our method of group supervision so it can be modified to accommodate different cultural contexts. This application still offers supervisees opportunities to express themselves freely, to honestly reflect on the discussions that take place, and therefore to develop informed solutions.

Our perspective concurs with basic principles of intercultural counseling and supervision (Haans, 2008). In our training of supervisors, we emphasize the concept of "cultural empathy" (Chung & Bemak, 2002; Rudolph, 2005). The intercultural sensitive supervisor recognizes relevant cultural issues of supervisees and their clients. The supervisor "... must be sensitive to the world orientation of the supervisee, how he/she experiences her/himself in the surrounding culture, which includes the whole field of attitudes, values, and world visions" (Rudolph, 2005, p. 45; translated by the authors). The supervisor's intercultural competence requires her or him to engage in different communication and learning styles (Gupta & Kumar, 2007).

Since many of our German supervisors belong to the "majority culture," we also emphasize the appropriate use of power. Holloway (1995) distinguished expert power and legitimate power from referent power. Expert power is based upon the specialized knowledge and skills an individual is perceived to have. Legitimate power is derived from the legal or organizational status someone has. Referent power results from the supervision process itself, and develops as supervisor and supervisees "learn to know each other's values, attitudes, beliefs and actions" (Holloway, 1995, p. 32). Our approach depends upon the supervisor achieving referent power. In intercultural supervision, the supervisor's referent power derives from her or his willingness and ability to raise cultural issues directly. "Thus, it is the duty of supervisors to raise the issues of racial and ethnic difference, of expectations and fears" (Estrada, Wiggings Frame, & Braun Williams, 2004, p. 314). If the supervisor is unable to address or ignores these topics, supervisees go into "survival mode." This means that "supervisees withhold information… and the frequency and type of nondisclosures are likely to differ as a function of the supervision alliance" (Hird, Cavalieri, Dulko, Felice, & Ho, 2001, p. 123).

A valuable tool in intercultural supervision is self-disclosure by the supervisor (Haans, 2008). "Self-disclosures of vulnerability and struggle by an experienced mentor can be comforting to supervisees, providing a model by which supervisees can address their own biases and assumptions as they understand and integrate multiculturalism. Furthermore, self-disclosure by one who is perceived to have "arrived" also "illustrates the ongoing process of identity and multicultural development" (Hird et al., 2001, p. 122).

Contracting for trauma-informed group supervision

Before engaging in supervision, the supervisor establishes a contract between herself or himself and the group as a whole and with each individual group member. This contracting phase (including an explanation of the method) takes two to three meetings. For the group as a whole, the supervisor must ensure "clarity of purpose. … [T]he group needs to be clear about [the group's purpose], checking to see that expectations are realistic" (Hawkins & Shohet, 2000, p. 131). In the group as a whole, the supervisor helps members identify shared goals and questions supervisees want to address in supervision. The supervisor also identifies, with the group's help, what members do *not* want to address. The supervisor clarifies what the purpose of the supervision will be; this includes informing members it is not a form of therapy, even though members will discuss their affective reactions to their work. Boundaries among group supervision, countertransference responses that arise in supervision, and personal counseling are clearly described.

The supervisor introduces the identification round method, explains its rationale and how it works, and clarifies that everyone in the group will present cases on a regular basis. Group members must understand and be willing to adhere to the seven-round format and commit to active participation. The supervisor also clarifies that part of her or his responsibility is to monitor members' participation and help members join in the discussion and present cases if they have problems doing so. Confidentiality always is an important issue, and it must be clarified. Refugee and trauma workers often know one another from other regional or study meetings and conferences. That is why the boundaries of the supervision process must be clearly formulated and understood and adhered to by all. In many cases, the final agreement relevant to confidentiality mirrors that which exists between supervisees and their clients, particularly in group therapy (Breeskin, 2011).

Sometimes supervisees come with potential conflicts of interest due to their agency affiliation. For example, nurses from a ward of a psychiatric hospital may be in the same supervision group with staff from local government responsible for admitting refugees to the hospital and shelters. These conflicts do not preclude the participation of both participants, but the nature of the potential conflict must be clarified and its resolution options determined.

Finally, we discuss practical and financial issues like location and frequency of meetings, length of group supervision sessions, fees, and what to do in case of absences of supervisor or a supervisee. Participants sign a written agreement confirming their understanding of these requirements and conditions.

In some instances, potential group members express learning needs specific to their practice. The supervisor considers whether these are in line with group goals and procedures. If so, these can be appended to the group contract, which is then shared with and agreed to by all members. For the supervision group to be effective, there can be no hidden agendas, and everyone—members and supervisor alike—must have a shared understanding of what will happen in the group. Once agreement among all parties has been achieved, the supervision sequence can begin.

Discussion

In our vignettes, we described individual and collective countertransference and social and cultural issues that might hamper a fruitful supervision process. These issues also occur in individual supervision between supervisee and supervisor. In group supervision, these issues often manifest themselves through subgrouping. As our vignettes revealed, this dynamic can undermine the supervision group's effectiveness. Therefore, it needs to be dealt with in a constructive way (Gantt & Agazarian, 2017). This requires the supervisor to be knowledgeable about and skilled at managing group dynamics. Unfortunately, this is not typically the case. The purpose of addressing group dynamics is to promote a culture of mutual exchange where differences are recognized and valued, as we discussed previously. Our method of using identification rounds in group supervision invites and gently "forces" the group members to gain empathic understanding and wisdom about the clients and the position and feelings of their colleagues *before* jumping to solutions.

Trauma-informed group supervision following our identification round format is applicable in many contexts. In European refugee trauma work, supervisees often work in remote areas and in different shifts. Supervisees in non-Western countries often have unexpected transportation problems. In both cases, participants often can only attend irregularly. Our TIGS model is the same in every session, and all supervisees are familiar with it. Therefore, they can easily acclimate to a particular session and join in the discussion when they can be present. Our structured model of group supervision also has the advantage of being economical. Nongovernmental organizations (NGOs) in Western and non-Western countries usually lack sufficient financial resources to provide individual supervision to staff. In low-income nations, group supervision is often the only option, given the scarcity of resources and the challenges associated with supervisees being able to attend all sessions (Haans, 2008).

In addition to these practical advantages, trauma-informed group supervision offers supervisees a number of benefits (Lansen & Haans, 2004; Hawkins & Shohet, 2000; Proctor, 2008). The group provides a supportive atmosphere where supervisees feel validated. Group supervision promotes independence and provides participants with varied points of view and therefore enhances their learning. Supervisees' insights and comments refine and enhance how the supervisor, the presenter, and the group as a whole think about the case. Given the variety of experiences that supervisees bring to the group, empathy for both presenter and client is enhanced, as is understanding. Participation in group supervision provides supervisees with experience that assists them in facilitating groups for their clients.

Despite the practical and professional benefits associated with our structured group supervision model, there are limitations. Chief among these are the need for the supervisor to attend to group dynamics and the more limited time that each supervisee receives. To avoid the drawbacks and maximize the benefits, the authors argue that the supervisor must explicitly identify expectations for supervision and ensure participants' understanding of, and agreement with, the approach (Hawkins & Shohet, 2000). The supervisor also needs to attend to potential participants' appropriateness for the group format. Supervisees who may need more direction and support might not benefit from this format. The supervisor also must possess an understanding of basic group dynamics and be prepared to intervene. Each round follows a prescribed format that assists the supervisor in understanding and managing group dynamics. The identification and solution rounds are designed to encourage supervisees to respect and therefore learn from different points of view. The supervisor's task is to ensure that the basic requirements of each round are being met; this may require her or him to be firm and at times directive. However, she or he also must refrain from being viewed as the expert, instead encouraging members to take primary responsibility for identifying solutions. In those instances when group dynamics threaten to undermine participants' learning, the supervisor must intervene directly. This will be easier to accomplish if the supervisor has achieved referent, personal power, rather than relying upon expert or legitimate power.

Challenges and future directions

The influx of traumatized refugees into European countries and their presence in war and low-income countries around the world have placed enormous pressures on social agencies and the professionals and volunteers they employ. The unpredictable, often chaotic, nature of the work and the nature of the trauma clients have experienced lead to professional isolation and burnout. Professionals easily forget about themselves and focus solely on the welfare of their clients. Our model of supervision, which reaches many people at the same time and provides a supportive environment, is suited to respond to these realities.

However, the use of our trauma-informed group supervision model requires training and preparation, as the vignettes presented at the outset of this article reveal. It has taken both authors and our colleagues a considerable amount of time to become proficient with the method. Feedback from our supervisees and supervisors-in-training has helped us refine the model. Future efforts should be directed toward how to reach and prepare considerable numbers of supervisors from around the world in a timely and efficient fashion. Internet technologies might be helpful; we use Skype to consult with supervisors who have gone through our training. But in remote areas Internet access is often interrupted, or too slow, which causes much confusion even with supervisees we know.

We often apply this identification round supervision method with *teams* in organizations in which patient care is undermined and staff communication compromised. Many trauma institutes develop these kinds of destructive interactions due to the nature of the work (Knight, 2013; Pross & Schweitzer, 2010). Trauma teams typically are hierarchical, with some professionals, like psychiatrists and managing directors, at the top and others, like psychologists, nurses, social workers, and volunteers, in lower positions. Communication tends to be top down, and often there is a founding "father" or "mother" who arbitrarily uses his or her coercive power. There often is a strong resistance among team members to *openly* examine how they work together. Through the identification rounds found in TIGS, staff members have to challenge their fixed, narrow views of clients and become more aware and sensitive of the involvement and dedication of their colleagues. This diminishes stereotyping and increases team cohesion.

Although there is a great deal of research on individual supervision, far less exists on the use of the group modality (Milne & Reiser, 2012). Research on trauma-informed supervision, particularly in a group format, is largely nonexistent. At this point, our method is based solely upon our observations and experiences from conducting supervision groups and training supervisors. Our experience suggests to us that we have developed an approach to supervision that is widely applicable in different cultural and intercultural contexts and with a complete range of trauma survivors, including those with complex needs. The model does reflect findings regarding what constitutes effective clinical supervision (e.g., Milne, Sheikh, Pattison, & Wilkinson, 2011; Tohidian & Mui-Teng Quek, 2017). However, what is needed is research that specifically examines the use of our structured group supervision format with trauma therapists.

Despite these shortcomings, we have experienced great enthusiasm for the application of this method. We are grateful to all the students who have followed our courses internationally; their enthusiasm and critical feedback has allowed us to refine and adapt the model to their specific needs and context. We hope readers/supervisors who want to use this approach will send us their feedback also.

References

Balke, N. (2015). *Supervisions ausbildung.* Retrieved from http://www.bzfo.de/images/stories/pdf/supervision_2015-2017.pdf

Bergerand, R., & Quiros, L. (2014). Supervision for trauma-informed practice. *Traumatology*, 20, 296–301. doi:10.1037/h0099835

Bernard, J. M., & Goodyear, R. K. (1992). *Fundamentals of clinical supervision.* Boston, MA: Allyn and Bacon.

Breeskin, J. (2011). *Procedures and guidelines for group therapy: Detailed procedures and rules members of group therapy must adhere to.* Retrieved from http://www.apadivisions.org/division-49/publications/newsletter/group-psychologist/2011/04/group-procedures.aspx

Chung, R., & Bemak, F. (2002). The relationship of culture and empathy in cross-cultural counseling. *Journal of Counseling & Development*, 80, 154–159. doi:10.1002/j.1556-6678.2002.tb00178.x

Enyedy, K., Arcinue, F., Nijhawan Puri, N., Carter, J. W., Goodyear, R. K., & Getzelman, M. A. (2003). Hindering phenomena in group supervision: Implications for practice. *Professional Psychology: Research and Practice*, 34, 312–317. doi:10.1037/0735-7028.34.3.312

Estrada, D., Wiggings Frame, M., & Braun Williams, C. B. (2004). Cross cultural supervision: Guiding the conversation toward race and ethnicity. *Journal of Multicultural Counseling and Development*, 32, 307–319.

Gantt, S. P., & Agazarian, Y. M. (2017). Systems-centered group therapy. *International Journal of Group Psychotherapy*, 67(Suppl 1), S60–S70. doi:10.1080/00207284.2016.1218768

Gupta, N., & Kumar P. (2007). Issues in cross-cultural supervision: some examples from community work settings in Australia. *International Journal of Business Strategy*, 7, 3, 67–75

Gurris, N. (2005). *Stellvertretende traumatisierung und behandlungseffizienz in der therapeutische arbeit mit traumatisierten flüchtlingen* (Vicarious traumatization and treatment efficiency in the care of traumatized refugees) (Unpublished doctoral dissertation). Ulm, Germany: Ulm University.

Haans, T. (2008). Culturally sensitive supervision by expatriate professionals: Basic ingredients. *Intervention*, 6(2), 140–146. doi:10.1097/WTF.0b013e328307ecd4

Haans, T., Lansen, J., & Ten Brummelhuis, H. (2007). Clinical supervision and culture: A challenge in the treatment of persons traumatized by persecution and violence. In J. Wilson & B. Drozdek (Eds.), *Voices of trauma across cultures: Treatment of posttraumatic states in global perspective* (pp. 339–366). New York, NY: Springer.

Hawkins, P., & Shohet, R. (2000). *Supervision in the helping professions.* Philadelphia, PA: Open University Press.

Hird, J. S., Cavalieri, C. E., Dulko, J. P., Felice, A. D. F., & Ho, T. A. (2001). Visions and realities: Supervisee perspectives of multicultural supervision. *Journal of Multicultural Counseling and Development, 29*, 114–130. doi:10.1002/j.2161-1912.2001.tb00509.x

Holloway, E. L. (1995). *Clinical supervision: A systems approach.* Thousand Oaks, CA: Sage.

Kaduvettoor, T., O'Shaughnessy, Y., Clyde, B. M., & Weatherford, R. D. (2009). Helpful and hindering multicultural events in group supervision. *The Counseling Psychologist, 37*, 786–820. doi:10.1177/0011000009333984

Kiesler, D. J. (2001). Therapist countertransference: In search of common themes and empirical referents. *Journal of Clinical Psychology, 57*, 1053–1063. doi:10.1002/(ISSN)1097-4679

Knight, C. (2013). Indirect trauma: Implications for self-care, supervision, the organization, and the academic institution. *The Clinical Supervisor, 32*, 224–243.

Lansen, J., & Haans, A. H. M. (2004). Clinical supervision. In J. P. Wilson & B. Drozdek (Eds.), *Broken spirits* (pp. 317–354). Philadelphia, PA: Bruner/Mazel.

Milne, D., & Reiser, R. P. (2012). A rationale for evidence-based clinical supervision. *Journal of Contemporary Psychotherapy, 42*, 139–149. doi:10.1007/s10879-011-9199-8

Milne, D., Sheikh, A., Pattison, S., & Wilkinson, A. (2011). Evidence-based training for clinical supervisors: A systematic review of 11 controlled studies. *The Clinical Supervisor, 30*, 53–71. doi:10.1080/07325223.2011.564955

Proctor, B. (2000). *Group supervision. A guide to creative practice.* London: Sage.

Proctor, B. (2008. 2nd edition). *Group supervision. A guide to creative practice.* London: Sage.

Pross, C., & Schweitzer, S. (2010). The culture of organizations dealing with trauma: Sources of work-related stress and conflict. *Traumatology, 16*(4), 97–108. doi:10.1177/1534765610388301

Ray, D., & Altekruse, M. (2000). Effectiveness of group supervision versus combined group and individual supervision. *Counselor Education and Supervision, 40*, 19–30. doi:10.1002/ceas.2000.40.issue-1

Rudolph, V. (2005). Interkulturalität und ihre bedeutung für supervision (Interculturalism and its consequences for supervision). *Supervision, 3*, 36–52.

Salinsky, J. (2009). *A very short introduction to Balint groups.* Retrieved from http://balint.co.uk/about/introduction/

Smith, A. J. M. (2009). *Listening to trauma: Therapists' countertransference and long term effects related to trauma work.* Heemstede, Netherlands: Arq.

Strohmeier, H., & Scholte, W. (2015). Trauma-related mental health problems among national humanitarian staff: A systematic review of the literature. *European Journal of Psychotraumatology, 6*, 28541. doi:10.3402/ejpt.v6.28541

Tay, A., & Silove, D. (2017). The ADAPT model: Bridging the gap between psychosocial and individual responses to mass violence and refugee trauma. *Epidemiology and Psychiatric Sciences, 26*, 142–145. doi:10.1017/S2045796016000925

Tohidian, N. B., & Mui-Teng Quek, K. (2017). Processes that inform multicultural supervision: A qualitative meta-analysis. *Journal of Marital and Family Therapy, 43*, 573–590. doi:10.1111/jmft.12219

Valentino, L., LeBlanc, L., & Sellers, P. (2016). The benefits of group supervision and a recommended structure for implementation. *Behavior Analysis in Practice, 9*, 320–328. doi:10.1007/s40617-016-0138-8

Wilson, J. P., & Lindy, D. J. (Eds.). (1994). *Countertransference in the treatment of PTSD.* New York, NY: Guilford.

When religion hurts: Supervising cases of religious abuse

Craig S. Cashwell and Paula J. Swindle

ABSTRACT

Clients who present in therapy having experienced abuse at the hands of a religious leader or religious community present a unique set of challenges for a therapist. Therapists treating such cases benefit from trauma-informed supervision that recognizes the power of the sacred to support client care and their own professional development. In this article, we define religious abuse, explore nuanced challenges of working with clients who present as survivors of religious abuse, and discuss ways in which supervisors, operating within a trauma-informed framework, can best support supervisees working with cases of religious abuse.

Clients often present in therapy with a religious or spiritual worldview, and it is incumbent on the therapist to understand and honor the beliefs and experiences of each client (American Counseling Association [ACA], 2014; Cashwell & Watts, 2010; Council for the Accreditation of Counseling and Related Educational Programs [CACREP], 2016). The Association for Spiritual, Ethical, and Religious Values in Counseling (ASERVIC) developed and promoted competencies for integrating religion and spirituality in counseling that state, in part, that an effective therapist "... recognizes that the client's beliefs (or absence of beliefs) about spirituality and/or religion are central to his or her worldview and can influence psychosocial functioning" (Cashwell & Watts, 2010, p. 5), acknowledging implicitly that the effect on psychosocial functioning can be either positive or negative. The competencies make this point more explicit in referencing diagnoses, suggesting that the religiously and spiritually sensitive therapist "recognizes that the client's spiritual and/or religious perspectives can a) enhance well-being; b) contribute to client problems; and/or c) exacerbate symptoms" (Cashwell & Watts, 2010, p. 5), further elucidating that the effects of religion and spirituality can be either positive or negative.

Although most scholars have focused on how religion and spirituality can enhance psychological functioning, a growing body of scholars are addressing the potential deleterious effects of religion and spirituality when they are misused or become abusive (Cashwell & Young, 2011). In particular, scholars have begun to examine the psychological implications of *religious abuse* (Swindle, 2017; Ward, 2011; Wood & Conley, 2014), defined by Gubi and Jacobs (2009) as the act of an individual in a position of religious leadership/authority to gain power and control over individuals or collective groups. As is elucidated in this article, we extend Gubi and Jacobs' definition of religious abuse to include abuse perpetrated by groups of people (e.g., religious communities) as well as individuals.

Religious abuse is a form of betrayal trauma, trauma in which "the people or institutions on which a person depends for survival significantly violates that person's trust or well-being" (Freyd, 2008, p. 76). Betrayal trauma theorists suggest that the extent to which the betrayal comes from a close or trusted other impacts how the experience is encoded and recalled (Sivers, Schooler, & Freyd, 2002) and, accordingly, has implications for the treatment process. Most scholars of betrayal trauma, however, have focused on betrayal from family, friends, and coworkers, with limited attention given to religious leaders and communities or to the sacred element of abuse that occurs within a religious context. Although we assume religious abuse can occur within any religious tradition, we are most familiar with religious abuse within Christian traditions and draw heavily from that background. The purpose of this article, then, is to explain religious abuse and the power of the sacred, highlight the traumatic impact of religious abuse and frame the importance of trauma-informed care, characterize religious abuse as a form of betrayal trauma, and discuss the importance of trauma-informed supervision in cases of religious abuse.

Categories of religious abuse

Religious abuse includes mental, physical, sexual, and/or emotional abuse that occurs within a religious context or setting, with results that can be traumatizing to the individual (Swindle, 2017). Although scholars tend to focus on religious abuse by religious leaders (i.e., clergy) and, in particular, clergy sexual abuse of children (Pargament, Murray-Swank, & Mahoney, 2009), religious abuse also may occur when the perpetrator is not a clergy member. For this article, we focus on more common forms of religious abuse, but it also is important to be mindful that more extreme forms of religious abuse occur within cults.

It seems important to explicate that religious abuse may be classified within three broad categories: Abuse perpetrated by religious leaders, abuse perpetrated by a religious group or person representing a religious group, or abuse with a religious or spiritual component (Swindle, 2017). Examples of *abuse perpetrated by a religious leader* are sexual abuse by a member of the clergy or emotional manipulation to force a parishioner to contribute more money to the religious community than he or she can afford (Doyle, 2003, 2006; Farrell, 2004). Examples of *abuse perpetrated by a religious group* include experiences in a religious community that engages in gender discrimination, promotes systemic racism, or engages in *othering* members of the gay, lesbian, bisexual, transgender, and questioning (GLBTQ) community (Super & Jacobson, 2011; Wood & Conley, 2014), resulting in a "legitimized inequality" (Greene, 2013, p. 41). *Abuse with a religious or spiritual component* involves a direct connection of religious beliefs to the abuse itself (Swindle, 2017). Examples of this include a clergy member who pressures a woman to remain in an abusive marriage due to religious beliefs against divorce (Swindle, 2017), a domestic violence or marital rape situation in which the husband justifies abusive behaviors with religious beliefs (Simonič, Mandelj, & Novsak, 2013), or the justification of child physical or sexual abuse (Horton & Williamson, 1988) using sacred texts. It is important to understand that these categories are not mutually exclusive, and that experiences of religious abuse may fall into multiple categories (Swindle, 2017). For example, a religious community that supports a clergy member who refuses to marry an interracial couple due to his interpretation of scripture would be an example of all three categories.

Impact of religious abuse

Although the impact of religious abuse is like other types of mental, physical, sexual, or emotional abuse, the element of the sacred is a unique component, especially when viewed through the lens of betrayal trauma. It is critical for therapists to understand that common experiences of trauma, betrayal, stigma, and confusion have the potential to take on amplified meaning when attached to the sacred. For people who believe in God, harm done to them in the name of God or by a representative of God carries enormous weight and power (Farrell, 2004). Victims who have previously found meaning in their religious beliefs may now face an existential crisis due to the use of the sacred in the abuse, such as when a clergy member grooms a potential sexual partner by referring to her or him as *chosen*. Understanding the *meaning* of the experience for the client, then, becomes of paramount importance. For example, some clients may continue to believe that the abuse they experienced was ordained by God; in other words, they conflate the abuser with God. In addition, therapists must consider potential factors such as grieving the loss of an important spiritual/religious community, a crisis of faith or anger at God, or an amplified feeling of powerlessness in the face of the abuse.

Furthermore, victims of religious abuse may experience emotional trauma, including feelings of anger, fear, depression, and decreased self-worth

(Swindle, 2017). In addition, feelings of betrayal are common and may be directed at a wide variety of people. These may include both the abuser and the religious community who may have failed to recognize or stop the abuse, may not support the voice of the victim, and who may even protect the abuser and engage in victim-blaming. For example, this type of betrayal was described by victims of sexual abuse in the Catholic Church scandals, due to the systemic cover-ups and protection of clergy perpetrators (Doyle, 2003, 2006; Goldner, 2004; Guido, 2008; Rossetti, 1995). Other examples of betrayal trauma would be a gay man who feels betrayed by the church in which he was raised that rejected him after he disclosed his affectional orientation, or a woman seeking counsel who is instructed by her clergy member to return home to an abusive husband and is blamed for her abuse by being told that she should submit more fully to her husband to stop the abuse. This trauma may be amplified as the victims were betrayed by the sacred system they thought would comfort them, and where they likely expected protection, acceptance, and positive experiences. That is, while the extent to which the experience induces terror and fear is critical, so too is the relationship with the abuser (Freyd, 1996), to the point that a strong relationship with the abuser, as is common in cases of religious abuse, can result in less persistent memories of the event through denial, forgetting, or dissociation (Freyd, DePrince, & Zurbriggen, 2001), none of which help the victim work through the experience.

Also, it is common for victims to conflate God with their religious abuser, and many describe feeling betrayed or abandoned by God (Farrell, 2004; Redmond, 1996; Rossetti, 1995; Swindle, 2017). This type of betrayal also may be connected to feelings of powerlessness. If the abuse is perceived as coming from God by someone who believes in an omnipotent God, there is nothing more powerful (Farrell, 2004). The power differential present in every type of abuse may be even stronger in religious abuse, as victims may see their abuser as having the ultimate supernatural power, particularly when the religious abuse is at the hands of clergy, who often are granted spiritual authority in their religious community. If abusers have God on their side, what chance do victims have?

Religious abuse also commonly occasions feelings of stigma among victims. This stigma may be a result of the abuse (such as when a woman is ostracized or blamed by members of the religious community for a sexual affair with a clergy, despite the clergy member's grooming of the affair and abuse of power). In other cases, though, the stigma may be the abuse in and of itself, such as in cases of religious communities systematically discriminating based on race, gender, or sexual orientation (Greene, 2013; Wood & Conley, 2014).

Finally, clients also may describe a loss of their spiritual community or support systems because of the abuse. This can be voluntary (i.e., the individual chooses to leave an abusive environment) or involuntary (the system forces the individual out). Examples of this include women being told they cannot be a member of a church anymore if they leave an abusive marriage, or a church that revokes the membership of a woman who seeks ordination (Mohl, 2015; Swindle, 2017).

Counseling needs of religious abuse survivors

It is important for supervisors to guide supervisees in understanding some of the unique needs of clients who have experienced religious abuse. It is likely that this work must be trauma-informed, with specific interventions to address the trauma, while also incorporating the sacred element. Therapists need to be aware of the impact of the trauma when the source of the trauma is a spiritual authority or community, however, and how experiences of sacred betrayal or the conflation of their abuser with God can impact or block the trauma work. Counselors should not ignore the potential spiritual needs or confusion connected to the religious abuse, and should broach the topic of how the involvement of the sacred has contributed to the trauma. It is imperative that therapists create safety around discussions of spirituality. Counselors should not assume a spiritual crisis is at play, but should provide space in case their clients do wish to discuss this element, or need to address their spiritual trauma to address other aspects of trauma.

In fact, simply participating in religious activities and rituals may trigger a trauma response. For example, if the religious abuse involved sexual abuse from a member of a clergy, the client may be triggered when attending religious services or receiving an invitation to a family baptism service. If a woman was pressured by her religious system to remain in an abusive marriage, attending a wedding where the vows include rigid gender roles may evoke feelings of anger and/or cause flashbacks to the abuse. In some cultures, religious attendance is expected and is a vital aspect of socialization and community, so family members or friends may not understand the victim's desire to avoid religious services or events. For victims, feeling as though they are speaking ill of the church or God may elicit feelings of extreme guilt and confusion as they work through the trauma, and these feelings should be validated and explored in the therapeutic process. Specifically, therapists must help clients (a) own the experience as abuse and traumatizing, (b) work through the impact on belief systems, (c) grieve losses, and (d) address issues of support for the client, particularly in situations where the support of the religious community is lost. Although the grief process is not unique to religious abuse, what is different in such cases is the difficulty survivors have in owning the experience as abuse, holding others accountable, and addressing the impact on religious beliefs (Park, Currier, Harris, & Slattery, 2017)

Owning the experience as abuse/traumatizing

Because religious abuse is a form of betrayal trauma, or trauma at the hands of one charged with care of the individual, there are cases where memories of the experience may be diminished (Freyd et al., 2001). In some cases, then, the client may not have sufficient memory of the experience to present it to the therapist. This presents the challenge of a hidden trauma that may emerge only with a careful, thorough, and compassionate assessment of the client.

In other cases, however, clients remember the experience but do not define the experience as abusive or traumatizing, despite their trauma symptoms. That is, some clients do not connect the experience to their current difficulties. As one example, Tina, a married woman, presents in therapy because of an affair with a married clergy member that has been discovered and discussed openly in church meetings, using her name freely. She may present initially with anxiety or depression and discuss the stress of her "sins" being discussed openly within this community of support. Because she was not forcibly raped, she may view the affair as consensual. Through careful exploration with her therapist, however, she may begin to discover the ways in which the clergy member was grooming her for the affair when he began meeting with her to discuss her marital problems, as well as grow in an understanding of the power dynamics at play in the situation. Furthermore, once the client begins to see the experience as abusive (both from the clergy member and the religious community that publicly judged and shamed her, including some who blamed her for "seducing" the clergy member), a trauma lens for therapy begins to help the client look at her symptoms (anxiety, feeling sad, self-blame, mood swings, and difficulty concentrating) as a normal response to the trauma she experienced.

Working through impact on religious and spiritual beliefs

Clients who have experienced religious abuse may find themselves in a spiritual crisis or crisis of faith. If the counseling setting is secular, they may not know whether addressing issues of religion and spirituality will be supported. In contrast, if the counseling setting has a religious affiliation, clients may either be triggered by the religious connection or question whether a religiously affiliated therapist will negatively judge the crisis of faith. Therefore, it is important that the counselor is comfortable broaching issues of religion and spirituality and providing a space to work through issues of faith and belief without imposing an agenda. Clients who have conflated the abuse with God may benefit from processing the conflation during counseling and separating the abuse from other aspects of their spirituality. Some clients will no longer want anything to do with God or religion and need to process the grief and loss or potential feelings of guilt or internal conflict around this termination. In addition, some may find that leaving a religious system or rejecting religious beliefs becomes a source of conflict within their family or culture if their family and/or culture expects religious practice. Some clients may express confusion about their religious and/or spiritual identity, and need a safe space to explore what role religion or spirituality will continue to have for them, if any. The challenges for therapists of doing this type of work are described later, but it is vitally important that supervisors attend to the comfort level of counselors in addressing religious and spiritual issues.

Grief/loss

Connected to struggling with issues of belief/faith is the potential for clients to present with issues of grief and loss. Although grief is a common experience for all trauma survivors, there are some nuanced experiences of religious abuse survivors that warrant attention. For example, some clients may choose to exit the religious system in which the abuse occurred. Many of these clients may acknowledge the abuse and trauma they have experienced, yet still feel a connection to the community, so they may be ambivalent about leaving their religious community. Although some of these individuals may look for another religious community, others may exit religion altogether (Swindle, 2017). Still others may choose to remain in their religious community but be more guarded or less involved, such as only attending social events or choosing not to go unless a friend goes with them. Each of these choices may include feelings of loss and a grieving process of denial, anger/blame, bargaining, depression, and acceptance (Kübler-Ross & Kessler, 2003) that warrant therapeutic support.

Some may not have made the choice to leave the community, but rather were forced out by the religious system. Religious communities can be important support systems for their members, and this forced loss of support has the potential to be devastating for the client. This can create complicated grief work, where feelings of loss are intermingled with feelings of anger, self-blame, and guilt. Some also may grieve a loss of the spiritual. That is, if the experience of religious abuse has resulted in a change in religious beliefs, clients may grieve the loss of this spiritual connection or miss the comfort the beliefs once brought.

In all the potential types of grief resulting from religious abuse, it is important for the therapist to provide space to process the loss, and it may be very comforting for clients to hear the word *grief* named and attached to their experience, as well as working through the stages and tasks of grief. The loss of faith, religious community, and/or personal relationships may feel especially heavy due to the sacred element attached to the loss. For some, their religious community may have been a large part of their social support, or may have provided meaning to their lives. Supervisors also should be aware of the potential for therapists with an anti-religious sentiment to disenfranchise this grief process for clients because they do not understand the salience of the religious community in the client's life. Similarly, an anti-religious bias may appear in a therapist who urges a client to exit the religious system rather than processing with the client and allowing the client to make these decisions, or the therapist may not fully understand or appreciate the depth of meaning and comfort the client was receiving from these religious institutions and activities, resulting in a dismissive attitude toward the experience (Pargament, 2001).

Community/support

People who have experienced religious abuse, especially those who experienced grief/loss, may find great comfort in seeking out new community (Swindle, 2017), which may come in the form of family or friends, a new religious community, or a support group. In some cases, family and friends can be a source of support and acceptance, and lessen the sting of betrayal. In other cases, however, family members and close friends may align with the religious community against the client, resulting in an additional layer of betrayal and loss.

It may be therapeutic for some clients to have a corrective experience in a religious setting where they experience a non-abusive community, while other clients may need support in their decision to leave organized religion temporarily or permanently as part of their healing. Others may find support in a therapy group or social activities that provide comfort and remind clients they are not alone. There are many ways clients may build community or support, and this is a common need for a survivor of religious abuse (Houck-Loomis, 2012).

Empowerment

Dynamics of power are present in any abuse situation and, accordingly, the experience of powerlessness or lack of control often are key aspects of trauma and trauma recovery. This power differential may feel amplified in cases of religious abuse due to the element of the sacred. Those who connect with strong religious beliefs often see God, or those who represent God, as the most powerful being or force imaginable, so those who feel they have been abused by God or in the name of God may feel the ultimate powerlessness (Berger & Quiros, 2016; Farrell, 2004). Even where there is not conflation with God, religious leaders often are elevated within their community such that the survivor can experience a strong power differential with the abuse perpetrator.

Challenges for therapists

Clients who present with issues of religious abuse may present unique challenges for therapists and their supervisors. Some therapists may not even assess for religion/spirituality in their clients (Cashwell et al., 2013) and, therefore, may miss the sacred element of the abuse, conceptualizing it as any other interpersonal trauma. Although religious abuse shares similarities with other types of trauma, for many clients there will be important nuances to their experience that could be missed by a therapist who is insensitive to religious and spiritual issues. Supervisors should be monitoring that their supervisees are assessing all developmental and cultural issues with clients, including client religion/spirituality, and assessing that supervisees can broach topics of religion.

The reluctance to broach or assess for religion or spirituality may be due to a therapist's fear of values imposition (Cashwell et al., 2016). Religion is powerful and personal and can create strong emotional reactions for both therapist and client. Consequently, discussions of religion can be difficult. In addition, some clients may be reticent to discuss their religious beliefs and experiences out of fear of therapist judgment (Worthington, 1988). Accordingly, client and therapist can implicitly collude in avoiding this critical content. For example, a client who feels deep shame about having an affair, compounded by being publicly shamed within her religious community by being required by church leadership to publicly confess her transgressions in detail, meets with a therapist who is disdainful of organized religion. The therapist acknowledges that religious abuse occurred, but does so in a way that is critical of the religious community without processing with the client the impact of this series of events, which shuts down client exploration. This example highlights how the personal biases of well-intentioned therapists can undermine full exploration, processing, and working through of issues related to religious and spiritual issues. In these instances, often therapists want to talk rather than listen and explain rather than explore. In the example above, given the level of shame the client was experiencing, it is likely that this therapist's approach would prevent further processing of the religious abuse.

Reluctance to discuss issues of religion may show up in the supervision relationship in a similar fashion or as a parallel process. Accordingly, supervisors also should be willing to broach the topic of religion/spirituality with supervisees and continually assess for their supervisees' comfort level in addressing these issues with clients. Supervision should be a safe place for counselors to process their own reactions and fears of imposing personal religious values.

Cases of religious abuse may elicit strong emotional reactions in the therapist, including the desire to defend God or religion among those who are religious, or feelings of anger or contempt among those who have their own negative experiences with organized religion. Therapists who treat clients with experiences of religious abuse also may feel confused about how to assess for and/or provide services due to the lack of research and guidance available on this topic (Ward, 2011). Due to the potential of these strong emotions and uncertainty about the best treatment, some therapists may be inclined to be more directive than is typical for them, even to the point of imposing values. It is critical for therapists to recognize how their own reactions may impact the therapeutic process, and to avoid a directive approach to therapy that could recapitulate the powerlessness already being experienced by the client. Accordingly, it is important to empower clients around the course of therapy and decisions related to their religious community rather than the therapists inserting their own experiences, personal beliefs, and assumptions about what is best for the client. Co-constructing the goals and tasks of therapy with an emphasis on deep respect and empowerment of the client ensures that this negative recapitulation of powerlessness does not occur (Giordano & Cashwell, 2012).

Therapist awareness of how the topic of religious abuse may stir up strong reactions, both within the client and the therapist, is critical to foster and maintain client autonomy. It is important in the treatment of religious abuse that the client feel empowered to set her or his own goals and direction for the therapy. Therapists should not make assumptions about what the client wants. For example, if the client is still attending the religious community in which the abuse occurred or is occurring, the counselor should not assume the client wants to work on leaving this system or direct the client to leave the system, but rather let the client direct the goal. The client may have many reasons for staying in this system, and may instead be seeking help with coping skills to remain in the system. Therapists may need to be reminded by supervisors of the importance of client autonomy, and may benefit from guidance to theoretical approaches/techniques such as Motivational Interviewing (Miller & Rollnick, 2012) to empower the client.

Despite efforts to maintain client autonomy, issues of religious abuse can present unique ethical challenges related to values imposition. For example, a therapist may have a client who was a longtime participant in a religious community until he disclosed his identity as a gay man. After the disclosure, church members ridiculed him and several beat him physically, saying they were driving out the demons that were making him gay. In an angry tone, this client declares in therapy that he is choosing to discontinue all religious and spiritual activity, including any personal spiritual practices. The therapist may genuinely believe that it would be therapeutic for the client to have a corrective experience by attending a church in his local community that is affirming of his sexual orientation. At the same time, introducing this idea may invalidate the client's choice to discontinue religious participation and disempower the client. This situation presents an opportunity for the therapist to consider whether introducing the idea of a different religious community is offering a possible support or imposing values. There are no easy answers to questions like this, and supervision provides a critical place for discussing such issues and keeping at the forefront of the discussion that client autonomy and empowerment are hallmarks of trauma-informed care. Supervision can be a place to explore whether counselors' desires to offer the option of a GLBTQ-friendly religious community is motivated by their own religious beliefs and values of the importance of religious community, or whether it might be an appropriate therapeutic intervention. Supervisors can model broaching issues of spirituality and creating a safe space to examine intricate nuances, emotions, and reactions related to religious abuse.

Implications for supervisors

When supervisees encounter cases of religious abuse, supervisors play a critical role in the well-being of both the supervisees and their clients. All the challenges faced by therapists discussed thus far in this article apply to supervisors as well, so supervisors need to engage in self-reflection and consultation when supervising cases of religious abuse. Just as a heavily biased and emotionally reactive therapist can do damage, so too can a supervisor harm both the supervisee and the client with strong biases, emotional reactions, and the imposition of personal values.

The potential tasks of the supervisor may be many, and careful assessment and conceptualization is important to work with intention. Although supervision strategies will be tailored to the unique needs of each supervisee, common focal points will be attending to the supervisory working alliance, attuning to supervisee needs, processing supervisee personal beliefs and experiences with organized religion, assessing supervisee vulnerabilities and resilience, modeling effective broaching, attending to supervisee emotionality, supporting supervisee bracketing, and addressing issues of transference and countertransference (Spero, 1994), resistance (Kehoe & Gutheil, 1984), and parallel process (Wells, Trad, & Alves, 2003), which are common in cases of therapy for religious abuse.

Attending to the supervisory working alliance

The supervisory working alliance (Bordin, 1983) is critical to effective trauma-informed supervision for cases of religious abuse and appears to be a protective factor for therapist experiences of vicarious trauma (Williams, Helm, & Clemens, 2012). In addition to the agreement on goals, tasks, and bond originally explicated by Bordin, it may be critical for the supervisor to discern the style of supervision warranted in each case. Friedlander and Ward (1984) identified three different supervisor styles: Attractive, Interpersonally Sensitive, and Task-Oriented. Supportiveness and friendliness characterize the collegial approach of the Attractive supervision style. Supervisors operating from the Interpersonally Sensitive Style are more relationship-oriented and might be characterized as therapeutic and invested. The Task-Oriented supervisor tends to be more goal-oriented, structured, and content (rather than process) focused. Although the developmental and experience level of the supervisee might dictate the extent to which a task-oriented approach might be needed (i.e., "What do I do in the next session?"), it is likely in cases of religious abuse that an effective supervisor will integrate aspects of the Attractive and Interpersonally Sensitive supervision styles to best meet the multifaceted needs of supervisees, particularly to create a sense of safety in discussing deeply personal religious and spiritual beliefs and experiences, and emotional reactions that may be occasioned by clients presenting with religious abuse.

Berger and Quiros (2014) suggested that there are five components (i.e., safety, trustworthiness, choice, collaboration, and empowerment) of effective trauma-informed supervision, further highlighting the necessity of the more relational and supportive approaches to supervision. The supervisory relationship in cases of religious abuse must be characterized by trust, clear boundaries and expectations, nonjudgment, encouraging supervisee self-reflection, giving clear feedback in a noncritical manner, and being fully present (Quiros, Kay, & Montijo, 2013). Effective trauma-informed supervisors demonstrate modesty, cultural humility, and acknowledgment of their own limitations (Berger & Quiros, 2016), all potentially critical in cases of religious abuse where personal biases and emotional reactions by therapists are important. Given the lack of scholarly writing on religious abuse (Ward, 2011), supervisors can express their own lack of training or experience on the topic, normalize the challenges of working with this issue, and share any personal reactions to the religious abuse, thereby providing important modeling to the supervisee, particularly related to cultural humility and creating safe conversations.

Attuning to supervisee needs

As is explored throughout the remainder of this article, supervisees presenting a case of religious abuse, like other trauma cases, often have myriad and multiple needs for supervision (Berger & Quiros, 2016). Within the context of the supervisory working alliance, it is important that the supervisor attend and attune to what is most pressing for the individual supervisee in the present moment (Berger & Quiros, 2014). It is only through attuning to the supervisee's narrative, nonverbal behaviors and emotions that the supervisor can effectively discern and respond to the needs of each supervisee.

Processing supervisee beliefs and experiences with organized religion

Each supervisee has a personal narrative around religious experiences that impact how the supervisee hears and makes meaning of the client's story. Although supervisors should maintain clear boundaries to ensure that the line between supervision and counseling is not crossed, it likely is not possible to provide effective supervision in cases of religious abuse without understanding the supervisee's personal experience with organized religion and trauma history. For example, consider the case of a female client who has been ostracized by her church and highly religious family after leaving a physically abusive marriage. Because therapists have very different life experiences and perspectives on organized religion (Cashwell & Young, 2011), it is important for the supervisor to process with therapists how their experiences and perspectives may influence the therapeutic process. This situation may create a wide range of reactions among therapists, including the extremes of one who is highly religious and has had highly positive experiences with religious communities and considers divorce to be sinful, in contrast to a second therapist, who has a history of negative experiences in organized religion, views religion as creating an unhealthy atmosphere of judgment and oppression, and has a strong negative anti-religion bias, to more moderate reactions of a therapist who is deeply religious but does not believe divorce is sinful and becomes angry at those she believes are misrepresenting her God to her client.

Although these types of values conflicts are not entirely unique to cases of religious abuse, the occurrence of religious abuse may evoke strong feelings and make values imposition of greater concern. Each of the three therapists discussed in the previous paragraph has the potential to impose personal values on the vulnerable client, albeit in very different ways. Supervision, then, becomes a place to model exploring and processing these reactions by broaching the therapist's experiences with religion and how that might affect how the therapist is viewing the experiences of the client. For example, the supervisor might ask the following:

- "How are the experiences with religion described by your client similar to or different from your own experiences?"
- What does talking with this client bring up for you?
- How do you think that is impacting your work with this client?"

Supervisors might help create safety by modeling their own processing:

"When I hear this client talk about how that pastor treated her, I notice I feel very angry. I just think 'that's not right; that's not what my God would say about a husband abusing his wife!' But then I realize, it's not the therapist's role to defend God here, even if I want to. What is the role of the therapist here?"

This self-disclosure could help to create a safe supervision environment for therapists to acknowledge their own reactions and process how to manage these reactions, thus keeping the focus on the needs of the client.

Assessing supervisee vulnerabilities and resilience

When the supervisor is attuned to supervisees' needs and understands their perspective on and experiences with organized religion, the supervisor is better prepared to assess supervisees' unique vulnerabilities and resilience, which informs the supervisory process. For example, consider the client discussed earlier whose sexual relationship with a clergy member became public in the church. A therapist who is pro-religion and has a history in religious communities that tend to "deify" clergy (i.e., they are always in the right and above reproach) may fail to see the manipulation and grooming that occurred. In this lens, the sexual relationship is viewed as consensual, which may leave the therapist struggling to see the traumatic aspects of the grooming and manipulation, and the public humiliation of being outed within her primary community of support. Consider the following exchange between this therapist and his supervisor:

Supervisor (S'or): As I hear you talking about this challenging case, I think I hear you suggesting that the pastor and your client had a consensual affair. Is that right?

Supervisee (S'ee): [Defensive tone] Well, she's a grown-up and there was no force involved.

S'or: I agree that she is an adult and the pastor didn't use any physical force. Help me if I'm missing something here [qualifier used in an effort to reduce s'ee defensiveness], but it sounds like the pastor was meeting with your client for pastoral counseling, and that she was talking about relationships difficulties, including feeling unloved by her husband.

S'ee: Yes, that's right.

S'or: Where I'm struggling here is that it seems like he had a counseling role with her, that she was in a very vulnerable position. If that is true [qualifier used to reduce s'ee defensiveness], I wonder if it was crossing professional boundaries to have a sexual relationship with her.

S'ee: [Silence as s'ee appears to be thinking]

S'or: I see you are really thinking this through. I am wondering what parts of your own experiences with religion might impact how you think this through.

This dialogue continues as the supervisee explores how his own narrative about religion and clergy influences how he thinks about this client and the abuse she experienced.

Modeling effective broaching

For many therapists, the topic of religion or spirituality is an uncommon topic of conversation. Indeed, many therapists do not broach the subject for fear of imposing values (Cashwell et al., 2013). In some cases, the religious abuse may be the primary presenting issue. In other instances, however, clients will present with other mental health concerns, such as anxiety or depression, but present the religious abuse secondarily, off-handedly, as if it is relatively unimportant or, in some cases, not present in the abuse at all. This may be because they do not recognize the experience as abusive and traumatic or they are trying to manage emotions related to the abuse experience (i.e., numbing; Horowitz, 2015). Because it is critical for the therapist to effectively broach topics of religion, spirituality, and religious abuse as appropriate to each case, with sensitivity to the worldview of the client (Cashwell & Watts, 2010), one important role for the supervisor is to model how to sensitively broach and engage in dialogue around topics of religion and spirituality.

Although most supervisors have the skill set to broach sensitive topics effectively, all supervisors must examine their own beliefs, values, and biases related to organized religion to recognize how their predilections could affect the supervision and, by extension, the therapy process. For example, if therapists are not comfortable with the general topic of religion, they may ask about religious affiliation in the intake, but not inquire further about salience or how clients' experiences in their religious community have been supportive or harmful. This omission could send the underlying message to the client that therapy is not the place to discuss religion or spirituality beyond the most basic identification. In addition, it may be necessary to remind supervisees to help clients explore religious beliefs and experiences rather than the therapist making assumptions.

For example, a therapist who identifies as Catholic notices that a client identifies as Catholic on intake paperwork. If the religious identity is salient for the client, this therapist will still want to explore what this means for the client rather than assuming they share the same beliefs, practices, and experiences. Supervisors also may guide supervisees in looking for places of how a similar background could be a place of connection and understanding, while still not assuming a shared experience. For example, it could be very therapeutic for a client who experienced childhood sexual abuse from a pastor to hear, "You know, in the church I grew up in, everyone treated the pastor almost like he was God, and nobody questioned him; nobody thought he could do anything wrong. I wonder if that was the case in your church and if that made it harder to tell someone what was going on?"

Attending to supervisee emotionality

Religion is a powerful topic that can evoke strong reactions. Because religion is intended to provide a safe haven for congregants, when treating cases of religious abuse, most therapists will experience an emotional reaction to the "abusive sanctuary." A devoutly religious counselor may have an emotional reaction of defensiveness, and may notice an urge to defend God or defend his faith, and run the risk of minimizing the client's experience and shutting down the therapeutic process. Conversely, a therapist who is anti-religion may have a very different reaction or way of imposing her own values, and may become angry, be highly critical of religion to the client, and encourage breaking all ties with this religious community, if not organized religion altogether. In addition, a therapist who has a personal history with religious abuse may be triggered and experience his own traumatic emotional reactions to the client's disclosure. Hearing experiences of religious abuse may bring up conflicting emotions or even a philosophical crisis of faith for the therapist. This discomfort could affect the therapeutic relationship with the client and lead the therapist to steer sessions away from the topic. Any of these reactions, driven by visceral emotional reactions of the therapist, can be harmful by not meeting clients where they are.

Accordingly, it is particularly critical for supervisors to attend to the nuanced emotional experiences of each supervisee (Tangen, 2017) in cases of religious abuse. Like other types of abuse, survivors of religious abuse may present with intense and complex emotions related to their betrayal trauma that may initially mirror pathology (Gómez, Lewis, Noll, Smidt, & Birrell, 2016), so it is critical to continually assess and develop the supervisee's capacity to experience multiple mixed emotions without becoming overwhelmed (Carsky & Yeomans, 2012; Lindquist & Barrett, 2008). (A detailed discussion of supervisee emotional awareness and complexity is beyond the scope of this article, but interested readers are encouraged to read Tangen [2017] for a comprehensive discussion of working with supervisee emotions.) Suffice it to say here that, in cases of religious abuse, supervision must be a safe place to process and work through personal emotional reactions to the religious abuse disclosed by the client so that the therapy session can focus solely on the needs of the client. One challenge for the supervisor in this process is how to balance validating the personal convictions of the supervisee with the ethical responsibilities of not imposing these beliefs on the client. To address this, a supervisor might engage in a role-play with the supervisee of "What do you really want to say to this client?" This approach allows therapists to process their own reactions, honor their own values and beliefs, and become clear about necessary boundaries to avoid values imposition.

Addressing transference, countertransference, and parallel process

In cases of religious abuse, there is the potential for many interpersonal processes to occur that can compromise the authenticity of either the therapy or the supervisory relationship. Because these dynamics may be unconscious, it is important for the supervisor to consider and explore these dynamics with the supervisee. For example, transference may occur in the therapeutic relationship when the client has a history of deferring to those in authority—whether spiritual authority or, in this instance, the therapist. Such transference requires the therapist to maintain a stance of empowering the client and championing the ethical principle of client autonomy, even as this may contradict the client's normal interactional pattern. Conversely, a client who is seeing a secular therapist may enter therapy with the projection that the therapist will be anti-religion or not understand her beliefs and experiences, and may be reticent to discuss issues related to the religious abuse. Such occurrences may require the therapist to explore client fears and issues of safety. This may include prompts such as, "It seems like you are reluctant to discuss religion with me. I wonder if you have been judged for this before, or if you worry about how I might react to this?"

Similarly, countertransference may occur in cases of religious abuse. Consider, for example, a therapist who holds a negative view of religion and has a sibling who is active in a community that the therapist considers a cult. The therapist has tried to discuss this with the sibling, but received a heated rebuke. A short time later, a client begins discussing her concerns about what she views as the "distorted theology" of her religious community, evoking in the therapist a strong emotional reaction. The supervisor notices the strong language in the case note (e.g., "perversion of religion," "mind control") and, in reviewing a recording of the session, the therapist's visceral reactions to this client. The supervisor gently inquires about how this client seems to be eliciting a different response from the supervisee than usual, and wonders aloud about whether the client reminds the supervisee of anyone, eliciting an exploration of the supervisee's relationship with her sibling, and an increased awareness from the supervisee about how countertransference is impeding the therapeutic process. Transference and countertransference also can be challenging when the therapist and client share religious beliefs (Peteet, 2009).

Finally, because religious abuse is a form of betrayal trauma that is inherently relational, both the therapeutic and supervisory relationships are important, as issues of parallel process may arise. One example occurs when both the client and the supervisee present as dependent on the therapist and supervisor, respectively, for how to move forward. That is, the client's anxious dependence on the therapist ("I don't know what to do!") is paralleled by the therapist's anxious dependence on the supervisor, reflecting an unconscious parallel process (Silberman, 2015). Another example occurs when the therapist, trapped in a "yes, but" interactional pattern with the client, unconsciously attempts to re-create this pattern in the supervisory relationship. In these instances, it is likely that "more is caught than taught" (Shulman, 2005, p. 24), as the supervisor models for the supervisee how to respond to this anxious dependent "other" or the "yes, but" pattern. In addition, supervisors can attend to parallel process by helping supervisees explore their trauma reactions to the client, including shock, anxiety, and ruminating about the client, thereby increasing supervisees' awareness of what the client might feel (Berger & Quiros, 2016).

Supporting supervisee bracketing

Finally, because issues of religious abuse may evoke strong emotional reactions and distorted relationships (e.g., transference, countertransference, and projection), it is important for the supervisor to support the supervisee to empower the client, prize autonomy, and avoid imposing values. Kocet and Herlihy (2014) introduced the concept of ethical bracketing. Drawn from qualitative research, where researchers must recognize and name their biases at the outset of the research so that the data are not contaminated by these biases, ethical bracketing refers to therapist awareness of biases and predilections, and the conscious and intentional setting aside of these so that client values and autonomy are honored in the therapeutic process. A safe supervisory relationship provides the perfect forum not only for exploration of biases, but also how these biases need to be bracketed to empower the client. Although this approach could be a helpful process in any supervisory relationship, it may be especially necessary and helpful when discussing issues of religion and spirituality, which form a core aspect of identity for some therapists. Even when therapists are properly trained to refrain from bringing their own experiences and biases into these topics with clients, a person's belief of religious matters can be extremely powerful and create reactions among the most ethical and highly trained therapists and supervisors. The intentional exercise of bracketing can be helpful in owning and honoring one's own beliefs while also focusing on the client's needs. While discussing the bracketing process in supervision, supervisors can acknowledge and validate the supervisees' right to hold their beliefs, their challenges in bracketing strongly held beliefs, and the primacy of empowerment and client autonomy in a trauma-informed approach (Berger & Quiros, 2014).

Conclusion

Cases of religious abuse can elicit strong emotional reactions and personal values from the therapist, and may present unique challenges from both a therapeutic and ethical perspective. Often, these clients present in therapy in highly vulnerable positions, having had their spiritual foundations compromised in some way by the abuse. Therapists charged with the care of these individuals face a myriad of relational, therapeutic, and ethical challenges that are best addressed within a framework of trauma-informed care that acknowledges the power of the sacred. Supervisors, also operating within a trauma-informed framework (Berger & Quiros, 2014), play a critical role in both client care and therapist development.

References

American Counseling Association. (2014). *2014 ACA code of ethics*. Retrieved from http://www.counseling.org/docs/ethics/2014-aca-code-of-ethics.pdf

Berger, R., & Quiros, L. (2014). Supervision for trauma-informed practice. *Traumatology, 20*, 296–301. doi:10.1037/h0099835

Berger, R., & Quiros, L. (2016). Best practices for training trauma-informed practitioners: Supervisors' voice. *Traumatology, 22*, 145–154. doi:10.1037/trm0000076

Bordin, E. S. (1983). A working alliance based model of supervision. *The Counseling Psychologist, 11*(1), 35–42. doi:10.1177/0011000083111007

Carsky, M., & Yeomans, F. (2012). Overwhelming patients and overwhelmed therapists. *Psychodynamic Psychiatry, 40*, 75–90. doi:10.1521/pdps.2012.40.1.75

Cashwell, C. S., & Watts, R. E. (2010). The new ASERVIC competencies for addressing spiritual and religious issues in counseling. *Counseling and Values, 55*, 2–5. doi:10.1002/(ISSN)2161-007X

Cashwell, C. S., & Young, J. S. (Eds.). (2011). *Integrating spirituality in counseling: A guide to competent practice* (2nd ed.). Alexandria, VA: American Counseling Association.

Cashwell, C. S., Young, J. S., Fulton, C., Willis, B. T., Giordano, A. L., Daniel, L. W.,… Welch, M. (2013). Clinical behaviors for addressing religious/spiritual issues: Do we "practice what we preach"? *Counseling and Values, 58*, 45–58. doi:10.1002/cvj.2013.58.issue-1

Cashwell, C. S., Young, J. S., Tangen, J. L., Pope, A. L., Wagener, A., Sylvestro, H., & Henson, R. A. (2016). Who is this God of whom you speak? Counseling students' concept of God. *Counseling and Values, 61*, 159–175. doi:10.1002/cvj.2016.61.issue-2

Council for the Accreditation of Counseling and Related Educational Programs. (2016). *2016 CACREP standards*. Retrieved from http://www.cacrep.org/wp-content/uploads/2016/02/2016-Standards-with-Glossary-rev-2.2016.pdf

Doyle, T. (2003). Roman Catholic clericalism, religious duress, and clergy sex abuse. *Pastoral Psychology*, *51*, 189–231. doi:10.1023/A:1021301407104

Doyle, T. P. (2006). Clericalism: Enabler of clergy sexual abuse. *Pastoral Psychology*, *54*, 189–213. doi:10.1007/s11089-006-6323-x

Farrell, D. (2004). An historical viewpoint of sexual abuse perpetrated by clergy and religious. *Journal of Religion & Abuse*, *6*, 41–80. doi:10.1300/J154v06n02_04

Freyd, J. J. (1996). *Betrayal trauma: The logic of forgetting childhood abuse*. Cambridge, MA: Harvard University Press.

Freyd, J. J. (2008). Betrayal trauma. In G. Reyes, J. D. Elhai, & J. D. Ford (Eds.), *Encyclopedia of psychological trauma* (pp. 76). New York, NY: Wiley.

Freyd, J. J., DePrince, A. P., & Zurbriggen, E. L. (2001). Self-reported memory for abuse depends upon victim-perpetrator relationship. *Journal of Trauma & Dissociation*, *2*, 5–15. doi:10.1300/J229v02n03_02

Friedlander, M. L., & Ward, L. G. (1984). Development and validation of the Supervisory Styles Inventory. *Journal of Counseling Psychology*, *31*, 541–557. doi:10.1037/0022-0167.31.4.541

Giordano, A. L., & Cashwell, C. S. (2012). Entering the sacred: Using motivational interviewing to address spirituality in counseling. *Counseling and Values*, *59*, 65–79. doi:10.1002/j.2161-007X.2014.00042.x

Goldner, V. (2004). Introduction: The sexual-abuse crisis and the Catholic church: Gender, sexuality, power and discourse. *Studies in Gender and Sexuality*, *5*, 1–9. doi:10.1080/15240650509349237

Gómez, J. M., Lewis, J. K., Noll, L. K., Smidt, A. M., & Birrell, P. J. (2016). Shifting the focus: Nonpathologizing approaches to healing from betrayal trauma through an emphasis on relational care. *Journal of Trauma & Dissociation*, *17*, 165–185. doi:10.1080/15299732.2016.1103104

Greene, B. (2013). The use and abuse of religious beliefs in dividing and conquering between socially marginalized groups: The same-sex marriage debate. *Psychology of Sexual Orientation and Gender Diversity*, *1*, 35–44. doi:10.1037/2329-0382.1.S.35

Gubi, P. M., & Jacobs, R. (2009). Exploring the impact on counsellors of working with spiritually abused clients. *Mental Health, Religion & Culture*, *12*, 191–204. doi:10.1080/13674670802441509

Guido, J. (2008). A unique betrayal: Clergy sexual abuse in the context of the Catholic religious tradition. *Journal of Child Sexual Abuse*, *17*, 255–269. doi:10.1080/10538710802329775

Horowitz, M. J. (2015). Effects of trauma on sense of self. *Journal of Loss and Trauma*, *20*, 189–193. doi:10.1080/15325024.2014.897578

Horton, A. L., & Williamson, J. A. (1988). *Abuse and religion: When praying isn't enough*. Lexington, MA: D. C. Heath.

Houck-Loomis, T. (2012). Good God?!? Lamentations as a model for mourning the loss of the good God. *Journal of Religion and Health*, *51*, 701–708. doi:10.1007/s10943-012-9581-1

Kehoe, N., & Gutheil, T. G. (1984). Shared religious belief as resistance in psychotherapy. *American Journal of Psychotherapy*, *38*, 579–585.

Kocet, M. M., & Herlihy, B. J. (2014). Addressing value-based conflicts within the counseling relationship: A decision-making model. *Journal of Counseling & Development*, *92*, 180–186. doi:10.1002/jcad.2014.92.issue-2

Kübler-Ross, E., & Kessler, D. (2003). *On death and dying: What the dying have to teach doctors, nurses, clergy and their own families*. New York, NY: Scribner.

Lindquist, K. A., & Barrett, L. F. (2008). Emotional complexity. In M. Lewis, J. M. Haviland-Jones, & L. F. Barrett (Eds.), *Handbook of emotions* (3rd ed., pp. 513–530). New York, NY: Guilford Press.

Miller, W. R., & Rollnick, S. (2012). *Motivational interviewing: Helping people change* (3rd ed.). New York, NY: Guilford Press.

Mohl, A. S. (2015). Monotheism: Its influence on patriarchy and misogyny. *The Journal of Psychohistory, 43,* 2–20.

Pargament, K. I. (2001). *The psychology of religion and coping.* New York, NY: Guilford Press.

Pargament, K. I., Murray-Swank, N. A., & Mahoney, A. (2009). Problem and solution: The spiritual dimension of clergy sexual abuse and its impact on survivors. In R. A. McMackin, T. M. Keane, & P. M. Kline (Eds.), *Understanding the impact of clergy sexual abuse: Betrayal and recovery* (pp. 200–223). New York, NY: Routledge.

Park, C. L., Currier, J. M., Harris, J. I., & Slattery, J. M. (2017). The intersection of religion/spirituality and trauma. In C. L.Park, J. M. Currier, J. I. Harris, & J. M. Slattery (Eds.), *Trauma, meaning, and spirituality: Translating research into clinical practice* (pp. 3–14). Washington, DC: American Psychological Association.

Peteet, J. R. (2009). Struggles with God: Transference and religious countertransference in the treatment of a trauma survivor. *The Journal of the American Academy of Psychoanalysis and Dynamic Psychiatry, 37,* 165–174. doi:10.1521/jaap.2009.37.1.165

Quiros, L., Kay, L., & Montijo, A. M. (2013). Creating emotional safety in the classroom and in the field. *Reflections: Narratives of Professional Healing, 18,* 39–44.

Redmond, S. A. (1996). God died and nobody gave a funeral. *Pastoral Psychology, 45,* 41–47. doi:10.1007/BF02251408

Rossetti, S. J. (1995). The impact of child sexual abuse on attitudes toward God and the Catholic church. *Child Abuse & Neglect, 19,* 1469–1481. doi:10.1016/0145-2134(95)00100-1

Shulman, L. (2005). The clinical supervisor-practitioner working alliance: A parallel process. *The Clinical Supervisor, 24*(1–2), 23–47. doi:10.1300/J001v24n01_03

Silberman, E. K. (2015). Parallel process and the evolving view of the therapeutic situation. *Psychiatry: Interpersonal and Biological Processes, 78,* 239–241. doi:10.1080/00332747.2015.1069649

Simonič, B., Mandelj, T. R., & Novsak, R. (2013). Religious-related abuse in the family. *Journal of Family Violence, 28,* 339–349. doi:10.1007/s10896-013-9508-y

Sivers, H., Schooler, J., & Freyd, J. J. (2002). Recovered memories. In V. S. Ramachandran (Ed.), *Encyclopedia of the human brain* (vol. 4, pp. 169–184). San Diego, CA: Academic Press.

Spero, M. H. (1994). Religious patients' metaphors in the light of transference and countertransference considerations. *Israel Journal of Psychiatry and Related Sciences, 31,* 145–161.

Super, J. T., & Jacobson, L. (2011). Religious abuse: Implications for counseling lesbian, gay, bisexual, and transgender individuals. *Journal of LGBT Issues in Counseling, 5,* 180–196. doi:10.1080/15538605.2011.632739

Swindle, P. J. (2017). *A twisting of the sacred: The lived experience of religious abuse* (Doctoral dissertation). Retrieved fromProQuest. (12186)

Tangen, J. L. (2017). Attending to nuanced emotions: Fostering supervisees' emotional awareness and complexity. *Counselor Education and Supervision, 56,* 65–78. doi:10.1002/ceas.12060

Ward, D. J. (2011). The lived experience of spiritual abuse. *Mental Health, Religion & Culture, 14,* 899–915. doi:10.1080/13674676.2010.536206

Wells, M., Trad, A., & Alves, M. (2003). Training beginning supervisors working with new trauma therapists: A relational model of supervision. *Journal of College Student Psychotherapy, 17,* 19–39. doi:10.1300/J035v17n03_03

Williams, A. M., Helm, H. M., & Clemens, E. V. (2012). The effect of childhood trauma, personal wellness, supervisory working alliance, and organizational factors on vicarious traumatization. *Journal of Mental Health Counseling, 34*, 133–153. doi:10.17744/mehc.34.2. j3l62k872325h583

Wood, A. W., & Conley, A. H. (2014). Loss of religious or spiritual identities among the LGBT population. *Counseling and Values, 59*, 95–111. doi:10.1002/cvj.2014.59.issue-1

Worthington, E. L. (1988). Understanding the values of religious clients: A model and its application to counseling. *Journal of Counseling Psychology, 35*, 166–174. doi:10.1037/0022-0167.35.2.166

Attending to racial trauma in clinical supervision: Enhancing client and supervisee outcomes

Alex L. Pieterse

ABSTRACT

This article is focused on racial trauma as a psychological outcome associated with experiences of racism. Guidelines for clinical intervention are presented and the role of the clinical supervisor is discussed, both as it relates to the therapy treatment and the process of supervision.

> … but our phrasing—race relations, racial chasm, racial justice, racial profiling, white privilege, even white supremacy—serves to obscure that racism is a visceral experience that dislodges brains, blocks airways…
>
> —Ta-Nehisi Coates, *Between the World and Me*

Clinical supervision is thought to serve two primary goals—increased supervisee competence (Westefeld, 2009) and the enhancement of psychotherapy outcomes (O'Donovan, Halford, & Walters, 2011). Reviews of the supervision outcome literature provide support for the role of clinical supervision in facilitating greater supervisee and trainee competence, including greater self-awareness, self-efficacy, improvement in therapy skills, and greater integration of theoretical orientation (Wheeler & Richards, 2007). Although research examining the relationship between clinical supervision and client outcome is less conclusive (Watkins, 2011), there is emerging evidence to suggest that, under certain conditions (e.g., type of therapy), client outcomes improve when the clinician is engaged in clinical supervision (Bambling, King, Raue, Schweitzer, & Lambert, 2006).

If improved client outcome and enhanced supervisee skills are indeed the primary goals of clinical supervision (Wheeler & Richards, 2007), then it becomes important to examine contextual factors that might influence the nature and quality of the supervisory relationship (Gatmon, Jackson, Koshkarian, & Martos-Perry, 2001). One contextual factor noted to have a direct bearing on the supervisory relationship is racial group membership and related constructs such as racism and racial trauma (Constantine & Sue, 2007; Jernigan,

Green, Helms, Perez-Gualdron, & Henze, 2010; Tummala-Narra, 2004). Racism, defined as an ideology of racial superiority, accompanied by prejudicial and discriminatory behavior in three domains (individual, institutional, and cultural), continues to be a ubiquitous and pervasive aspect of American life (Feagin, 2014; Hemmings & Evans, 2018). Within the field of mental health, much has been written about the need to understand the psychological impact of racism, and the need to attend to race as an important variable in counseling and psychotherapy (e.g., Miller & Garran, 2017; Thompson & Neville, 1998). The supervision literature has also highlighted the need to be attentive to race-related factors within the supervisory relationship (e.g., Chang, Hays, & Shoffner, 2004), with experiencing racism within the supervisory process/relationship now being understood as a type of harmful supervision (Ellis et al., 2014). Given the growing appreciation of the negative psychological outcomes associated with experiences of racism (Pieterse & Powell, 2016), the current discussion focuses on how racial trauma is an outcome of racism. First, an overview of racial trauma is presented, followed by a set of guidelines that supervisors can use in facilitating an effective clinical response to racial trauma. The discussion will conclude by describing approaches to reducing the possibility of racial trauma occurring within the supervisory process.

Racial trauma and supervision

Racial trauma

In powerful prose, Ta-Nehisi Coates (2015) at the beginning of this discussion reminds us of the power of racism on individual lives. Indeed, his comment, drawn from his autobiographical discussion of race in America, has been supported by a substantial body of empirical literature establishing a positive relationship between experiences of racism, psychological distress, and adverse health outcomes (e.g., Carter, Lau, Johnson, & Kirkinis, 2017; Paradies et al., 2015). In seeking to further understand the more specific effects of racism, racial trauma has emerged as an important area of focus (Carter, 2007).

Simply stated, racial trauma, otherwise referred to as race-based traumatic stress, is understood to be the emotional and psychological response to racial incidents that are unexpected, experienced as threatening, and result in significant psychological stress (Carter, 2007; Comas- Diaz, 2016; Bryant-Davis & Ocampo, 2006). More specifically, Bryant-Davis (2007) outlined the breadth of racial trauma by identifying the following elements:

a) an emotional injury that is motivated by hate or fear of a person or group of people as a result of their race; b) a racially motivated stressor that overwhelms a person's capacity to cope; c) a racially motivated, interpersonal severe stressor that causes bodily harm or threatens one's life integrity; or d) a severe interpersonal or institutional stressor motivated by racism that causes fear, helplessness or horror. (p. 135)

In keeping with the widely accepted definition of racism as including individual, cultural, and institutional components (Feagin, 2014), racial trauma, unlike more traditional notions of trauma, incorporates stressors that are associated with an individual's membership in a racial group and the status of that group within society. Furthermore, experiences of racism associated with trauma symptoms do not necessarily have to be experienced as life-threatening. In Carter, Forsyth, Mazulla, and Williams' seminal 2005 study that laid the groundwork for the Race-Based Traumatic Stress Symptom Scale (RBTSSS; Carter et al., 2013), racial incidents that participants identified as being associated with trauma symptoms included such categories as having a hostile work environment, experiencing verbal assaults, being denied access or service, and being racially profiled. It is important to note that, unlike typical incidents associated with traumatic stress (e.g., acts of physical violence, threats of harm to one's self, natural disasters, sexual, verbal, and emotional abuse), racial incidents associated with racial trauma are predicated on an individual belonging to a specific racial group. Simply stated, one is denied service or accused of criminal activity, not based on the merits or characteristics of oneself as an individual, but based on one's perceived membership in a particular racial group. As such, the emotional responses to racial incidents that have been noted to be reflective of trauma (Carter et al., 2005) include responses that are conditioned by the particular racial group's history within the United States.

In view of the history of racism and racial oppression within the United States (Feagin, 2014), an individual's experience of racism needs to be understood within the historical context of the individual's racial group. As such, scholars have highlighted the role of intergenerational trauma as an important consideration when seeking to understand the experiences of people of color within the United States (Evans-Campbell, 2008; Sotero, 2006). Stamm, Stamm, Hudnall, and Higson-Smith (2004) captured this phenomenon when stating, "It is important to remember that, to some extent, all members of a group share the history or experiences of that group. Thus, a member of a group subjected to past trauma might view current traumatic experiences (whether as victim, perpetrator, or bystander) through a particular lens tempered by that history" (p. 96). As such, a racial group's history within the United States, such as enslavement and Jim Crow segregation for Black Americans (Feagin, 2014) or genocide and forced relocation for Native Americans (Whitbeck, Adams, Hoyt, & Chen, 2004), might exacerbate symptoms associated with experiences of racism, or might frame an individual's perception of a racial incident as being traumatic.

The development and subsequent validation of the RBTSSS (Carter et al., 2013; Carter, Muchow, & Pieterse, 2017) has provided an important window into the experience of racial trauma. The RBTSSS is a self-report measure in which individuals describe a memorable racial encounter, and then indicate the accompanying emotional response to the encounter. Based on this measure, there is now empirical evidence to suggest that stressful racial encounters are indeed associated with a range of emotional responses that are reflective of a trauma response, including avoidance, intrusive thoughts, hypervigilance, confusion, anger, depression, and low self-esteem (Carter et al., 2017). These findings build on earlier studies that identified a relationship between experiences of racism and trauma symptoms (Loo et al., 2001; Pieterse, Carter, Evans, & Walter, 2010).

In sum, race-based traumatic stress is an emerging model within which to understand those racial experiences that rise to the level of trauma. Furthermore, given the ubiquitous and ongoing nature of racism within American society, it is highly likely that psychotherapy supervisees will encounter cases of racial trauma at some point during their training. As such, the following sections outline guidelines for attending to racial trauma in clinical practice and the supervisory relationship.

Supervisor responsibilities for attending to racial trauma

It should be noted initially that the supervisor's responsibility for attending to racial trauma applies to both the clinical case as well as the supervisory relationship (Pendry, 2012). In keeping with multicultural counseling guidelines (Ratts, Singh, Nassar-McMillan, Butler & McCullough, 2016), Harrell (2014) identified racial self-awareness as the most important starting point for racial competence in clinical practice and supervision. In order to effectively guide a supervisee when working with racial trauma in a clinical setting, and to decrease the possibility of racial trauma within the supervisory process, it is essential that supervisors address their own racial self-awareness by engaging in reflection on their personal experience as a racial being. When working with racial trauma, supervisors might initially gravitate to specific techniques or interventions, not unlike novice counselors who tend to prioritize counseling techniques over self-awareness (Hill, Sullivan, Knox, & Schlosser, 2007). The approach being offered in this discussion, however, prioritizes a commitment to racial self-awareness and an antiracism stance as pre-requisites for effective supervision dealing with racial trauma (Mackenzie-Mavinga, 2016; Ridley, 2005). As such, supervisors are encouraged to engage in thoughtful reflection guided by the following questions taken from various approaches for elevating racial awareness gleaned from the training literature (see Carter, 2003; Mackenzie-Mavinga, 2016; Pendry, 2012; Pieterse, 2009).

- When did I first become aware of my racial group membership?
- How do I identify racially, and what is the identification based on? (e.g., physical features? cultural values?)
- How has my racial background influenced my life experiences?

- What beliefs do I have about myself and others based on my racial group membership?
- How do I feel about my racial group membership?
- How do I acknowledge racial difference and similarity when beginning the work with my supervisee?
- How do I explore race-related experiences with my supervisee?
- Am I comfortable discussing race-related topics with my supervisee? What is my discomfort/comfort level based on?
- How might my racial background facilitate or impede interactions with my supervisee?
- How am I attentive to potential experiences of racism that my supervisees might be experiencing?
- Do I allow my supervisees to address their clients' experience of racism?
- How do I confer a sense of safety and trust to my supervisee when addressing race and racism?

Although these prompts might appear simplistic and possibly intuitive, there is evidence to suggest that supervisors might ignore or minimize racial content, largely due to their own discomfort with their racial identity or discomfort with their participation in a racialized society (Chang, Hays, & Shoffner, 2004; Jernigan et al., 2010; Utsey, Bernat & Groth, 2005). Without racial self-awareness, supervisors run the risk of engaging in ineffective supervisory behaviors, such as not discussing racial differences with supervisees, being inattentive and insensitive to supervisees' insecurities in addressing racism, not attending to or addressing a supervisee's own racial identity development, and becoming too preachy about racism/prejudice (Dressel, Consoli, Kim, & Atkinson, 2007). On the contrary, there is evidence to suggest that when supervisors attend to racial variables in supervision, the supervisory alliance is strengthened, and supervisees of color are more likely to engage more openly in the supervisory process (Gatmon et al., 2001; Hird, Cavalieri, Dulko, Felice, & Ho, 2001).

Supervisor guidelines for attending to racial trauma in clinical cases

Racial incidents associated with racial trauma have been noted to be not as discrete and specific as those experiences traditionally associated with traumatic stress (e.g., combat, natural disasters, life-threatening injuries, sexual, physical, and emotional abuse; Nadal, 2018). Furthermore, the experience of racial trauma has to be understood within the larger context of historical racism and the accompanying phenomenon of intergenerational trauma. As such, the guidelines presented here focus on the essential knowledge needed to work effectively with racial trauma and review specific therapeutic interventions that have been outlined in the literature.

Effective work with racial trauma requires requisite knowledge that will guide the choice of intervention and will inform the case conceptualization. Harrell (2014) outlined a number of content areas that supervisors should be familiar with when providing supervision for cases of racial trauma. These content areas include the following: racial identity theory, which focuses on individual variations associated with thoughts and feelings about one's racial group (Carter, 1995); racial socialization, the process of transmitting positive messages about one's racial heritage (Hughes et al., 2006); White privilege, the unearned social advantages afforded to Whites based only on their race (Neville, Worthington, & Spanierman, 2001); the history of race within psychology (Yee, Fairchild, Weizman, & Wyatt, 1993); racism-related stress and mental health (Harrell, 2000); aversive and contemporary racism, which refers to covert and indirect actions of discrimination, subtle endorsement of negative racial stereotypes, and the experience of negative emotions in the presence of people of color (Dovidio & Gaertner, 2004); prejudice reduction and antiracism strategies (Ridley, 2005); and Liberation Psychology, which focuses on a psychology of empowerment and self-worth in the face of oppression (Duran, Firehammer, & Gonzalez, 2008).

Not every case of racial trauma will require knowledge in all of the domains outlined by Harrell (2014); however, it is important to note that, without a theoretical framework with which to understand racial trauma, the supervisor might downplay or delegitimize the client's experience of racism, and possibly exacerbate the effects of racial trauma.

Clinical interventions for racial trauma

Supervisors should be aware that many clients of color might not identify racial material as their primary concern; however, supervisees should be instructed to be attentive to those aspects of a client's experience that could be reflective of racial trauma. As such, an assessment of racial trauma should be included as part of the initial intake or initial assessment procedure, analogous to inquiries of emotional, verbal, or sexual trauma. When clients endorse an experience of racial trauma, a more extensive interview can be undertaken, drawing on such instruments as the RBTSSS (Carter et al., 2013). This instrument allows a client to outline and describe a racial incident in-depth, and then identify accompanying emotional reactions, as well as the duration of these reactions. Examples of items include "As a consequence of the memorable encounter I had with racism, I tend to overreact to situations" and "As a consequence of the memorable encounter I had with racism, I tend to stay away from people/places who remind me of the event" (see Carter & Sant-Barket, 2015). In cases in which racial trauma is clearly identified, the following therapeutic interventions have been suggested by a number of authors (e.g., Bryant-Davis & Ocampo, 2006; Harrell, 2014; Helms, Nicolas,

& Green, 2010) and should guide supervisors' approach to assisting their supervisee in their work with clients experiencing racial trauma.

Acknowledgment and validation

Notable responses to experiences of racism include shame, anger, and low-ered sense of self-worth. Supervisees should be instructed not to challenge the client's perception of the experience, but provide empathic acknowl-edgment. Supervisees can facilitate this process by normalizing the client's response and acknowledging the larger social context of racism within American society. Clients' emotional responses to a race-based incident should always be accepted as valid, irrespective of whether the event is objectively confirmed or not.

Assessment of impact

Carter and Forsyth (2010) outlined varying psychological responses based on the type of racist incident experienced. Their findings suggested that hostile racist experiences (e.g., verbal, physical threat, communications that convey devaluing, racially based insults) are more likely to be associated with hypervigilance and anxiety, while racist experiences that are more reflective of avoidant behaviors (e.g., being denied service, being overlooked for a promotion) are associated with feelings of shame, guilt, depression, and general distress. An accurate assessment of the predominant affective response enables the supervisee to provide empathic validation, and to explore/identify the coping strategies that clients employ in response to traumatizing racial experiences, as well as the extent to which the strategies are effective. Coping strategies identified in the literature include seeking social support, taking direct action, trying to address outcomes associated with the racist event using problem-solving approaches, and avoidance strategies such as denial or rationalization (Forsyth & Carter, 2012).

Working with cognitive distortions

After having facilitated a space of safety through accurate assessment and empathic validation, supervisees can explore with their clients the impact of the traumatic experience in regard to assumptions and beliefs that the client might be holding as a result of the racist incident. An important and harmful aspect of racial trauma is the notion of internalized shame and self-blame. For clients of color, the phenomenon of internalized racism, the process of internalizing negative stereotypes of one's racial group (Speight, 2007), might exacerbate feelings of shame, guilt, and self-blame that accompany experi-ences of racial trauma. A simple distortion with far-reaching consequences could be "It was my fault" or "I did something wrong." When the working alliance is secure, a supervisee can collaboratively test those assumptions with the client, with the goal of facilitating a more realistic set of cognitive assumptions, and thereby assisting clients in recognizing the external source of their distress.

Processing strong emotions

For many supervisees, the experience of clients' strong emotions such as anger can be discomforting and threatening. Recognizing anger as an important and healthy emotion in response to a racist incident is a central aspect of working with racial trauma. For White supervisees, emotions such as anger displayed by clients of color might feel threatening, especially if supervisees have some awareness of privileged aspects of their own racial experience (Utsey, Gernat, & Hammar, 2005). Supervisors play an important role in normalizing supervisees' responses of fear or discomfort, and supporting them as they work with their clients to facilitate healthier expression of the anger. The goal of supervisors is to facilitate in their supervisee a nondefensive, nonjudgmental, and supportive stance as the supervisee attempts to provide clients a safe place for emotional expression. For clients, the need to learn strategies for effective regulation of their emotions is an important aspect of their recovery. Here, Dialectical Behavior Therapy (DBT) techniques (see McKay, Wood, & Brantley, 2010), such as nonjudgmental acceptance, mindfulness practice, skills training for increasing distress tolerance, acting opposite to emotion, and teaching problem-solving techniques, will allow the client not to be consistently overwhelmed by emotions associated with the traumatic racial incident.

Responding to loss

The experience of loss is seen as an integral aspect of trauma (Boden, Kulkarni, Shurick, Bonn-Miller, & Gross, 2014). Loss can reflect actual physical loss of health and belongings; however, loss can also refer to loss of identity, loss of self-concept, or loss of trust. As such, it is helpful to consider the emotional response to trauma as also a type of grief reaction (Utsey & Payne, 2000). When working with individuals who have experienced a traumatizing racial incident, the supervisee should be mindful that losing a sense of self, safety, and trust occurs in the context of the larger racial group's experience of trauma, and therefore can exacerbate feelings of powerlessness, anger, and depression. Furthermore, in cross-racial dyads, clients of color might be hesitant to identify their experience as racial trauma, fearing that White therapists might not understand, might minimize their experience, or be defensive. This phenomenon, identified as cultural mistrust (Whaley, 2001), has been implicated in the manner in which people of color seek out or participate in mental health treatments. Given findings associated with the racial identity literature, clients who are more deeply connected to their racial group are most likely the clients who will understand individual racist experiences in the context of the larger racial groups experience (see Iwamoto & Liu, 2010; Shelton & Sellers, 2000). Here, clients might connect their individual experience to the larger group experience in ways that might intensify feelings of anger, distrust, feelings of depression and hopelessness, and feeling disempowered. The supervisees/therapists who are willing to explore this aspect of the client's experience will likely be perceived as more competent and therefore more trustworthy by a client of color (Knox, Burkard, Johnson, Suzuki, & Ponterotto, 2003).

Strategies for coping and resistance

Supervisees should have some familiarity with the range of interventions associated with stress reduction and management of anxiety, such as mindfulness-based practices, relaxation exercises, and grounding techniques (Davis, Eshelman, & McKay, 2008). A more focused intervention is EMBRace, an acronym for Engaging, Managing, and Bonding through Race, a therapeutic approached specifically designed to address racial trauma by drawing on collective cultural experiences associated with race among Black Americans (Anderson & Stevenson, 2016). EMBRace utilizes racial socialization as a means to provide positive messages of racial heritage, and facilitate empowerment through the identification of effective coping responses associated with experiencing racism. The intervention is family based, targeting adolescents between the ages of 10 and 14 and at least one parent. Emphasis is placed on understanding family history, instilling pride in one's racial culture, providing psychoeducation on how to convey positive racial messages to children, and balancing hope for racial equality in the future with examining the current experience of hopelessness and demoralization experienced by many Blacks. The intervention is also designed to provide social support and bonding around a common experience of racism and racial trauma (Anderson, McKenny, Mitchell, Koku, & Stevenson, 2017).

An important aspect of coping is regaining a sense of control and mastery. For individuals who have experienced racial trauma, empowerment is facilitated when individuals find ways to address the traumatic experience. Bryant-Davis and Ocampo (2006) stressed the role of empowering individuals after experiences of racial trauma. Empowering strategies include becoming politically active, engaging in antiracism activism, filing racial harassment charges where applicable, educating others about racism, and finding ways to share one's stories. As such, supervisors should be familiar with the types of opportunities clients can engage in (e.g., becoming involved in racial justice organizations; see http://www.racialequityre sourceguide.org) that would promote a sense of self-efficacy, and should encourage supervisees to explore these opportunities with their clients.

Supervisor guidelines for attending to racial trauma within the supervisory process

There is evidence to indicate that graduate students of color (potential supervisees) experience individual and institutional racism, which leaves them feeling negatively stereotyped and subject to racial microaggressions, which in turn are associated with anger, low self-efficacy, self-doubt, and anxiety (Gildersleeve, Croom,

& Vasquez, 2011; Truong, Museus, & McGuire, 2016). The experience of racial microaggressions, defined by Sue and colleagues (2007) as "brief and commonplace daily verbal, behavioral, and environmental indignities, whether intentional or unintentional, that communicate hostile, de-rogatory, or negative racial slights and insults to the target person or group" (p. 271), is now being understood within the larger framework of traumatic stress (Nadal, 2018). Microaggressions experienced in the context of clinical supervision could increase the possibility of a trauma response experienced by the supervisee, given the interpersonal nature of super-vision and the inherent power imbalance that resides within the supervisory relationship.

The discussion of racial trauma within supervision in this article is noteworthy for its lack of focus on explicitly traumatic incidents perpetrated by a supervisor such as physical assault or threats of intimidation. In supervision, these types of incidents are rare and infrequent (Ellis et al., 2014); however, the more uninten-tional incidents that convey a devaluing message of supervisee's race or the client's experience of racism could be experienced as a racial microaggression (Constantine, 2007; Constantine & Sue, 2007), with findings now suggesting that racial microaggressions are positively associated with trauma symptoms (Torres & Taknint, 2015).

In thinking about racial microaggressions as a subtle communication of deva-luation, perhaps the most pernicious antecedent of racial trauma in the supervisory experience is when the supervisor diminishes or dismisses race-related experiences and dynamics (Knox, Burkard, Johnson, Suzuki, & Ponterotto, 2003). To illustrate, a supervisee of color is working with a client of color who has started sharing experiences of racism that have resulted in anxiety-related symptoms. In working with the client, the supervisee seeks to provide empathic validation of the client's racial trauma, reframe the experience such that the client understands that some-thing indeed has happened to them, as opposed to the client feeling responsible and disempowered, and review coping strategies that facilitate a sense of agency, such as direct confrontation, spiritual and social support, and increased sense of racial consciousness (see Forsyth & Carter, 2012). The supervisor, however, instructs the supervisee to focus on the anxiety symptoms as reflective of an underlying attachment disorder, and suggests either dynamic approaches to attend to the attachment disorder or cognitive-behavioral approaches to respond to the anxiety symptoms. As such, the supervisee receives the message that the client's experience of racism is not important, and that the client's psychological response is primarily reflective of intrapsychic dysfunction. Furthermore, the supervisee most likely assumes that the supervisory space is not one in which race-related material is valued, thereby also experiencing a sense of personal invalidation and minimization (Mackenzie-Mavinga, 2016).

Another potential source of racial trauma for a supervisee is when the supervisor chooses not to address racial dynamics that occur within the supervisory relation-ship. Although this dynamic is most often associated with a cross-racial dyad, depending on the supervisor's racial identity status, it might also occur in same-race supervisory dyads in which supervisees might be at a more mature racial identity status; that is, the supervisee might display a greater level of comfort and understanding of their racial background than does the supervisor (Chang et al., 2004). Harrell (2014) noted that processes reflective of racial dynamics, or supervisees wanting to respond to clients' sense of invalidation based on their racial group membership, may potentially be more salient for supervisees of color. When supervisors therefore choose not to attend to race-related material, supervisees of color could feel silenced, which could result in feelings of anger, disappointment, a lowered sense of self-efficacy, and a likely rupture in the supervisory alliance (Chopra, 2013). It is important to note that experiencing a lowered sense of self-worth and a diminished sense of personal agency are defining characteristics of racial trauma (Carter et al., 2005). When these attributes are triggered in clinical supervision, there could be a corresponding increase in the risk of harmful supervision (see Ellis, 2017). It is therefore critical that supervisors consider inattention to race-related dynamics, both in relation to client material and the supervisory relationship, as indicative of harmful supervision (Ellis et al., 2014), in view of the possible trauma response that could be produced. Furthermore, given that micro-invalidations are considered a type of racial microaggression (Nadal, 2018), behaviors and communications that convey a sense of invalidation based on a supervisee's racial group membership could be perceived as threatening and unsafe by supervisees, and could also elicit unacknowledged trauma symptoms associated with prior traumatic experiences (Helms et al., 2010).

Attending to power in the supervisory relationship

Inherent in any supervisor/supervisee relationship are dynamics of power. In the training environment, the role of the supervisor includes both the facilitation of therapy skills as well as a gatekeeping role associated with a supervisee's ability to practice (Lichtenberg et al., 2007). The dynamics of race within the supervisory relationship mean that issues of power and authority take on a larger meaning. Given current racial demographics in counseling and psychotherapy training, trainees of color are much more likely to have White supervisors than supervisors of color (see Hipolito-Delgado, Estrada, & Garcia, 2017). This racial arrangement is situated in a societal context in which being a person of color is afforded less power and devalued. As such, it is imperative for supervisors to address the power dynamic both as it relates to the role of the supervisor as well as the manner in which race might influence supervisees' experience of the supervisory role. One approach to attending to the power dynamic is for supervisors to be deliberate and intentional in initiating discussions of race with their supervisees (Tummala-Narra, 2004). Given that supervisees are in a position of less power, relying on the supervisee to initiate discussions of race conveys a message that the supervisory space is not one of safety. Indeed, a supervisor's willingness to discuss racial similarities and differences has been noted to be of greater importance for effective supervision than merely matching a supervisee with a racially similar supervisor (Duan & Roehlke, 2001).

It is important to note that these suggestions, offered as a means of reducing the potential for racial trauma, are fully situated in the best practice guidelines for supervision (see Borders et al., 2014). The need for the supervisor to embody cultural sensitivity, to initiate dialogues on racial diversity, to maintain a commitment to ongoing racial self-awareness, and to be attentive to dynamics of power has been clearly documented in the best practice guidelines. As such, the focus on racial awareness and attending to the potential for racial trauma should not be viewed as an area of specialization in clinical supervision, but should be viewed as a central and core aspect of supervision.

Concluding thoughts

Given the ongoing role of race and racism in American society, the need to be attentive to racial dynamics in the therapeutic setting is well-accepted in the clinical literature (Mackenzie-Mavinga, 2016). Within the context of clinical supervision, racism experienced by the supervisees is considered to be harmful supervision (Ellis, 2017; Ellis et al., 2014), and supervisors have been encouraged to establish the supervision relationship as a safe space wherein issues of power and racial experiences can be addressed and processed (Hernândez & McDowell, 2010). It would be amiss, however, to conclude the current discussion without a reminder that the supervisor can also experience racial trauma, either through direct interactions of racial hostility perpetrated by a supervisee or experiences of racial invalidation perpetrated by institutions of higher learning and/or mental health settings (see Butler-Byrd, 2010). For supervisors of color, having one's competencies questioned, having supervisees respond to one's interventions with fear and suspicion, having supervisees be dismissive of needing to focus on race and culture (see Burkard, Knox, Clarke, Phelps, & Inman, 2014), feeling that one lacks institutional support, and noting that, as a faculty member or supervisor of color, the expectation of multicultural competence is higher than that of White colleagues, are all ways in which supervisors of color are first and foremost seen and evaluated based on their racial group membership as opposed to their individual experiences and competencies in supervision. Butler-Byrd (2010) captured these dynamics in a compelling manner by stating, "Some of my students initially question my knowledge and experience.... Some students have admitted that they were skeptical about my knowledge or ability to help them learn because I am not European American like the teachers they have known all of their lives. I have often felt that I have to 'work twice as hard' to prove I am as good as or better than European American supervisors or faculty" (p. 12).

Race and racism continue to be a real aspect of the American landscape. Given that the field of mental health reflects larger social dynamics, the endeavor of clinical supervision will continue to be shaped and informed by racial dynamics. In order to minimize the possibility of these dynamics evolving to racial trauma, supervisors are charged with the responsibility of ensuring that the supervisory experience is one of safety, acceptance, racial sensitivity, and racial affirmation. Supervisees in turn need to be open to their experience as racial beings, and work through those negative racial assumptions that impede their ability to fully enter the supervisory experience with openness and vulnerability.

References

Anderson, R. E., McKenny, M., Mitchell, A., Koku, L., & Stevenson, H. C. (2017). EMBRacing racial stress and trauma: Preliminary feasibility and coping responses of a racial socialization intervention. *Journal of Black Psychology*. Advance online publication. doi: 0095798417732930.

Anderson, R. E., & Stevenson, H. (2016). *EMBRace training manual*. Unpublished training manual prepared for the University of Pennsylvania–Graduate School of Education's Racial Empowerment Collaborative, Philadelphia, PA.

Bambling, M., King, R., Raue, P., Schweitzer, R., & Lambert, W. (2006). Clinical supervision: Its influence on client-rated working alliance and client symptom reduction in the brief treatment of major depression. *Psychotherapy Research, 16*, 317–331. doi:10.1080/ 10503300500268524

Boden, M. T., Kulkarni, M., Shurick, A., Bonn-Miller, M. O., & Gross, J. J. (2014). Responding to trauma and loss: An emotion regulation perspective. In M. Kent, M. C Davis, & J. W. Reich (Eds.), *The resilience handbook: Approaches to stress and trauma* (pp. 86–99). New York, NY: Routledge.

Borders, L. D., Glosoff, H. L., Welfare, L. E., Hays, D. G., DeKruyf, L., Fernando, D. M., & Page, B. (2014). Best practices in clinical supervision: Evolution of a counseling specialty. *The Clinical Supervisor, 33*, 26–44. doi:10.1080/07325223.2014.905225

Bryant-Davis, T. (2007). Healing requires recognition: The case for race-based traumatic stress. *The Counseling Psychologist, 35*, 135–142. doi:10.1177/0011000006295152

Bryant-Davis, T., & Ocampo, C. (2006). A therapeutic approach to the treatment of racist-incident-based trauma. *Journal of Emotional Abuse, 6*, 1–22. doi:10.1300/ J135v06n04_01

Burkard, A. W., Knox, S., Clarke, R. D., Phelps, D. L., & Inman, A. G. (2014). Supervisors' experiences of providing difficult feedback in cross-ethnic/racial supervision. *The Counseling Psychologist, 42*(3), 314–344. doi:10.1177/0011000012461157

Butler-Byrd, N. M. (2010). An African American supervisor's reflections on multicultural supervision. *Training and Education in Professional Psychology, 4*, 11–15. doi:10.1037/a0018351

Carter, R. T. (1995). *The influence of race and racial identity in psychotherapy: Toward a racially inclusive model*. Hoboken, NJ: Wiley.

Carter, R. T. (2003). Becoming racially and culturally competent: The racial-cultural counseling laboratory. *Journal of Multicultural Counseling and Development, 31*, 20–30. doi:10.1002/jmcd.2003.31.issue-1

Carter, R. T. (2007). Racism and psychological and emotional injury: Recognizing and assessing race-based traumatic stress. *The Counseling Psychologist, 35*, 13–105. doi:10.1177/ 0011000006292033

Carter, R. T., & Forsyth, J. (2010). Reactions to racial discrimination: Emotional stress and help-seeking behaviors. *Psychological Trauma: Theory, Research, Practice, and Policy*, 2, 183–191. doi:10.1037/a0020102

Carter, R. T., Forsyth, J. M., Mazzula, S. L., & Williams, B. (2005). Racial discrimination and race-based traumatic stress: An exploratory investigation. In R. T. Carter (Ed.), *Handbook of racial-cultural psychology and counseling: Training and practice* (pp. 447–476). Hoboken, NJ: Wiley.

Carter, R. T., Lau, M. Y., Johnson, V., & Kirkinis, K. (2017). Racial discrimination and health outcomes among racial/ethnic minorities: A meta-analytic review. *Journal of Multicultural Counseling and Development*, 45, 232–259. doi:10.1002/jmcd.12076

Carter, R. T., Mazzula, S., Victoria, R., Vazquez, R., Hall, S., Smith, S.,… Williams, B. (2013). Initial development of the Race-Based Traumatic Stress Symptom Scale: Assessing the emotional impact of racism. *Psychological Trauma: Theory, Research, Practice, and Policy*, 5, 1–9. doi:10.1037/a0025911

Carter, R. T., Muchow, C., & Pieterse, A. L. (2017). Construct, predictive validity, and measurement equivalence of the Race-Based Traumatic Stress Symptom Scale for Black Americans. *Traumatology*. Advance online publication. doi:10.1037/trm0000128

Carter, R. T., & Sant-Barket, S. M. (2015). Assessment of the impact of racial discrimination and racism: How to use the Race-Based Traumatic Stress Symptom Scale in practice. *Traumatology*, 21(1), 32–39. doi:10.1037/trm0000018

Chang, C. Y., Hays, D. G., & Shoffner, M. F. (2004). Cross-racial supervision: A developmental approach for White supervisors working with supervisees of color. *The Clinical Supervisor*, 22(2), 121–138. doi:10.1300/J001v22n02_08

Chopra, T. (2013). All supervision is multicultural: A review of literature on the need for multicultural supervision in counseling. *Psychological Studies*, 58, 335–338. doi:10.1007/s12646-013-0206-x

Coates, T. N., (2015). *Between the world and me*. New York, NY: Random House.

Comas- Diaz, L. (2016). Racial trauma recovery: A race informed therapeutic approach to racial wounds. In A. N. Alvarez, C. T. H. Liang, & H. A. Neville (Eds.), *The cost of racism for people of color: Contextualizing experiences of discrimination* (pp. 249–272). Washington, DC: American Psychological Association.

Constantine, M. G. (2007). Racial microaggressions against African American clients in cross-racial counseling relationships. *Journal of Counseling Psychology*, 54, 1–16. doi:10.1037/0022-0167.54.1.1

Constantine, M. G., & Sue, D. W. (2007). Perceptions of racial microaggressions among Black supervisees in cross-racial dyads. *Journal of Counseling Psychology*, 54, 142–153. doi:10.1037/0022-0167.54.2.142

Davis, M., Eshelman, E. R., & McKay, M. (2008). *The relaxation and stress reduction workbook*. Oakland, CA: New Harbinger Publications.

Dovidio, J. F., & Gaertner, S. L. (2004). *Aversive racism. Advances in experimental social psychology*, 36, 4–56.

Dressel, J. L., Consoli, A. J., Kim, B. S., & Atkinson, D. R. (2007). Successful and unsuccessful multicultural supervisory behaviors: A Delphi poll. *Journal of Multicultural Counseling and Development*, 35, 51–64. doi:10.1002/j.2161-1912.2007.tb00049.x

Duan, C., & Roehlke, H. (2001). A descriptive "snapshot" of cross-racial supervision in university counseling center internships. *Journal of Multicultural Counseling and Development*, 29, 131–146. doi:10.1002/jmcd.2001.29.issue-2

Duran, E., Firehammer, J., & Gonzalez, J. (2008). Liberation psychology as the path toward healing cultural soul wounds. *Journal of Counseling & Development*, 86, 288–295. doi:10.1002/j.1556-6678.2008.tb00511.x

Ellis, M. V. (2017). Narratives of harmful clinical supervision. *The Clinical Supervisor, 36,* 20–87. doi:10.1080/07325223.2017.1297753

Ellis, M. V., Berger, L., Hanus, A. E., Ayala, E. E., Swords, B. A., & Siembor, M. (2014). Inadequate and harmful clinical supervision: Testing a revised framework and assessing occurrence. *The Counseling Psychologist, 42,* 434–472. doi:10.1177/0011000013508656

Evans-Campbell, T. (2008). Historical trauma in American Indian/Native Alaska communities: A multilevel framework for exploring impacts on individuals, families, and communities. *Journal of Interpersonal Violence, 23,* 316–338. doi:10.1177/0886260507312290

Feagin, J. R. (2014). *Racist America: Roots, current realities, and future reparations.* New York, NY: Routledge.

Forsyth, J., & Carter, R. T. (2012). The relationship between racial identity status attitudes, racism-related coping, and mental health among Black Americans. *Cultural Diversity and Ethnic Minority Psychology, 18,* 128–140. doi:10.1037/a0027660

Gatmon, D., Jackson, D., Koshkarian, L., & Martos-Perry, N. (2001). Exploring ethnic, gender, and sexual orientation variables in supervision: Do they really matter? *Journal of Multicultural Counseling and Development, 29,* 102–113. doi:10.1002/j.2161-1912.2001.tb00508.x

Gildersleeve, R. E., Croom, N. N., & Vasquez, P. L. (2011). "Am I going crazy?!": A critical race analysis of doctoral education. *Equity & Excellence in Education, 44,* 93–114. doi:10.1080/10665684.2011.539472

Harrell, S. P. (2000). A multidimensional conceptualization of racism-related stress: Implications for the well-being of people of color. *American Journal of Orthopsychiatry, 70,* 42–57. doi:10.1037/h0087722

Harrell, S. P. (2014). Compassionate confrontation and empathic exploration: The integration of race-related narratives in clinical supervision. In C. A. Falender., E. P. Shafranske, & C. J. Falicov (Eds.), *Multiculturalism and diversity in clinical supervision: A competency-based approach* (pp. 83–110). Washington, DC: American Psychological Association.

Hemmings, C., & Evans, A. M. (2018). Identifying and treating race-based trauma in counseling. *Journal of Multicultural Counseling and Development, 46,* 20–39. doi:10.1002/jmcd.12090

Helms, J. E., Nicolas, G., & Green, C. E. (2010). Racism and ethnoviolence as trauma: Enhancing professional training. *Traumatology, 16*(4), 53–62. doi:10.1177/1534765610389595

Hernández, P., & McDowell, T. (2010). Intersectionality, power, and relational safety in context: Key concepts in clinical supervision. *Training and Education in Professional Psychology, 4,* 29–36. doi:10.1037/a0017064

Hill, C. E., Sullivan, C., Knox, S., & Schlosser, L. Z. (2007). Becoming psychotherapists: Experiences of novice trainees in a beginning graduate class. *Psychotherapy: Theory, Research, Practice, Training, 44,* 434–449. doi:10.1037/0033-3204.44.4.364

Hipolito-Delgado, C. P., Estrada, D., & Garcia, M. (2017). Counselor education in technicolor: Recruiting graduate students of color. *InterAmerican Journal of Psychology, 51,* 73–85.

Hird, J. S., Cavalieri, C. E., Dulko, J. P., Felice, A. A., & Ho, T. A. (2001). Visions and realities: Supervisee perspectives of multicultural supervision. *Journal of Multicultural Counseling and Development, 29,* 114–130. doi:10.1002/j.2161-1912.2001.tb00509.x

Hughes, D., Rodriguez, J., Smith, E. P., Johnson, D. J., Stevenson, H. C., & Spicer, P. (2006). Parents' ethnic-racial socialization practices: A review of research and directions for future study. *Developmental Psychology, 42,* 747–770. doi:10.1037/0012-1649.42.5.747

Iwamoto, D. K., & Liu, W. M. (2010). The impact of racial identity, ethnic identity, Asian values, and race-related stress on Asian Americans and Asian international college students' psychological well-being. *Journal of Counseling Psychology, 57,* 79–91. doi:10.1037/a0017393

Jernigan, M. M., Green, C. E., Helms, J. E., Perez-Gualdron, L., & Henze, K. (2010). An examination of people of color supervision dyads: Racial identity matters as much as race. *Training and Education in Professional Psychology, 4,* 62–73. doi:10.1037/a0018110

Knox, S., Burkard, A. W., Johnson, A. J., Suzuki, L. A., & Ponterotto, J. G. (2003). African American and European American therapists' experiences of addressing race in cross-racial psychotherapy dyads. *Journal of Counseling Psychology, 50,* 466–481. doi:10.1037/0022-0167.50.4.466

Lichtenberg, J. W., Portnoy, S. M., Bebeau, M. J., Leigh, I. W., Nelson, P. D., Rubin, N. J., … Kaslow, N. J. (2007). Challenges to the assessment of competence and competencies. *Professional Psychology: Research and Practice, 38,* 474–478. doi:10.1037/0735-7028.38.5.474

Loo, C. M., Fairbank, J. A., Scurfield, R. M., Ruch, L. O., King, D. W., Adams, L. J., & Chemtob, C. M.(2001). Measuring exposure to racism: Development and validation of a Race-Related Stressor Scale (RRSS) for Asian American Vietnam veterans. *Psychological Assessment, 13,* 503–520. doi:10.1037//1040-3590.13.4.503

Mackenzie-Mavinga, I. (2016). *The challenge of racism in therapeutic practice: Engaging with oppression in practice and supervision.* New York, NY: Palgrave.

McKay, M., Wood, J. C., & Brantley, J. (2010). *The dialectical behavior therapy skills workbook: Practical DBT exercises for learning mindfulness, interpersonal effectiveness, emotion regulation and distress tolerance.* Oakland, CA: New Harbinger Publications.

Miller, J., & Garran, A. M. (2017). *Racism in the United States: Implications for the helping professions.* New York, NY: Springer Publishing Company.

Nadal, K. (2018). *Microaggression and traumatic stress.* Washington, DC: American Psychological Association.

Neville, H. A., Worthington, R. L., & Spanierman, L. B. (2001). Understanding White privilege and color-blind racial attitudes. In J. G. Ponterotto, J. M. Casas, L. A. Suzuki, & C. M. Alexander (Eds.), *Handbook of multicultural counseling* (pp. 257–288). Thousand Oaks, CA: Sage.

O'Donovan, A., Halford, W. K., & Walters, B. (2011). Towards best practice supervision of clinical psychology trainees. *Australian Psychologist, 46,* 101–112. doi:10.1111/j.1742-9544.2011.00033.x

Paradies, Y., Ben, J., Denson, N., Elias, A., Priest, N., Pieterse, A., … Gee, G. (2015). Racism as a determinant of health: A systematic review and meta-analysis. *PLoS ONE 10(9)*: e0138511. doi:10.1371/journal.pone.0138511

Pendry, N. (2012). Race, racism and systemic supervision. *Journal of Family Therapy, 34,* 403–418. doi:10.1111/j.1467-6427.2011.00576.x

Pieterse, A. L. (2009). Teaching anti-racism in counselor training: Reflections on a course. *Journal of Multicultural Counseling and Development, 37,* 141–152. doi:10.1002/j.2161-1912.2009.tb00098.x

Pieterse, A. L., Carter, R. T., Evans, S. A., & Walter, R. A. (2010). An exploratory examination of the associations among racial and ethnic discrimination, racial climate, and trauma-related symptoms in a college student population. *Journal of Counseling Psychology, 57,* 255–263. doi:10.1037/a0020040

Pieterse, A. L., & Powell, S. (2016). A theoretical overview of the impact of racism on people of color. In A. N. Alvarez, C. T. H. Liang, & H. A. Neville (Eds.), *The cost of racism for people of color* (pp. 11–30). Washington, DC: American Psychological Association.

Ratts, M. J., Singh, A. A., Nassar-McMillan, S., Butler, S. K., & McCullough, J. R. (2010). Multicultural and social justice counseling competencies: Guidelines for the counseling profession. *Journal of Multicultural Counseling and Development, 44,* 28–48. doi:10.1002/jmcd.12035

Ridley, C. R. (2005). *Overcoming unintentional racism in counseling and therapy: A practitioner's guide to intentional intervention* (vol. 5). Thousand Oaks, CA: Sage.

Shelton, J. N., & Sellers, R. M. (2000). Situational stability and variability in African American racial identity. *Journal of Black Psychology, 26,* 27–50. doi:10.1177/0095798400026001002

Sotero, M. (2006). A conceptual model of historical trauma: Implications for public health practice and research. *Journal of Health Disparities Research and Practice, 1,* 93–108.

Speight, S. L. (2007). Internalized racism: One more piece of the puzzle. *The Counseling Psychologist, 35,* 126–134. doi:10.1177/0011000006295119

Stamm, B. H., Stamm, H. E., Hudnall, A. C., & Higson-Smith, C. (2004). Considering a theory of cultural trauma and loss. *Journal of Loss and Trauma*, *9*, 89–111. doi:10.1080/15325020490255412

Thompson, C. E., & Neville, H. A. (1999). Racism, mental health, and mental health practice. *The Counseling Psychologist*, *27*, 155–223. doi:10.1177/0011000099272001

Sue, D. W., Capodilupo, C. M., Torino, G. C., Bucceri, J. M., Holder, A., Nadal, K. L., & Esquilin, M. (2007). Racial microaggressions in everyday life: Implications for clinical practice. *American Psychologist*, *62*, 271–286. doi:10.1037/0003-066X.62.4.271

Torres, L., & Taknint, J. T. (2015). Ethnic microaggressions, traumatic stress symptoms, and Latino depression: A moderated mediational model. *Journal of Counseling Psychology*, *62*, 393–401. doi:10.1037/cou0000077

Truong, K. A., Museus, S. D., & McGuire, K. M. (2016). Vicarious racism: A qualitative analysis of experiences with secondhand racism in graduate education. *International Journal of Qualitative Studies in Education*, *29*, 224–247. doi:10.1080/09518398.2015.1023234

Tummala-Narra, P. (2004). Dynamics of race and culture in the supervisory encounter. *Psychoanalytic Psychology*, *21*, 300–311. doi:10.1037/0736-9735.21.2.300

Utsey, S. O., Gernat, C. A., & Hammar, L. (2005). Examining White counselor trainees' reactions to racial issues in counseling and supervision dyads. *The Counseling Psychologist*, *33*, 449–478. doi:10.1177/0011000004269058

Utsey, S. O., & Payne, Y. (2000). Psychological impacts of racism in a clinical versus normal sample of African American men. *Journal of African American Men*, *5*, 57–72. doi:10.1007/s12111-000-1004-9

Watkins, Jr., C. E. (2011). Does psychotherapy supervision contribute to patient outcomes? Considering thirty years of research. *The Clinical Supervisor*, *30*, 235–256. doi:10.1080/07325223.2011.619417

Westefeld, J. S. (2009). Supervision of psychotherapy: Models, issues, and recommendations. *The Counseling Psychologist*, *37*, 296–316. doi:10.1177/0011000008316657

Whaley, A. L. (2001). Cultural mistrust and mental health services for African Americans: A review and meta-analysis. *The Counseling Psychologist*, *29*, 513–531. doi:10.1177/0011000001294003

Wheeler, S., & Richards, K. (2007). The impact of clinical supervision on counsellors and therapists, their practice and their clients. A systematic review of the literature. *Counselling and Psychotherapy Research*, *7*, 54–65. doi:10.1080/14733140601185274

Whitbeck, L. B., Adams, G. W., Hoyt, D. R., & Chen, X. (2004). Conceptualizing and measuring historical trauma among American Indian people. *American Journal of Community Psychology*, *33*, 119–130. doi:0091-0562/04/0600-0119/0. doi:10.1023/B:AJCP.0000027000.77357.31

Yee, A. H., Fairchild, H. H., Weizmann, F., & Wyatt, G. E. (1993). Addressing psychology's problem with race. *American Psychologist*, *48*, 1132–1140. doi:10.1037/0003-066X.48.11.1132

Trauma-informed supervision in the disaster context

Carole Adamson

ABSTRACT
Supervision is increasingly defined by reflection and traumain-formed knowledge and practice. When faced with a disaster, the role and function of supervision is changed by the scale of events, with psychosocial support for traumatic stress often side-lined by, or subsumed within, emergency interventions. Disasters, however, need a longitudinal focus on recovery for many years following; this focus provides the logic for super-vision at every stage of a disaster. In this article, the author defines disaster and its phases, and raises issues for supervision within the disaster context. Hypothetical examples are used both from the author's location in Aotearoa New Zealand and from disasters more internationally familiar.

Supervision in a disaster context is under-addressed in the supervision litera-ture, which largely focuses on the establishment and building of safe, reflective relationships with the goals of professional development, effective practice, and organizational accountability. Disasters, however, are by definition com-munity-level events of such scale that "normal" processes of professional practice (including those of supervision) may be severely compromised or inappropriate. Disasters are bigger than trauma, bigger than supervision, and have the potential to challenge or develop supervision practice. Disasters can be conceived, as Hoffman and Kruczek (2011) suggested, as bioecological experiences that require not only addressing the psychological effects of trauma within supervision, but consideration of the community-wide reach of both individual and shared exposure and recovery

In this article, I address some of the key issues for supervision in the context of disaster. I begin by defining and exploring the definition and dimensions of disaster in which to embed an understanding of trauma-informed practice. Because of the pervasive nature of disasters, I consider not only the potential for trauma-informed practice and secondary traumatization of supervisors and supervisees by the impact of client stories, but also the shared impact of disasters on supervisees' and supervisors' own lives, and the necessity that supervision practice is able to respond at both the individual and systemic levels. Key issues for supervision are discussed within the phases of disaster response and recovery. Self-care for supervisors is acknowledged, and recommendations for practice are considered throughout. Practice examples and brief scenarios are introduced as illustration.

The disaster dimensions: Magnitude, origin, and time

In defining disasters, we link to our immediate context for definitional understanding. I am a social work educator living on the Pacific Ring of Fire, teaching a course on stress and trauma within a postgraduate qualification in professional supervision. Ask any supervisor in Aotearoa New Zealand to give an example of a disaster, and they will name Christchurch (the Canterbury earthquake sequence of 2010-2011) or perhaps Kaikoura (a less globally known but incredibly disruptive earthquake in November 2016). A United States supervisor may immediately identify 9/11 or Hurricanes Katrina, Andrew, Harvey, or Maria as contexts for trauma-informed supervision practice. For social and humanitarian workers responding to a refugee experience, there is yet a different context in which to define the disaster experience, one where "disaster" has occurred elsewhere and "survivors" now must settle in someone else's space. It is therefore important that we develop a conceptual understanding of what we mean by disaster with which to explore the risk of traumatization, and the role of trauma-informed supervision practice.

The United Nations Office for Disaster Risk Reduction (UNISDR) defines disaster as follows:

> A serious disruption of the functioning of a community or a society at any scale due to hazardous events interacting with conditions of exposure, vulnerability and capacity, leading to one or more of the following: human, material, economic and environmental losses and impacts. (UNISDR, 2009)

The UNISDR definition acknowledges that the impact of a disaster may be localized (for example, a landslide that blocks access to a rural community) or widespread (such as the effects of Hurricane Maria in Puerto Rico). Disasters may occur without specific warnings (sudden-onset events such as earthquakes) or may have years of antecedents (such as the slow-onset impact of sea-level rises on small island states in the Pacific Ocean). I have suggested elsewhere that a useful definitional framework for understanding disasters is one with a consideration of the three factors of *magnitude and impact, origin,* and *time* (Adamson, 2014). Of these three factors, it is the magnitude, scale, or severity of an event (or sequence of events) that often suggest the most immediate risk of traumatic impact to those caught up in the disaster; however, the origin of the disaster, preexisting vulnerabilities, and how the disaster plays out over time, also emerge as determinants of impact. All people caught up in such an event may be vulnerable to traumatic impact, as the protective factors of training and the opportunity to perform a prescribed role may be overwhelmed by the scale and intensity of the events. From

$$\text{Impact} = \frac{\text{hazard} \quad \times \quad \text{vulnerability}}{\text{exposure}}$$

Figure 1. The dimensions of disaster.

our understanding of both trauma and resilience, however, comes an appreciation of the complex interaction of factors that may contribute to impact. Although traumatic impact is clearly a risk factor in the overwhelming experience of (for instance) an earthquake or a terrorist attack, trauma symptoms or a trauma diagnosis are by no means certain outcomes of disaster. Many other factors contribute to risk of traumatization. As Figure 1 suggests, that impact results from the interplay between what, in the concept of disaster risk reduction management (DRRM), is termed the "hazard" (or, in stress and trauma literature, the "stressor") in relation to levels of vulnerability of those experiencing the events, and their degree of exposure.

Using the Christchurch earthquake as an example: A practitioner at work in the center of the city, where most of the casualties occurred due to falling masonry or collapsing buildings, was exposed to sights, sounds, and smells beyond her previous experience. All her senses engaged in the attempt to cope; traumatic symptoms were present for many days or weeks past the initial earthquake, with the frequent and often strong aftershocks viscerally triggering her into alarm responses that also kicked in when other loud, but benign, noises occurred. As a clear example of the overwhelming *scale* of the experience, her risk of trauma impact was (and remains) high, and will likely be evident in supervision.

Within the intersecting factors cited in Figure 1, a person's vulnerability to impact may also be determined by preexisting exposure to trauma, or by the high levels of stress within the home and work environment. A post-earthquake supervision session with this social worker may reveal that the earthquakes have exacerbated ongoing relationship tensions, the balancing act that she maintains in responsibilities for her children and her elderly mother, and new challenges that disaster creates by competition for rental accommodation, fuel, and transport. Although these stressors may not in themselves be traumatic, such stress compounds to undermine opportunity for resilience and posttraumatic growth, and therefore needs to be acknowledged within supervision. Appreciation of the intersection of disaster scale, exposure, and preexisting vulnerabilities therefore adds to a more nuanced appreciation of trauma-informed supervision within a disaster context.

The cause and origin of disasters further add to the complexity of our understanding. Aotearoa New Zealand expectation is that of a vulnerability to events originating in the natural world—those which the International Federation of Red Cross and Red Crescent Societies (IFRC) categorize as geophysical, hydrological, climatological, or biological—as distinct from technological and "manmade" hazards (International Federation of Red Cross and Red Crescent Societies [IFRC], n.d.). In Aotearoa New Zealand, we are schooled to expect earthquakes such as the earthquake sequence that saw Canterbury hit by more than 4,300 tremors of more than magnitude 3 on the Richter scale in the five years from September 2010(Earthquake Commission, n.d.), and which created major damage and brought loss of life in the city of Christchurch. Our beaches have tsunami warning systems in place; our North Island volcanoes periodically rumble and remind us of the lava beneath. There is often a distinction made between these "natural" disasters and those of human origin perpetrated by humans through political action, industrial malfeasance, or poor engineering. For events of human origin, we like to think we can exert some control, perhaps prevent them from occurring; there are people we may blame, social and political changes that we may attempt to create through military intervention, change of government, or through legislation. Disasters of human origin play out as much along moral and ethical lines as they do through disaster relief. However, our understanding of the phases of disaster will, in this article, illustrate that even natural disasters follow lines of human vulnerability and interaction, important factors for trauma-informed supervision practice.

To illustrate this interplay of factors, another Christchurch example is used. Our houses in Aotearoa New Zealand are usually wooden, and tend to bend and buckle in earthquakes rather than shatter, as would brick. Insurance assessors for one supervisee may have considered his house repairable: out of alignment and off its foundations, it could be rebuilt. However, one of the big post-earthquake problems was the liquefaction and strength of the ground itself, and the geological surveys may have considered the land under this supervisee's house to be unsafe for any construction. The potential trauma here is not from the earthquake but the limbo created by institutional inter-mediaries in his insurance claim, adding a relational dimension informed by trauma research that considers the human origin of the stressors and the breaches of trust that may ensue (Ratcliffe, Ruddell, & Smith, 2014). In this instance the supervisee is locked into the anger and frustration of wrangling with bureaucracies, and is at risk of both emotional exhaustion and an over-identification with clients in a similar situation. Any trauma that he may have experienced in the actual quakes has morphed into blame, recrimination, and a bitter comparison between himself and others in a similar situation. Recovery processes explored within supervision must therefore consider not only the physical impact of a natural disaster, but the subsequent relational processes in which survivors (supervisees and clients alike) are engaged.

Conversely, disasters created by human negligence or malfeasance may have physical or environmental consequences that may be explored within super-vision. In Aotearoa New Zealand in 2011, the container ship *Rena* struck a reef and sank in the Bay of Plenty in the North Island, a result of human error and poor judgment. It had a devastating effect on beach environments and seafood, and impacted social and cultural domains as well as the natural environment (Hunt, Smith, Hamerton, & Sargisson, 2014). The definitional distinction between human and natural causation is therefore one that perhaps masks the complexity of the human experience of disaster that may be addressed within a supervision context.

As supervisors, we have a range of accessible theories with which to understand the impact of disasters on ourselves, on supervisees, and on the client communities in which we work. Unlike most trauma-informed supervision that focuses on the impact of life events experienced by individual clients and their families, the trauma lens that we use in a disaster context therefore needs to be informed by the recognition that recovery from trauma may be a shared, community-wide endeavor affecting clients, supervisees, and supervisors alike. Supervision practice can incorporate the possibilities of posttraumatic growth (Westphal & Bonanno, 2007), strengths and recovery perspectives, resilience (Bottrell, 2009), and cultural meaning-making in the face of adverse events (Tummala-Narra, 2007; Ungar, 2008). Social capital principles of bonding, bridging, and linking (Aldrich, 2012) connect relational and ecological understanding with a community-level opportunity for sense-making and action within supervision. Alongside the psychological impact of disasters, trauma-informed supervision in a disaster context needs also to be framed by issues of equity and marginalization, access to support and resources, institutional and organizational functioning, and the relationships among national, regional, and local governance (Alipour et al., 2015; Dionisio & Pawson, 2016; Finch, Emrich, & Cutter, 2010; Quiros & Berger, 2015). The challenge for anyone supervising the two Christchurch supervisees in the previous scenarios may be to find active supports (conceptual or practical) by which they can regain a sense of agency and efficacy, and separate the impact on themselves from that on their clients. Trauma-informed supervision in a disaster context is therefore a challenge of working in complexity; the origin of the stressor, the marginalization that may result for both supervisees and their clients, and the environmental conditions post-disaster are therefore also of key importance in our understanding of disasters within supervision.

I now turn to a consideration of the role of supervision in the disaster context, utilizing an understanding of the phases of disaster, and employing a systems perspective of supervision that assists in unpacking the different roles and tasks of supervision that may be utilized within each disaster phase.

The location, role, and function of supervision practice in the disaster context

DRRM can be portrayed simplistically as a sequential and cyclical process of prevention and mitigation, preparation, response, and recovery (Figure 2), alongside a recognition that recovery for individuals and communities is not linear and

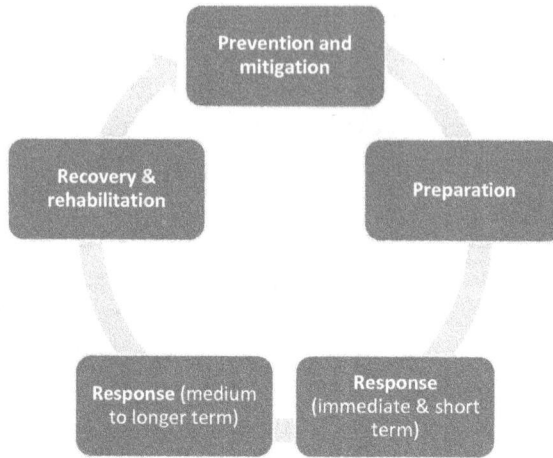

Figure 2. The phases of disaster.

is subject to a complex interaction of factors (Norris, Tracy, & Galea, 2009; Wisner & Adams, 2002). Models of disaster response do not usually contain expectations of the role of supervision, being characterized more by the physical management of the disaster (building collapse, threats to physical safety, movement of peoples and resources, for instance) and by a "command and control" approach to disaster management that does not suggest an easy integration with preexisting, developmental support structures such as clinical supervision (Harrald, 2006; Manyena, 2006; van Heugten, 2014). Similar fields (critical incident stress management [CISM], and the humanitarian aid field) have evolved differing relationships with supervision: within CISM, supervision is located in the preparation and follow-up phases rather than in active crisis intervention (Adamson, 2013; Pack, 2012). Supervisory support for humanitarian workers has relatively recently been constructed as a core requirement to prepare staff for the field while deployed and post-deployment (Ehrenreich & Elliott, 2004; Sphere, 2011). The role of supervision as a stress management tool—clearly of importance from a trauma-informed perspective—may drop off at times of crisis, either as an expedient focus on immediate survival and resource needs, or because other models of support, such as psychological first aid, are more tailored to a crisis and emergency context (World Health Organization, 2011). The principle, however, upon which I base this article is that supervision has a role to play within all phases of a disaster, but that it will be more active and visible in the before-and-after periods of DRRM, when the immediacy of physical risks and survival have either not yet occurred or have given way to more relational processes of human recovery in the changed environment.

In order to make sense of the relationship between supervision and DRRM, I utilize a systems perspective of a developmental model of supervision from the social work profession, which incorporates an understanding of supervision

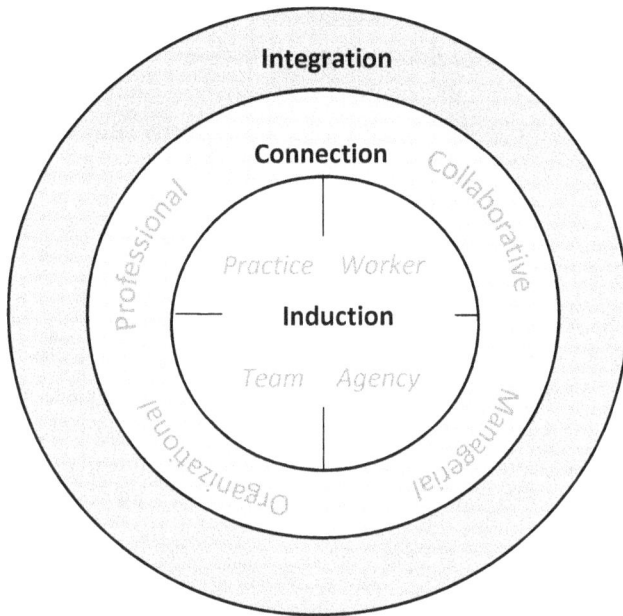

Figure 3. Developmental model of supervision (Brown & Bourne, 1996).

within organizational and practice contexts and addresses the development of the supervision relationship over time. Brown and Bourne's (1996) systemic model of supervision development (Figure 3) depicts the three conceptual stages of supervision from the induction phase for a new supervisee (where learning about roles and contexts is discrete), through a stage of making connection (where different aspects of the systemic process emerges), into an integration phase representative of the non-directive, reflective, and challenging roles of supervision with an experienced practitioner. This model enables a nuanced appreciation of how crisis and environmental events may alter the supervisee-supervisor relationship.

Brown and Bourne (1996) compared and contrasted the requirements of supervision in the induction and integration phases of the supervision journey, suggesting that orientation and settling into a new environment require supervision to be relatively directive and didactic, with a focus on information-giving and skills. In contrast, an experienced practitioner's "helicopter view" of practice enables the development of self-directed, creative, abstract, and reflective thinking, with the supervisor's role more challenging and focused on process. Fundamental assumptions about the roles and tasks of supervision may be challenged when trauma, acute stress, and crisis enter into the supervision space through disaster. Integration is no longer possible in a markedly disintegrated environment; supervisees' thinking, decision making, and problem solving may be rigid under stress. Professional, managerial, organizational, and collaborative practices cannot be assumed in disaster settings (van Heugten, 2014) because the factors that ground supervisees in their practice may have radically shifted: it is not "business as usual." New roles and tasks are required to adapt to both the external environment and to personal and professional impacts that may include traumatic reactions. In response, the supervisee and supervisor will both experience the need to revisit their own comprehension of their practice, their roles within and outside of supervision, and the tasks and functions of their immediate team and organization. Regardless of the level of experience of the supervisee, the "new normal" may require the use of practices and processes within supervision that may be more resonant of an induction and early developmental phase, as new experiences, responses, and pathways are explored. Adaptations to supervision practice may therefore be required in response to the immediate crisis and in the downstream period of response and recovery.

For both our Christchurch supervisees in the previous examples, one faced with stressors within her home and relationships, the other battling the bureaucratic processes that are preventing him from addressing the fundamental needs of adequate shelter and a place to belong, their abilities to integrate the roles and tasks of their occupation have been inhibited, despite being experienced practitioners. The disaster has, in a very real sense, dis-integrated their sense of agency, affected their decision-making processes, and over-emphasized emotion-based coping over a problem-solving coping style. The supervisor response may, as Brown and Bourne (1996) suggested, need to revert to a more directive mode of engagement more reminiscent of an induction phase of supervision.

Preparation for disaster does, of course, begin in the classroom. Cunningham (2004), Carello and Butler (2015), and Weine and colleagues (2002) called for trauma-informed education to increase practice effectiveness, to reduce the risks of secondary traumatization, and to allow for the maximization of learning opportunities within conditions of emotional safety. These suggestions parallel calls for the curriculum in human service disciplines to be disaster-informed and disaster-aware (e.g., Adamson, 2014; Dominelli, 2013; Yutrzenka & Naifeh, 2008). Topics taught in qualifying courses may predict the knowledge bases required across the phases of disaster. Where attachment theory is taught, for instance, the impact of disasters can be used as a case example of a child growing up in stressful environments; where community development is taught, so can notions of social capital be illustrated through the development of networking skills and the examination of social supports. Within supervision, the supervisor can ask supervisees to make links with their professional education and to utilize these links within the current disaster-recovery context. A knowledge focus can continue into post-qualifying supervision, with a supervisee's awareness of burnout, secondary and vicarious traumatic stress and trauma, compassion fatigue, and resilience theories (perhaps with a clinical focus on the needs of individual clients) refocused in relation to their workload, work-life balance, and ongoing well-being and performance.

What follows is an overview of the role and function of supervision, as demonstrated through the main phases of disaster response (Figure 2) and summarized within Table 1. Whilst there is a conceptual and practical

Table 1. The role and function of supervision in the disaster context.

Phases of Disaster			
Prevention and Mitigation Preparation		Response	Recovery
Focus on self-care, self-knowledge, reflection, enhancement of emotional intelligence, stress management.			
Relationship between supervision and other organizational supports (emergency plans, debriefing, etc.).			
Ensuring adequate psycho-education regarding trauma, disaster, impact, and intervention. "Audits" for awareness of personal and systemic resources. Creation, monitoring, and updating of stress management plans for both ambient and acute stress. Awareness of disaster plans (personal, organizational, and community). Tabletop exercises with disaster scenarios.		Changes of role for supervisor and supervisee. Coping with personal and professional impact. Is supervision available? Is it appropriate? Are supervisors affected as well as supervisee? Are the supervisory spaces intact? Is there still risk?	Reflection on new ways of coping, new learning, post-traumatic growth. Systems planning in response to the "new normal." Identifying triggers. Creating safe space within supervision.
		Implementation of stress management strategies for acute stress and crisis. Are traditional or usual forms of supervision adequate or appropriate? Awareness of grief and healing processes (individual, community, and cultural). Skills for assessing and addressing traumatized and stressed behavior (e.g., rigid decision making, emotional versus problem-focused coping). Responding to outsiders.	

difference between the first phase (prevention and mitigation of harm) and the second phase of preparation and planning, I have collapsed both into a discussion of the role of supervision prior to a disaster occurring.

Planning for the unpredictable: Prevention, mitigation, and preparation

Much effective practice from a systems perspective can be underpinned by attention to the first two phases of the cycle, those of prevention and mitigation, and of preparation. Prior to disaster, other roles and responsibilities of a supervision agenda will dominate: attention to casework, organizational processes, professional development, and so on, may appear as more pressing topics. Even a trauma-informed process may focus upon the individual client, worker, and team as opposed to the community-level focus of a disaster. Supervisions may focus on "what's on top" rather than planning for future occurrences. Thus, one of the responsibilities of supervision is to equip both supervisors and supervisees with the systemic analysis that both alerts and strengthens future responses to community-wide disaster.

A practical example of a tool to increase disaster awareness and planning is the stress and trauma audit. (*Audit* is somewhat actuarial term, and may be reimagined as an informal survey, a guided conversation, or a piece of creative whiteboard drawing. It can be structured as a flexible list of questions or intersessional homework.) Attention in an audit process can be paid not only to the knowledge bases for professional practice in disaster, but also to supervisees' and clients' individual levels of preparedness. Developed initially as a supervision tool to prepare for the occurrence of critical incidents, an audit can serve to develop a shared understanding of supervisees' levels of awareness and the ecology of their own support systems and coping responses to stress that they can then mirror in work with clients. Both informal and formal supports can be explored, through reflection on past experience ("How have you coped when this has happened in the past?"), to consideration of a supervisee's knowledge of formal organizational responses within a critical incident stress management framework (Adamson, 2013). An audit can be used in the early stages of a supervision relationship, or perhaps at a significant point where issues of stress, trauma, and resilience occur, or when news of a global disaster has triggered reflection on community vulnerability. Part of a supervision session can be devoted to exploring where supervisees' supports come from, in their individual home and work situations, and their knowledge of community and workplace resources. A new lens of crisis, stress, and trauma can be introduced with questions such as "Where do you turn when you are under stress?" or "What supports are available in the neighbourhood/organisation?" Although from a trauma-informed perspective we need to be alert to the risks inherent in the disclosure of past traumas, opening up conversations about current processes of self-care and support can allow for a platform of preparation for resilience in regard to the likelihood of trauma-related impacts, including the advent of disaster. From a systemic perspective such as that which Brown and Bourne (1996) espoused, a trauma-informed preparation for the impact of disaster will require consideration of both individual and contextual knowledge and skills.

Following Brown and Bourne's (1996) developmental approach to supervision, both induction and integration phases of supervision can accommodate preparation for disaster. Alongside agency orientation, team roles, and professional tasks, contextual awareness of disaster risk can be introduced. Corin (2011) described the preparation of Christchurch hospital social workers to respond to mass emergencies, which anticipated their role within a coordinated incident response, focusing on the provision of psychosocial support to patients and their families. This occurred prior to the earthquakes of 2010–2011. Although Corin did not explicitly mention supervision's contribution to this preparation, the accepted role of the social worker as part of the emergency team, on call for such events, would have created a platform within supervision for the exploration of trauma-informed and disaster-aware discussion.

Disaster research universally suggests that individuals and communities are more resilient after disasters if they are more connected (in terms of social capital) prior to the event (United Nations, 2015; UNISDR, 2015). Prevention and mitigation of disasters may take supervision outside of its traditional roles and clinical focus. Supervisors may have management and leadership roles in their profession and in the organization; this means that they can be active in systems preparedness through the raising of issues introduced by supervision sessions in a leadership or management forum. Engaging the supervisee in a scoping of organization and community resources (e.g., "What are our disaster plans? Where is the emergency kit? How do we prepare the clients for an evacuation? Where do we find an animal-friendly shelter?") can be a step toward trauma mitigation for agencies when conducting planning cycles, re-structuring, or in team development processes, that can introduce a systemic alertness to the mitigation of disaster risk and its resultant risk of traumatization. Case studies of experiences within the disaster context can be introduced (for instance) into staff development planning, journal clubs, leadership coaching, or the critical incident stress management plans for an organization. Supervisors can construct group activities with supervisees to do "tabletop" or whiteboard exercises using "what if" scenarios involving, for instance, an apartment building fire or the aftermath of a terrorist attack. Such exercises integrate knowledge of clients' needs, supervisees' own professional development and skills, trauma awareness, and the organizational environment.

Responding to disasters: The limits to the role of supervision

Supervision is not a mainstay of disaster response and may, indeed, not be available in a disaster situation. Supervision is often one of the first supports to be underutilized in crisis, either due to re-prioritization of tasks or for resourcing reasons (Pulido, 2007; van Heugten, 2014). Supervision's role may change, but its status and networked location within, or between, organizational settings can contribute to new and fast-changing demands. Of prime importance in a disaster event is whether supervisors are able to function as supervisors *and* in their other roles, or whether they are temporarily forced by the exigencies of the emergency to attend to their own individual, family, and community needs. The "airline principle" of self-care (as in airplane safety briefings; putting on your own oxygen mask before that of others) applies here.

Assuming one's own safety has been regained, it may still be some considerable time before "normal service" of supervision sessions can be resumed, during which time roles, responsibilities, locations, and even client groups may have changed. Nonetheless, a preexisting supervisory relationship can become a tool for disaster response: brief encounters with supervisees, reminding them of their trauma and community knowledge, may assist with crisis management; new roles forced upon all workers by the disaster may be expedited by established working relationships. Supervision may morph into debriefing roles, utilizing trauma-informed supervisory skills to defuse and debrief from particular incidents within the disaster (Pulido, 2007). Group supervision methods may be utilized as an alternative to individually focused exploration of impact. Supervisors who remain working in the same locality as their supervisees can use the supervisory relationship to advantage by providing creative stress-reducing activities for individuals or groups: for example, the introduction of 30-minute breaks for groups of workers to sing or dance (neither activity being a customary activity for supervision). The prior relationships and a trauma-informed awareness of the need for stress release enables a supervisor to provide respite—and some light relief—within a potentially overwhelming situation.

Disaster recovery and supervision

It is in the immediate and longer term processes of recovery from disaster that the opportunities for clinical supervision become most apparent, and where the process focus of the reflective space can be most easily identified as trauma-informed. Our awareness of the element of time within the definition of disaster is crucial here. Not only will the tasks and demands of an early recovery stage be different from the needs of the organizational, worker, and client needs several years later; in later recovery periods, too, there is a risk that a disaster- and trauma-informed lens may be subsumed within the everyday pressures without recognition of the pervasiveness of adaptive patterns and resource issues stemming from the disaster events.

The caveat that supervision under these conditions needs to be trauma-informed rather than trauma-centred (Knight, 2015) suggests that supervisors may be in a position to identify and assess traumatic impact—to triage, name, and support rather than to work predominantly from within a therapeutic lens of trauma practice. A supervisor of a community agency in London, assisting family support workers in low-income areas, may not predominantly be supervising from a trauma-informed perspective; other frames of reference such as social justice, domestic violence, or addiction knowledge may take center stage. When the Grenfell Tower fire occurred in London in June 2017, the practice within this agency would need to deliver the family support—perhaps being involved in re-housing, reestablishing financial security, or locating food and clothing grants —but the workers' supervision and practice would need to be trauma-informed because of the ongoing community sensitivity to this disaster. Mindful that resilience will be supported by community and social processes outside of super-vision, supervisors in a disaster recovery stage may utilize a bifocal approach of being able to assess distress, avoidant, or hyper-vigilant responses of clients and supervisees, or rigid decision making, within a broader awareness of social justice and psychosocial issues in the community. A practitioner in this London agency, for example, may have been verbally attacked by a family made homeless by the fire and traumatized by losing neighbors and playmates to the flames. For a supervisee hurt and distressed by the anger of the family, supervision may afford a safe space in which to process the reasons for the anger, and to locate these trauma-induced emotions within an analysis of tenants' relationships with the local authority housing department, or the council policy of placing refugee and asylum seeker families within run-down, high-rise apartment blocks.

In considering the role of supervision in recovery from disasters, I address the following factors: supervision in a shared traumatic reality; the importance of culture for recovery; challenges to adaptation and coping in recovery; and the importance of taking a long-term view in our understanding of recovery after disaster.

Supervision in a shared traumatic reality

Supervision has been described as a buffer to trauma impact and a support for worker resilience in a non-disaster context (Mor Barak, Travis, Pyun, & Xie, 2009; Toren, 2008). This buffer becomes even more crucial in a community-wide disaster. Not only will disaster-affected supervisees be working directly with survivors; supervisors may be sharing their supervisees' traumatic realities (Baum, 2010, 2013). The relational space carries risk of secondary or vicarious traumatization. Although risks (the "wounded healer" being one psychodynamic concept, for example) abound in this shared exposure to disaster, one of the processes of healing is that of social connectedness and social capital (Aldrich, 2012). Shared understandings can provide a bond from which to develop deeper and trauma-informed consideration of recovery. The early days after resumption of supervision may feel a very fragile experience, with the challenge of creating safety while the disaster is still playing out, and, as with Brown and Bourne's (1996) model, reconnecting with roles and tasks in the new and perhaps unrecognizable organizational environment. Not having to justify changes in emotional and physical reactiveness, behavioral patterns such as keeping a mobile phone switched on, lateness in attendance due to slowed or rerouted traffic, or changes in office location, all are foundations upon which to reflect on experience and practice. The (well-supervised) supervisors' awareness of their own reactivity can heighten awareness of a supervisee's emotional well-being, with disaster and its potentially traumatizing effects no longer being an elephant in the room, but as a named and very obvious element in supervision, checking in and identifying concerns may be facilitated. Rituals of creating safety may be important here, developed in a shared understanding of disaster and its impact.

Differential experience may produce challenges. One supervisee from Christchurch, out of town for the most devastating earthquake, experienced an "insider/outsider" divisiveness with a supervisor who was actually present, suggesting that (as the supervisee had not been present) she had no right to express distress, despite her house being badly damaged. A trauma-informed explanation of this lies in the as yet unresolved emotional impact on the supervisor, and suggests that the supervisor too required some further support. The intrusion of outsiders into the liminal space of a disaster may be fraught with unintended pitfalls. Both in 9/11 and in Aotearoa New Zealand's Canterbury earthquakes, media reports highlighted an influx of counselors immediately following the disaster. Aside from the inadvisability of interpreting all disaster impact as traumatic and all survivors as victims needing therapy, the presence of outsiders offering professional services such as counseling or supervision requires sensitivity on the part of the outsiders, and considerable explanation by insiders, who may initially prefer a supervision process with someone who shares their experience.

Culture, supervision, and recovery

Traditional, Western-based models of supervision, while acknowledging the opportunity for group supervision practice, tend to emphasize the professional development and well-being of the individual supervisee, who is often engaged in a casework relationship with, perhaps, individuals, couples, or families. Supervision in a disaster context has much to learn from models of supervision from indigenous and non-Western cultures such as Māori (Eruera, 2005; Hair & O'Donoghue, 2009; Lipsham, 2012). Collective cultures may offer models appropriate for the recognition of community-wide trauma and stress, as well as collective approaches to resilience-building that both supervision and its associated practice may utilize. For instance, workers within one agency, all equally involved and affected by their work in assisting fire survivors, such as those in the Grenfell Tower disaster in London, may use group supervision and activities such as team meals, singing, and time-out, as an organized response to issues identified within supervision. Two relational processes familiar to those in Aotearoa New Zealand, that of *karakia* (prayer or call to wider spiritual realities) at the opening and closing of a session, and of *whanaungatanga* (checking in/the making of connections) may develop greater significance and be paralleled within other cultures (Eruera, 2005; Lipsham, 2012). A *karakia* can be either religious or secular, and such an adaptation to the beginning process of a supervision can call attention to altered realities outside of the supervision: similarly, asking after the well-being of friends and family, perhaps not usually included within the professional space, links the supervision environment to the wider community context in which disaster recovery is occurring.

Challenges to adaptation and coping in recovery

On a practical basis, the shape and processes of supervision may need to adapt to a post-disaster environment. Resources, practicalities, and a keener sense of shared group identity and bonding may suggest the use of group supervision processes as opposed to a one-on-one model. Distance processes such as online supervision may be more feasible for regular supervision (Augusterfer, 2012). Relocation of staff, and new agency roles and multidisciplinary relationships, may become both barriers and opportunities. Supervisors and supervisees alike may be faced with the competing demands for resources and the diminishing of the perceived importance of supervision by organizations facing financial and resourcing challenges (Pulido, 2007; van Heugten, 2014).

Within supervision sessions, the disaster experience will not always be the focal point of supervision in a time of recovery, and the supervisor's task may resemble a balancing act between remembering and moving on, when both home lives and work pressures are experiencing high levels of adaptation demands (Palm, Polusny, & Follette, 2004). Supervision's positioning as a relational process can assist in identifying concerns such as grief and loss (Harms et al., 2015), and anxiety and depression presentations. Thus, supervision of our two workers in Christchurch may, on an ongoing basis, incorporate a trauma-informed and disaster-aware approach that allows for periodic check-ins on the meaning-making process that is continuing to undergo change and growth in the months and years following the disaster. Supervision in a disaster context may be constructed as a "liminal" space, a transitional, fluctuating zone that navigates thresholds between continuity and change in an unsettled and evolving environment, with the supervisor's challenge being a cognitive-behavioral task of working with a supervisee to see what can be changed. Supervision can work toward the acceptance of those things over which the supervisee has no control and assistance in consolidating a sense of agency and hope. I use a three-stage model that assists supervisees in identifying the personal impact on themselves ("What are you experiencing right now?"), then a separation of the things that are theirs to work on from the things that cannot be resolved by their own (or their allies') actions ("What control do you have over this? Who will assist in finding those necessary resources?"), and finally a re-integration process that may involve planning courses of action for changes that can be achieved ("What steps are you going to take before our next meeting?").

Imagine a supervision occurring in the aftermath of a terrorist attack, perhaps any one of the recent knife or vehicle attacks in Europe. A supervisee is working in the community, responding to the anger of local residents (often expressed as anti-immigrant sentiment), alongside supporting immigrant families who are justifiably fearful of an escalation of racist attacks in the neighborhood. The supervisee expresses frustration and despair at the enormity of the political and social realities that have led to these attacks. The supervision session offers the supervisee, in this disaster-recovery context and in keeping with Brown and Bourne's (1996) model, the opportunity to reexamine the professional role, to reevaluate assumptions and knowledge about the situation, to reassess skills and interventions, and perhaps to reconsider strategies for change. A decision to engage with different religious communities, or to learn more about the refugee and migrant experience, may provide a sense of forward movement and hope for the workers, as they regain a sense of agency.

The importance of taking a long-term view in our understanding of recovery after disaster

Finally in this discussion of recovery from disaster, I wish to acknowledge that, within supervision, there is no recognizably finite end to the need to be disaster-informed. Our knowledge of the generational impact of trauma informs us that echoes of distress, disenfranchisement, and horror can reverberate across genera-tions. An outsider view of the Canterbury earthquakes of 2010–2011, for instance, is that the city of Christchurch is being rebuilt, that almost all insurance claims are settled, and the majority of people have their homes back; and yet the dynamics of disaster impact continue to play out in the marginalization of vulnerable people, the dislocation of whole suburbs and communities, school closures, and the mental health presentations as a result of six years of continuing stress. Children born in 2010 have known no other environment. Trauma-informed supervision in a recovery environment needs to be vigilant for disaster impact. While the earthquake sequences used as examples of disasters in this article appear to be lessening in intensity, they have not gone away; the sensitivities for new shakes remain. For those in other disaster contexts around the world, community vigilance for the next terror threat mirrors the hypervigilance of traumatic expo-sure, and thus shapes the manner in which supervision can be most effective. A simple check-in asking the supervisee to locate, on a scale of 1 to 10, the influence of the disaster on their current experiences (and that of their clients) may be a simple snapshot of well-being that assists in remembering and accepting the impact of the disaster.

Self-care and the supervisor

Palm and colleagues (2004) suggested that disaster and trauma workers are often inclined to neglect their own well-being in the face of the overwhelming needs outside of themselves. The magnitude and scale of the disaster may seem as if there is unending need that may appear to surmount the individual needs of both the supervisee and supervisor. Supervision will be a chain reaction; supervisors will also bear witness and there is a professional obligation to attend to self-care so that damage from traumatic exposure does not result. Pulido (2007) talked about the impact of clients' stories on social workers, who mirrored feelings of being over-whelmed, helplessness in the face of immense suffering, and the consequent emotional and psychological impact on themselves. Compassion fatigue is a very real risk for supervisors (Chung & Davies, 2016; Creamer & Liddle, 2005; Dekel, Hantman, Ginzburg, & Solomon, 2007) and our self-care and stress management practices can therefore serve as a mirror to supervisees. Exploration of the processes of self-care can be a useful adjunct to the auditing of stress, trauma, resilience, and coping repertoires in the planning for disaster.

Supervisors in a disaster context may well be survivors of the disaster themselves. It is more than likely that they too will be living and working within a disaster-infused reality, and responding to the pressures that are playing out over time—relationally, systemically, and structurally. Bearing witness, listening to narratives of distress and the voicing of frustrations at bureaucratic ineptitude or insensitivity, has to be managed, perhaps by limiting exposure and certainly by having supervision oneself. Virtue developed the concept of multiple holding (Virtue & Fouché, 2010): the work that the supervisors do with supervisees must also be supported by their own supervision and other supports, both formal and informal, thus forming a chain of support that has as many links in it as necessary. The greater the length of the chain from the trauma, the greater the opportunity for an overview of systemic and structural responses and reflections to support the relational processes of the actual supervision. Although the supervision of a frontline worker in a disaster context may need to be trauma-informed about the physical, emotional, and psychological impact of the disaster (on supervisees, on clients, on supervisees' listening to clients' stories), the narratives may reverberate with the supervisor, who may be exposed to many similar stories. The disaster impact may therefore provide opportunity for a nuanced analysis of what can be done to support *all* supervisees affected by the disaster, thus providing an action-focused potential for posttraumatic growth after their own disaster experience.

Conclusion

Supervision can become an extraordinarily pivotal process between the processing of individual responses to traumatic exposure within a disaster context, and the forging of new, systemically and community-based opportunities for recovery and rebuilding. It is a site for the development of trauma and disaster awareness, for linking supervisees to wider community recovery, raising awareness of the social justice and psychosocial issues in community, and for encouraging the growth of resilience both individually and systemically. In order to effectively supervise in a trauma-informed disaster context, we need an equally complex knowledge base that spans both clinical interventions and community-level awareness. We work from the value base that the impact of disasters can vary from person to person, and that the appraisal of traumatic stress is potentially individual (Hobfoll, 2001) and open to cultural interpretation (Ungar, 2008). Supervision needs to be trauma-alert and trauma-informed without always being trauma-centered. Supervisors negotiate a balancing act between establishing supervision as a site for resilience and hope, and becoming vulnerable to secondary traumatization through exposure to wider stress levels than they themselves are experiencing; self-care and the modeling of this for supervisees is paramount.

Disasters can fracture networks and communities; supervision practice can actively contribute to strengthening narratives of hope and to "resilience moves" for supervisee practice. Trauma-informed supervision in the disaster context requires us to maintain continuity in our supervision practice while adapting flexibly to the demands of a new order. New and adapted processes will emerge out of the changes that the external events and our personal, professional, and systemic responses have determined. Disasters, like any traumatic experience, can shatter assumptions but can also lead to new possibilities, altered configurations of alliances and networks, new organizational awareness of the needs of employees and clients, and a heightened appreciation for the importance of the reflective space.

References

Adamson, C. (2013). Stress, resilience and responding to civil defence emergencies and natural disasters: An ecological approach. In L. Beddoe & J. Maidment (Eds.), *Social work practice for promoting health and wellbeing: Critical issues* (pp. 63–75). Abingdon, UK: Routledge.

Adamson, C. (2014). A social work lens for a disaster-informed curriculum. *Advances in Social Work and Welfare Education, 16*, 7–22.

Aldrich, D. P. (2012). *Building resilience: Social capital in post-disaster recovery.* Chicago, IL: University of Chicago Press.

Alipour, F., Khankeh, H., Fekrazad, H., Kamali, M., Rafiey, H., & Ahmadi, S. (2015). Social issues and post-disaster recovery: A qualitative study in an Iranian context. *International Social Work, 58*, 689–703.

Augusterfer, E. F. (2012). Telemental health: Clinical, technical, and administrative foundations for evidence-based practice. In K. Myers & C. L. Turvey (Eds.), *Clinically informed telemental health in post-disaster areas* (pp. 347–366). London, UK: Elsevier.

Baum, N. (2010). Shared traumatic reality in communal disasters: Toward a conceptualization. *Psychotherapy: Theory, Research, Practice, Training, 47*, 249–259.

Baum, N. (2013). Professionals' double exposure in the shared traumatic reality of wartime: Contributions to professional growth and stress. *British Journal of Social Work, 44*(8), 2113–2134. doi:10.1093/bjsw/bct085

Bottrell, D. (2009). Understanding "marginal" perspectives: Towards a social theory of resilience. *Qualitative Social Work, 8*, 321–339.

Brown, A., & Bourne, I. (1996). *The social work supervisor.* Buckingham, UK: Open University Press.

Carello, J., & Butler, L. D. (2015). Practicing what we teach: Trauma-informed educational practice. *Journal of Teaching in Social Work, 35*, 262–278.

Chung, J., & Davies, N. (2016). A review of compassion fatigue of nurses during and after the Canterbury earthquakes. *Australasian Journal of Disaster and Trauma Studies, 20*, 69–80.

Corin, C. (2011). The Christchurch hospital social work service response in the first hours after the Christchurch earthquake of 22nd February 2011. *Aotearoa New Zealand Social Work, 23*(3), 58–62.

Creamer, T. L., & Liddle, B. J. (2005). Secondary traumatic stress among disaster mental health workers responding to the September 11 attacks. *Journal of Traumatic Stress, 18*, 89–96.

Cunningham, M. (2004). Teaching social workers about trauma: Reducing the risks of vicarious traumatization in the classroom. *Journal of Social Work Education, 40*, 305–317.

Dekel, R., Hantman, S., Ginzburg, K., & Solomon, Z. (2007). The cost of caring? Social workers in hospitals confront ongoing terrorism. *British Journal of Social Work, 37*, 1247–1261.

Dionisio, M. R., & Pawson, E. (2016). Building resilience through post-disaster community projects: Responses to the 2010 and 2011 Christchurch earthquakes and 2011 Tōhoku tsunami. *Australasian Journal of Disaster & Trauma Studies, 20*, 107–115.

Dominelli, L. (2013). Social work education for disaster relief work. In M. Gray, J. Coates, & T. Hetherington (Eds.), *Environmental social work* (pp. 280–297). Abingdon, UK: Routledge.

Earthquake Commission. (n.d.). *Scorecard.* Retrieved from http://www.eqc.govt.nz/canter bury-earthquakes/progress-updates/scorecard

Ehrenreich, J. H., & Elliott, T. L. (2004). Managing stress in humanitarian aid workers: A survey of humanitarian aid agencies' psychosocial training and support of staff. *Peace and Conflict: Journal of Peace Psychology, 10*(1), 53–66.

Eruera, M. M. (2005). *He kōrero kōrari: Supervision for Māori: Weaving the past, into the present for the future* (Unpublished master's thesis). Palmerston North: Massey University.

Finch, C., Emrich, C., & Cutter, S. (2010). Disaster disparities and differential recovery in New Orleans. *Population & Environment, 31*, 179–202.

Hair, H. J., & O'Donoghue, K. (2009). Culturally relevant, socially just social work supervision: Becoming visible through a social constructionist lens. *Journal of Ethnic and Cultural Diversity in Social Work, 18*, 70–88.

Harms, L., Block, K., Gallagher, H. C., Gibbs, L., Bryant, R. A., Lusher, D., & Waters, E. (2015). Conceptualising post-disaster recovery: Incorporating grief experiences. *The British Journal of Social Work, 45*, i170–i187.

Harrald, J. R. (2006). Agility and discipline: Critical success factors for disaster response. *The Annals of the American Academy of Political and Social Science, 604*, 256–272.

Hobfoll, S. E. (2001). The influence of culture, community, and the nested-self in the stress process: Advancing conservation of resources theory. *Applied Psychology, 50*, 337–421.

Hoffman, M. A., & Kruczek, T. (2011). A bioecological model of mass trauma: Individual, community, and societal effects. *The Counseling Psychologist, 39*, 1087–1127.

Hunt, S., Smith, K., Hamerton, H., & Sargisson, R. J. (2014). An incident control centre in action: Response to the Rena oil spill in New Zealand. *Journal of Contingencies and Crisis Management, 22*(1), 63–66. doi:10.1111/1468-5973.12036

International Federation of Red Cross and Red Crescent Societies (IFRC). (n.d.). *Types of disasters: Definition of hazard.* Retrieved from http://www.ifrc.org/en/what-we-do/disaster-management/about-disasters/definition-of-hazard/

Knight, C. (2015). Trauma-informed social work practice: Practice considerations and challenges. *Clinical Social Work Journal, 43*, 25–37.

Lipsham, M. J. H. (2012). Āta as an innovative method and practice tool in supervision. *Aotearoa New Zealand Social Work Review, 24*, 31–40.

Manyena, S. B. (2006). The concept of resilience revisited. *Disasters, 30*, 434–450.

Mor Barak, M., Travis, D. J., Pyun, H., & Xie, B. (2009). The impact of supervision on worker outcomes: A meta-analysis. *Social Service Review, 83*(1), 3–32.

Norris, F. H., Tracy, M., & Galea, S. (2009). Looking for resilience: Understanding the longitudinal trajectories of responses to stress. *Social Science & Medicine, 68*, 2190–2198.

Pack, M. J. (2012). Critical incident stress management: A review of the literature with implications for social work. *International Social Work, 56*, 608–627.

Palm, K. M., Polusny, M. A., & Follette, V. M. (2004). Vicarious traumatization: Potential hazards and interventions for disaster and trauma workers. *Prehospital and Disaster Medicine, 19*, 73–78.

Pulido, M. L. (2007). In their words: Secondary traumatic stress in social workers responding to the 9/11 terrorist attacks in New York City. *Social Work, 52*, 279–281.

Quiros, L., & Berger, R. (2015). Responding to the socio-political complexity of trauma: An integration of theory and practice. *Journal of Loss and Trauma, 20*, 149–159.

Ratcliffe, M., Ruddell, M., & Smith, B. (2014). What is a "sense of foreshortened future?" A phenomenological study of trauma, trust, and time. *Frontiers in Psychology, 5*, 1026.

Sphere. (2011). *Humanitarian charter and minimum standards in humanitarian response.* Retrieved from http://www.spherehandbook.org/en/core-standard-6-aid-worker-performance/

Toren, A. L. (2008). Supervision as a buffer to vicarious trauma among counselors-in-training (Dissertation). *Abstracts International Section A: Humanities and Social Sciences, 69*(5-A), 1683.

Tummala-Narra, P. (2007). Conceptualizing trauma and resilience across diverse contexts: A multicultural perspective. *Journal of Aggression, Maltreatment & Trauma, 14*, 33–53.

Ungar, M. (2008). Resilience across cultures. *British Journal of Social Work, 38*, 218–235.

United Nations. (2015). *Sendai framework for disaster risk reduction 2015–2030.* Retrieved from http://www.preventionweb.net/files/43291_sendaiframeworkfordrren.pdf

United Nations Office for Disaster Risk Reduction (UNISDR). (2009). *Terminology.* Retrieved from https://www.unisdr.org/we/inform/terminology

United Nations Office for Disaster Risk Reduction (UNISDR). (2015). *Hyogo framework for action (HFA).* Retrieved from http://www.unisdr.org/we/coordinate/hfa

van Heugten, K. (2014). *Human service organizations in the disaster context.* Basingstoke, UK: Palgrave Macmillan.

Virtue, C., & Fouché, C. (2010). Multiple holding: A model for supervision in the context of trauma and abuse. *Social Work Review, 21*, 64–72. Retrieved from http://anzasw.nz/wp-content/uploads/SWR-Issue-4-2009-and-Issue-1-2010-Mental-health-and-well-being-Virtue-and-Fouche.pdf

Weine, S., Danieli, Y., Silove, D., Van Ommeren, M., Fairbank, J. A., & Saul, J. (2002). Guidelines for international training in mental health and psychosocial interventions for trauma exposed populations in clinical and community settings. *Psychiatry, 65*, 156–164.

Westphal, M., & Bonanno, G. A. (2007). Posttraumatic growth and resilience to trauma: Different sides of the same coin or different coins? *Applied Psychology, 56*, 417–427.

Wisner, B., & Adams, J. (2002). *Environmental health in emergencies and disasters: A practical guide.* Geneva, Switzerland: World Health Organization.

World Health Organization. (2011). *Psychological first aid: Guide for field workers.* Geneva, Switzerland: Author. Retrieved from http://www.who.int/mental_health/publications/guide_field_workers/en/

Yutrzenka, B. A., & Naifeh, J. A. (2008). Traumatic stress, disaster psychology, and graduate education: Reflections on the special section and recommendations for professional psychology training. *Training and Education in Professional Psychology, 2*(2), 96–102. doi:10.1037/1931-3918.2.2.96

Index

Note: **Bold** page numbers refer to tables and *italic* page numbers refer to figures.

action-oriented approach 75
acute trauma centers: ACS 84; alcohol-related injuries 86; Centers for Disease Control and Prevention 84; clinical skills 92; comorbid conditions 85; counseling approach 92; cultural orientation 90; dose–response relationship 86; dynamic fluid process 91; education preparation programs 88; individual supervisory relationships 93; intentional and unintentional mechanisms 84; intervention services 87–8; mental health comorbidity 89; mental health symptoms and diagnoses 85; National Center for Injury Prevention and Control 84; patient categories 89; patient identification process 88; personal trauma history 90; physical and mental traumas 90; responsibilities 88; robust training program 87; SAMHSA 92, 93; secondary trauma responses 90; self-awareness 91; substance abuse training and feedback 92; supervision history 90; support perceptions 90; training and skills 90; trauma-informed clinical supervision, definition 90; trauma-informed screening 87; trauma-informed supervisory approach 91; trauma settings 97–8; vicarious trauma 90
Adams, C. E. 115
Adamson, C. 4
alcohol-related injuries 86
Allen, A. B. 115
American College of Surgeons (ACS) 84
anti-religious bias 187
Antle, B. 3
articulated model 78
Association for Spiritual, Ethical, and Religious Values in Counseling (ASERVIC) 180
Ausbrooks, A. R. 77
authoritative group supervision 170

Balke, N. 4
Bartlett, J. D. 67
behavioral health providers 71

behavioral health workers 50
Benavidez-Hatzis, J. R. 3
Berger, R. 3, 20–1, 91, 92, 102, 112, 114, 191
Bernard, J. M. 22; discrimination model 19
betrayal trauma 181, 183, 197
biochemical changes 10
Black Lives Matter ideology 129
Bogo, M. 69
Bostock, L. 65
Bourne, I. 225, 226, 228, 231, 233
Bride, B. E. 75, 108
Brown, A. 225, 226, 228, 231, 233
Bryant-Davis, T. 203
Burnes, R. 122
Burn Intensive Care Unit 94
Butler-Byrd, N. M. 213
Butler, L. D. 226

Carello, J. 226
Carpenter, J. 65
Carter, R. T. 204, 208
case: presentation 166–7; selection of 165
case presenter, role and position of 172; selection of 165
Cashwell, C. S. 4
Centers for Disease Control and Prevention 84
Center, The 147, 148
Chau, S. 77
Cherpitel, C. J. 85
childhood trauma 9, 12
childhood victimization 26
child welfare (CW) supervision 3; behavioral health providers 71; case planning process 71; clinical intervention 64; compassion fatigue 66; data analysis 68; descriptive analysis 68, **69**; educational preparation 65; elements 69, 70; evidence-informed continuous quality improvement 74–5; goals 70; indirect trauma 75–7; interpersonal interaction 65; life-work balance 65; meta-analysis 65; National Child Welfare Resource Center on Organizational

Improvement 69–70; organizational climate 66; organizational factors 66; out-of-home placement 71–2; physical and psychological safety 67; protective factors 71; public and private agencies 64; reflective supervision 72–3; risk factors 71; social/emotional support 65; standardized scales 67–8; STS 66; task assistance 65, 74; tools development 66; trauma-informed support, supervisors 77–8; trauma screening procedures 69; vicarious traumatization 66, 69

Chu, J. A. 49

client: autonomy 189, 196; communities 223; empowerment 17; satisfaction 17; trauma disclosure 52

clinical practice treatment guidelines (CPG) 54

clinical supervision model 18; Bernard's discrimination model 19; childhood victimization 26; egalitarian approach 25; organizational demands *vs.* responsibilities 25; safety 20–1; sharevision concept 25; supervisees' learning responsibility 20; supervisory relationship 27; trauma-informed supervisors 25; trust 21–2; *see also* racial trauma, clinical supervision

Clinical Supervisor, The 2, 5, 7

Coates, T. N. 203

cognitive-behavioral approach 45, 211

cognitive needs 146

cognitive schema 9, 12

collaborative approach 16

Collins-Camargo, C. 3

"command and control" approach 224

community-level awareness 235

community levels 9; events 219; focus of disaster 227; opportunities 223

compassion fatigue 11, 12, 66, 75, 109, 110

competence constellation approach 111

competency-based approach 41

Complex Posttraumatic Stress Disorder (CPTSD) 54

confidentiality protection 15

Conrad, D. 66

Constantine, M. G. 126–7

contemporary research and theory 8

Cook, J. M. 39

cooperative group supervision 170

core components: child welfare 3; clinical practice 2; *Clinical Supervisor, The* 2, 5; commonalities 5; *in-extremis* practice 3; natural disasters 1, 4; organizational environment 2; practice contexts and situations 2; racial trauma 4; religious community 4; short- and long-term impact 1; social and cultural identities 3; social media 1

Corin, C. 228

Council on Social Work Education (CSWE) 38

counterresilience 58

Courtney, M. E. 66

Courtois, C. A. 2

cross-cultural contexts 173

cultural awareness 15

cultural competence 16

cultural empathy 173

cultural humility 191

cultural identities 128

Cunningham, M. 226

Dalenberg, C. 55

Dancy, T. E. 122

Davis, T. E. 47

DD *see* dissociative disorder (DD)

degree of responsibility 43

Delima, J. 10

Delworth, U. 48

deployed mental health professionals 105; compassion fatigue 109; competence constellation approach 111; experiential reflections 109–10; *in extremis* 107; risk factors 108; STS 108; traumatic events 108; VT 108–9

deployed military settings: clinical supervision 102–6; deployment cycle 105; educative function 103; ethical obligation (*see* ethical obligation); *in extremis* clinical work 106–7; interpersonal skills 103; MHPs 102; relational dynamics 103; supportive function 103

deployment cycle, phase of 105

Diagnostic and Statistical Manual of Mental Disorders (DSM) 11

Dialectical Behavior Therapy (DBT) 209

Dill, K. 69

disaster-aware approach 233

disaster context: Christchurch earthquake 221, 222, 226; client communities 223; clinical interventions 235; "command and control" approach 224; community-level awareness 235; definition 219; deployed and post-deployment 224; developmental model 225, *225*; dimensions 221, *221*; disaster-aware approach 233; distance process 232–3; DRRM 223–5; Grenfell Tower disaster 232; IFRC 221–2; magnitude and impact 220; organizational awareness 236; origin 220; phases 223–4, *224*; physical management 224; planning 227–9; political and social realities 233; recovery 230–1; re-integration process 233; role and function, supervision 226, **227**; self-care 220, 234–5; shared traumatic reality 231–2; social capital principles 223; stress management tool 224; supervision role limitations 229–30; time 220; trauma impact 234; trauma-informed education 226; traumatization risk 220, 221; UNISDR 220; Western-based models 232

discrimination model 21

dissociative disorder (DD) 11, 54, 56, 59

dissociative process 52–3

education preparation programs 88
educative function 103
egalitarian approach 25
emotional distress 117, 150
emotional dysregulation 50
emotional functioning 10
emotional intelligence 76
emotional needs 146
emotional resilience 56
emotional responses 10
empathy failure 109–10
emphasis 11; on precipitating events 8;
    on trauma effects 8–9
empowerment 16, 113, 187–8
Engaging, Managing, and Bonding through
    Race (EMBRace) 210
ethical dilemmas 104
ethical obligation: choice 113; collaboration
    113; countertransference reactions 113;
    empowerment 113; human self-assessments
    112; professional ethical codes 111; safety
    113; self-assessing competence levels 111;
    supervisory/training ethos 113; trauma-
    informed supervision 112; trustworthiness 113
evidence-based supervision 48
evidence-based treatment 54
evidence-informed continuous quality
    improvement 74–5
exposure therapy 134
eye movement desensitization and reprocessing
    (EMDR) therapy 163, 164

Falender, C. A. 121
Falicov, C. J. 121
Fallot, R. 2, 15
Figley, C. R. 78, 108
Fontes, L. 25
Forsyth, J. M. 204, 208
Friedlander, M. L. 191

Gabbard, G. 113
gay, lesbian, bisexual, transgender, and
    questioning (GLBTQ) community 182
Geeseman, R. 47
gender distribution 162
Goldberg, G. 108
Goodyear, R. K. 22
Grenfell Tower disaster 232
group supervision methods 165, **165**, 230
Gubi, P. M. 181
Guidelines and Principles of Accreditation 41
*Guidelines for Clinical Supervision of Health
    Service Psychologists* 41

Haans, T. 4
Hancock, J. 115
Harrell, S. P. 207, 212

Harris, M. 2, 15
Healing the Incest Wound (Courtois) 41
health care service providers 103
Heckman-Stone, C. 48
Herlihy, B. J. 197
Hernandez, P. 129
Hess, P. 78
Higson-Smith, C. 204
Hoffman, M. A. 219
Holloway, E. L. 173
Howe, P. 77
Hrostowski,S. 66
Hudnall, A. C. 204
Hughes, J. 108

impulsive behaviours 10
indirect trauma 14, 17–19, 21, 23; childhood
    trauma 12; compassion fatigue 11, 12; CW
    supervision 75–7; organizational climate 12;
    outcomes 13; personal history 12; secondary
    traumatic stress 11–2; self-care activities 12;
    vicarious trauma 11, 12
in extremis: clinical work 106–7; definition 107;
    practice 3
informed consent 15, 46
intercultural supervision 174
intercultural trauma-informed supervision 173–4
intergenerational trauma 206
International Federation of Red Cross and Red
    Crescent Societies (IFRC) 221–2
International Society for the Study of Trauma and
    Dissociation (ISST-D) 38
interpersonal dynamics 121
interpersonal victimization 8, 10, 14, 23, 130
intervention techniques 21

Jacobs, R. 181
Jean-Marie, G. 122
Johnson, M. 3
Johnson, W. B. 3, 103, 109, 117
Jones, J. L. 75

Kadushin, A. 65
Kellar-Guenther, Y. 66
Knight, C. 2
Kocet, M. M. 197
Kolditz, T. A. 107
Kruczek, T. 219
Kruzich, J. M. 66

Landsinger, K. L. 3
leadership: Center, The 148; characteristics
    147; emotional distress 150; international
    news agency 150; organizational skills 147;
    Red Cross mental health care 147; roles 149;
    volunteer helping professionals 147
learning supervision sessions 158

Leary, M. R. 115
Lee, J. 66
Leslie, B. 77
level I hospital trauma center, counselors: acute
    trauma centers 84–6 (*see also* acute trauma
    centers); case study 94–7; integrated care
    settings 86–7; psychological and physical
    trauma 83
liability insurance 46
licensing board 46
life-work balance 65
Lindy, D. J. 161
Linnerooth, P. J. 105

McCann, I. 9
McPherson, R. H. 47
maladaptive brain process 11
Mazulla, S. L. 204
Mensah, J. 122
mental health care 42
mental health comorbidity 89
mental health disorders 10, 11
Miehls, D. 25
Mienko, J. A. 66
military mental health professionals (MHPs)
    102, 112; deployed 105, 107–11; *in extremis*
    clinical work 106–7; licensed 105; trainees 105;
    uniformed 103–4 (*see also* uniformed mental
    health professionals, clinical supervisors);
    unlicensed 105
Mills, S. M. 72
mixed-agency ethical conflict 107
Moore, B. A. 105
Mor Barak, M. E. 65, 73–4
Mrdjenovich, A. J. 105
multicultural counseling guidelines 205
multifaceted treatment 7
multi-session counseling models 151

National Center for Injury Prevention and
    Control 84
National Child Welfare Resource Center on
    Organizational Improvement 69–70
natural disasters 1, 4
neurobiological changes 10, 11, 48
Newman, E. 39
non-abusive community 187
nongovernmental organizations (NGOs) 176
non-trauma-focused treatments 42

organizational approach 13
organizational awareness 236
organizational change 74
organizational climate 12, 66, 74; and
    leadership 17
organizational culture 74, 77
organizational process 227

organizational skills 147
Osborn, C. J. 47

Palm, K. M. 234
participative group supervision 170
patient identification process 88
Pearlman, L. A. 9, 42, 52, 56, 108–9
personal psychotherapy 54–5
personal transformation responses 51
personal trauma history 50
Pieterse, A. L. 4
political violence 157
posttraumatic distress 52
post-traumatic stress disorder (PTSD) 11, 40, 51,
    54, 56, 75, 85–7, 133, 163
practitioner-client relationships 125
professional development plan 131
professional ethical codes 111
professional practice guidelines (PPGs) 39, 54
psychiatry-grounded biomedical trauma
    conceptualization 132
psychological distress 107
psychological reactions 48–9
psychosocial-oriented counseling approach 86
Pulido, M. L. 234
Pyun, H. 65

quasi-therapy 18
Quiros, L. 3, 20–1, 91, 92, 102, 112, 114, 191

Race-Based Traumatic Stress Symptom Scale
    (RBTSSS) 204
race-related attitudes 121
racial microaggressions 211–12
racial trauma, clinical supervision 4; client
    outcome 202; elements 203; emotional
    responses 204, 205; goals 202; psychological
    stress 203; race-related factors 203;
    racism, definition 203; RBTSSS 204; self-
    awareness 202; self-efficacy 202; supervisor
    responsibilities (*see* supervisor responsibilities,
    racial trauma)
Rankin, P. 129
Red Cross 143, 144, 147, 154, 155
reflective supervision 131
Regehr, C. 77, 108, 109
religious abuse cases: abuse/traumatizing
    185; ASERVIC 180; assessment and
    conceptualization 190; betrayal trauma
    181, 183, 197; broaching 194–5; categories
    181–2; church leadership 188; client
    autonomy 189, 196; client experience 182;
    community/support 187; countertransference
    196; "distorted theology" 196; emotional
    reactions 189; empowerment 187–8; grief/
    loss 186–7; interpersonal process 196;
    leadership/authority 181; personal beliefs

189; psychosocial functioning 180; religious values 189; self-reflection 190; services/events 184; sexual abuse 184; spiritual authority 183–4, 196; spiritual beliefs 185–6; supervisee beliefs and experiences 192–3; supervisee bracketing support 197–8; supervisee emotionality 195–6; supervisee needs 191–2; supervisee vulnerabilities and resilience 193–4; supervisory working alliance 190–1; therapeutic intervention 190; therapist awareness 189; victims of 182–3
religious affiliation 185
religious community 186, 195
Risking Connection (Saakvitne, Gamble, Pearlman and Lev) 42
romantic/sexual relationships 47

Saakvitne, K. 9, 42, 48, 52, 56, 108–9
safety 15, 17
Schore, A. N. 48
secondary traumatic stress (STS) 11–2, 66, 75, 108
secondary traumatization 130
self-assessing competence levels 111
self-assessment 41, 57
self-awareness 57, 91, 115, 202, 205
self-care 76, 78, 97, 132, 220, 234–5; activities 12; elements 116
self-compassion 57
self-development 9
self-disclosure 192–3
self-efficacy 9, 10, 18, 74, 202, 212
self-exploration 45, 127–9
self-identities 127
self-monitoring 51
self-regulation 10
sexual abuse 8
Shackelford, K. K. 76
Shafranske, E. P. 121
sharevision concept 25
Shilling, E. H. 3
Singh, L. 122
social determinants 86
social media 142, 146
social service agencies 38
social support 9
socio-political occurrences 8
somatosensory channels 48
spiritual authority 183–4, 196
Stamm, B. H. 204
Stamm, H. E. 204
Strolin-Goltzman, J. 66
Substance Abuse and Mental Health Services Administration (SAMHSA) 92, 93
Sue, D. W. 126–7, 211
Super, J. 3
supervisee/consultee behaviors 48

supervision/consultation, trauma treatment: awareness 56–7; balance 57; boundaries and methods 47; client's trauma disclosure 52; cognitive-behavior paradigm 45; competency-based approach 41; connection 57; containment 57; counseling psychology 41; counterresilience 58; countertransference responses 55; CPG 54; CPTSD 54; DDs 54, 59; degree of responsibility 43; dissociative process 52–3; eclectic and psychodynamic psychotherapy 40; emotional resilience 56; evidence-based treatment 54; formal supervision contract 43; *Guidelines and Principles of Accreditation* 41; *Guidelines for Clinical Supervision of Health Service Psychologists* 41; *Healing the Incest Wound* 41; informed consent 46; liability insurance 46; licensing board 46; malpractice coverage 47; mental health care 42; non-trauma-focused treatments 42; personal psychotherapy 54–5; posttraumatic distress 52; posttraumatic growth 40, 58, 59; posttraumatic symptoms 56; PPGs 54; process 47–51; professional disciplines 41; psychotherapy 45; PTSD 40; responsibilities and liabilities 43; *Risking Connection* 42; romantic/sexual relationships 47; self-assessment 41; self-compassion 57; self-exploration 45; sequenced/stage-oriented treatment 53; signed placement contract 46; "supervision of supervision" training 41; trauma, definition 51–2; traumatic memory 53; vicarious liability concept 44; vicarious resilience 40, 58; VT 55–6; workable contract 39
"supervision of supervision" training 41
supervisor responsibilities, racial trauma: acknowledgment 208; clinical interventions 207–8; cognitive distortions 208–9; coping and resistance 210; EMBRace 210; guidelines 206–7; impact assessment 208; loss experience 209–10; multicultural counseling guidelines 205; racial identity 206, 207; self-awareness 205; strong emotions 209; supervisor/supervisee relationship 212–213; supervisory process 206, 210–12; validation 208
supervisory alliance 20
supervisory beliefs 153
supervisory techniques 28
supervisory/training ethos 113
supervisory working alliance 190–1
supportive function 103
Sutter, E. 47
Swindle, P. J. 4

task assistance 65, 74
Task-Oriented supervisor 191
Tate, E. B. 115
transformational (mentoring-oriented) supervisory relationship 116

trauma-focused services 17
trauma-informed care (TIC) 8, 13, 16–17; APA
    39; behavioral health facilities 38; behavioral
    health settings 39; clinical practice 39; CSWE
    38; CW supervision (*see* child welfare (CW)
    supervision); definition 16; elements 18;
    ISST-D 38; knowledge and skills 39; medical
    settings 38; professional practice guidelines
    39; social service agencies 38; supervision/
    consultation, trauma treatment (*see*
    supervision/consultation, trauma treatment);
    traumatic stress 39; trauma treatment
    organizations 39
trauma-informed group supervision (TIGS):
    advantages 176; authoritative group
    supervision 170; case and case presenter
    selection 165; case presentation 166–7;
    case presenter, role and position 172;
    clarification questions 167; communication
    163; contracting 174–5; cooperative group
    supervision 170; countertransference 160–2;
    cultural and intercultural contexts 177–8;
    disadvantages 176; enthusiasm 178; factual
    questions 171; features 158; feedback 178;
    group members roles 162–4; group supervision
    sequence 165, **165**; identification rounds 171;
    identification with client 168, 172; intercultural
    trauma-informed supervision 173–4;
    learning supervision sessions 158; NGOs 176;
    participative group supervision 170; political
    violence 157; psychological trauma 165;
    refugees 158; self-help capacities 170; social
    agencies 177; solutions 172–3; supervision
    principles 165; supervision question 172; task
    and position, case presenter 168–9; trauma-
    related impediments 158
trauma-informed orientation 27

uniformed mental health professionals, clinical
    supervisors: competence constellation 117;
    deployment and post-deployment phases 114;
    empty chair technique 115; equip supervisees
    115; inoculation and training 115; intentional
    role-modeling, supervisees 117; qualitative
    interviews 114; self-awareness 115; self-care,
    elements 116; self-compassion 115; training
    phase 114; transference dynamics 116–117;
    transformational (mentoring-oriented)
    supervisory relationship 116
United Nations Office for Disaster Risk
    Reduction (UNISDR) 220

Veach, L. J. 3
Vespia, K. M. 48
vicarious liability concept 44
vicarious resilience 12–13, 40, 58
vicarious traumatization (VT) 11, 12, 51, 55–6,
    75, 90, 108–9
Vimpani, G. 10
volunteer supervisor's perspective, Pulse in
    Orlando: brief therapy model 150; Center,
    The 142–4; cognitive and emotional responses
    152–3; confidentiality 152; emotional needs
    142; grieving process 141; identification
    process 144; leadership (*see* leadership); long-
    term effects 154; multi-session counseling
    models 151; professionals 144–7; Red Cross'
    training protocol 144, 154, 155; social media
    142; supervision training and experience
    151; supervisory beliefs 153; thoughts and
    emotional reactions 142; vicarious trauma 154

Walker, M. 24
Ward, L. G. 191
Weaver, C. 66
Webb, C. M. 65
Weine, S. 226
Western-based models 232
Williams, B. 204
Wilson, J. P. 161
Wissow, L. S. 86
work-related distress 108

Xie, B. 65

For Product Safety Concerns and Information please contact our EU
representative GPSR@taylorandfrancis.com
Taylor & Francis Verlag GmbH, Kaufingerstraße 24, 80331 München, Germany

www.ingramcontent.com/pod-product-compliance
Lightning Source LLC
Chambersburg PA
CBHW081100220326
41598CB00038B/7169